STUDY GUIDE

Maternal Child Nursing Care

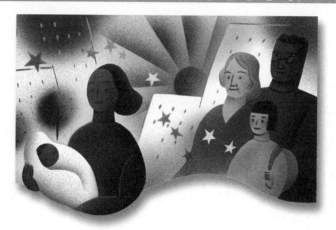

THIRD EDITION

Donna L. Wong, PhD, RN, PNP, CPN, FAAN
Marilyn J. Hockenberry, PhD, RN-CS, PNP, FAAN
David Wilson, MS, RNC

Shannon E. Perry, RN, CNS, PhD, FAAN
Deitra Leonard Lowdermilk, RNC, PhD, FAAN

By

Karen A. Piotrowski, RNC, MSN
Associate Professor of Nursing
D'Youville College
Buffalo, New York

Anne Rath Rentfro, MSN, RN
Associate Professor of Nursing
The University of Texas at Brownsville
Texas Southmost College
Brownsville, Texas

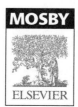

MOSBY

ELSEVIER

11830 Westline Industrial Drive
St. Louis, Missouri 63146

STUDY GUIDE FOR MATERNAL CHILD NURSING CARE, ED 3   ISBN-13: 978-0-323-03201-8
Copyright © 2006, 2002, 1998 by Mosby, an affiliate of Elsevier Inc.   ISBN-10: 0-323-03201-X

NOTICE

Knowledge and best practice in this field are constantly changing. As new research and experience broaden our knowledge, changes in practice, treatment, and drug therapy may become necessary or appropriate. Readers are advised to check the most current product information provided (i) on procedures featured or (ii) by the manufacturer of each product to be administered, to verify the recommended dose or formula, the method and duration of administration, and contraindications. It is the responsibility of the practitioner, relying on their own experience and knowledge of the patient, to make diagnoses, to determine dosages and the best treatment for each individual patient, and to take all appropriate safety precautions. To the fullest extent of the law, neither the Publisher nor the Authors assume any liability for any injury and/or damage to persons or property arising out or related to any use of the material contained in this book.

ISBN-13: 978-0-323-03201-8
ISBN-10: 0-323-03201-X

Acquisitions Editor: Catherine Jackson
Managing Editor: Michele D. Hayden
Senior Developmental Editor: Laurie K. Gower
Publishing Services Manager: Jeff Patterson
Senior Project Manager: Anne Konopka
Designer: Julia Dummitt

Printed in the United States of America

Last digit is the print number: 9 8 7 6 5 4 3

Introduction

Maternal Child Nursing Care, third edition, is a comprehensive textbook of maternity and pediatric nursing. This Study Guide is designed to help students use the textbook more effectively. In addition to reviewing content of the text, this Study Guide encourages students to think critically in applying their knowledge.

Organization

Each chapter in this Study Guide is designed to incorporate all of the learning activities that will help students meet the objectives of the corresponding textbook chapter. The content is organized as follows:

- **Learning Key Terms**—Matching or fill-in-the-blank questions give students the opportunity to test their ability to define all key terms highlighted in the corresponding textbook chapter.

- **Reviewing Key Concepts and Content**—A variety of questions (matching, fill-in-the-blank, true/false, short answer, and multiple choice) are used to provide students with ample opportunity to assess their knowledge and comprehension of the information covered in the text. These activities are specifically designed to help students identify the important content of the chapter and test their level of knowledge and understanding after reading the chapter.

- **Thinking Critically**—Students are required to apply concepts found in the chapter to solve problems, make decisions concerning care management, and provide responses to patients' questions and concerns.

- **Answer Key**—Answers to all questions are provided at the end of this Study Guide.

Contents

INTRODUCTION iii

PART I   MATERNITY NURSING

UNIT 1: INTRODUCTION TO MATERNITY NURSING

1   Contemporary Maternity Nursing 1
2   The Family and Culture 5
3   Community and Home Care 10

UNIT 2: REPRODUCTIVE YEARS

4   Health Promotion and Prevention 14
5   Health Assessment 20
6   Common Health Problems 29
7   Infertility, Contraception, and Abortion 41

UNIT 3: PREGNANCY

8   Genetics, Conception, and Fetal Development 49
9   Assessment for Risk Factors 55
10   Anatomy and Physiology of Pregnancy 61
11   Nursing Care during Pregnancy 68
12   Maternal and Fetal Nutrition 78
13   Pregnancy at Risk: Preexisting Conditions 83
14   Pregnancy at Risk: Gestational Conditions 94

UNIT 4: CHILDBIRTH

15   Labor and Birth Processes 107
16   Management of Discomfort 112
17   Fetal Assessment during Labor 120
18   Nursing Care during Labor and Birth 126
19   Labor and Birth at Risk 136

UNIT 5: POSTPARTUM PERIOD

20   Maternal Physiologic Changes 147
21   Nursing Care during the Fourth Trimester 150
22   Transition to Parenthood 157
23   Postpartum Complications 162

UNIT 6: NEWBORN

24   Physiologic Adaptations of the Newborn 172
25   Nursing Care of the Newborn 179
26   Newborn Nutrition and Feeding 187

27   Infants with Gestational Age-Related Problems   196

28   The Newborn at Risk: Acquired and Congenital Problems   205

PART II   PEDIATRIC NURSING

UNIT 7: CHILDREN, THEIR FAMILIES, AND THE NURSE

29   Contemporary Pediatric Nursing   213

30   Community-Based Nursing Care of the Child and Family   219

31   Family Influences on Child Health Promotion   222

32   Social, Cultural, and Religious Influences on Child Health Promotion .   226

33   Developmental Influences on Child Health Promotion   231

UNIT 8: ASSESSMENT OF THE CHILD AND FAMILY

34   Communication and Health Assessment of the Child and Family . .   237

35   Physical and Developmental Assessment of the Child   241

UNIT 9: HEALTH PROMOTION AND SPECIAL HEALTH PROBLEMS

36   The Infant and Family   245

37   The Toddler and Family   248

38   The Preschooler and Family   251

39   The School-Age Child and Family   255

40   The Adolescent and Family   258

UNIT 10: SPECIAL NEEDS, ILLNESS, AND HOSPITALIZATION

41   Chronic Illness, Disability, and End-of-Life Care   263

42   Cognitive and Sensory Impairment   267

43   Family-Centered Home Care   272

44   Reaction to Illness and Hospitalization   274

45   Pediatric Variations of Nursing Interventions   278

UNIT 11: HEALTH PROBLEMS OF CHILDREN

46   Respiratory Dysfunction   283

47   Gastrointestinal Dysfunction   289

48   Cardiovascular Dysfunction   296

49   Hematologic and Immunologic Dysfunction   302

50   Genitourinary Dysfunction   305

51   Cerebral Dysfunction   309

52   Endocrine Dysfunction   313

53   Integumentary Dysfunction   317

54   Musculoskeletal or Articular Dysfunction   323

55   Neuromuscular or Muscular Dysfunction   327

ANSWER KEY   331

Contemporary Maternity Nursing 1

I. REVIEWING KEY CONCEPTS AND CONTENT

MATCHING: Match the definition in Column I with the appropriate descriptive term from Column II.

COLUMN I	COLUMN II

1. _____ Number of live births in 1 year per 1000 population.

2. _____ Infant whose age at birth is less than 38 weeks of gestation.

3. _____ Number of maternal deaths from births and complications of pregnancy, childbirth, and the puerperium (the first 42 days after termination of the pregnancy) per 100,000 live births.

4. _____ An infant who, at birth, demonstrates no signs of life, such as breathing, heartbeat, or voluntary muscle movements.

5. _____ Number of stillbirths and the number of neonatal deaths per 1000 live births.

6. _____ Number of births per 1000 women between the ages of 15 and 44 years (inclusive), calculated on a yearly basis.

7. _____ Infant whose weight at birth is less than 2500 g (5 lb, 8 oz).

8. _____ Number of deaths of infants under 1 year of age per 1000 live births.

9. _____ Number of deaths of infants under 28 days of age per 1000 live births.

COLUMN II

a. Fertility rate

b. Infant mortality rate

c. Birth rate

d. Maternal mortality rate

e. Neonatal mortality rate

f. Perinatal mortality rate

g. Low-birth-weight infant

h. Preterm infant

i. Stillbirth

FILL IN THE BLANKS: Insert the term that corresponds to each of the following definitions or descriptions.

10. _____ Specialty area of nursing practice that focuses on the care of childbearing women and their families through all stages of pregnancy and childbirth, as well as the first 4 weeks after birth.

11. _____ Approach to health care that encompasses complementary and alternative therapies in combination with conventional Western modalities of treatment.

12. _____ A set of goals that reflects the nation's agenda for improving health with the ultimate aims to increase the quality and years of healthy life and to eliminate health disparities.

13. _____ A comprehensive standardized language that describes the contributions of generalist or specialist nurses to patient care.

14. _____ Statements of the expected effectiveness of interventions and quality of care.

15. _____ A program or service that has been recognized for excellence—one that provides a better or a new way to achieve goals and to be sound from operational, clinical, and financial perspectives.

16. _____ A process used to compare one's own performance against the performance of the best in an area of service. This process supports and promotes continual quality improvement and helps the organization remain competitive in the health care market.

17. _____ Guidelines for nursing practice that reflect current knowledge, represent levels of practice agreed on by leaders in the specialty, and can be used for clinical benchmarking.

18. _____ Health care that is based on information gained through research and clinical trials.

19. Identify the factors that contribute to higher infant mortality in the United States.

20. State several changes that have occurred in maternity care. Discuss your thoughts concerning the effect these changes have had or could have on the health of women, their infants, and families.

21. Cite the four predominant causes of maternal mortality.

22. List the most common barriers to early and ongoing prenatal care in the United States today.

TRUE OR FALSE: Circle T if true or F if false for each of the following statements. Correct the false statements.

23. T F The neonatal period refers to the first 3 months of an infant's life.

24. T F Currently the highest birth rates are for women between 18 and 25 years of age.

25. T F Abortion refers to the expulsion/removal of an embryo/fetus from the uterus at 26 weeks of gestation or less, weighing 1000 g or less, or measuring 30 cm or less.

26. T F The birth rate for women in their forties continues to increase.

27. T F Births to unmarried women are frequently related to less favorable outcomes because there are typically a large number of teenagers in this group.

28. T F The infant mortality rate for African-American babies is more than three times higher than for Hispanic babies.

29. T F In 2002, one third of all births in the United States were to unmarried women.

30. T F The number of low-birth-weight infants can be substantially reduced through the perfection of advanced technology.

31. T F The greatest risk for giving birth to a low-birth-weight infant occurs among African-American women.

32. T F The United States ranks twenty-third for infant mortality among industrialized nations.

33. T F The infant mortality rate is a common indicator of the adequacy of prenatal care and the health of the nation as a whole.

34. T F In the United States, the maternal mortality rate among African-American women is twice the rate for Caucasian women.

35. T F The most significant barrier to accessible health care is minority status.

36. T F In 2002, the number of pregnant women beginning prenatal care during their first trimester was approximately 75%.

37. T   F   The cesarean birth rate has continued to decrease since 2000.

38. T   F   Violence is a major factor affecting pregnant women and may increase during pregnancy.

II. THINKING CRITICALLY

1. Imagine that you are the nursing director of an inner-city prenatal clinic that serves a large number of minority women, many of whom are younger than 20 years of age. Describe five nursing services you would provide for these women that would help reduce the potential for maternal and infant morbidity and mortality and low birth weight. Use the statistical data and risk behaviors presented in Chapter 1 to support the types of services you propose.

2. Support the accuracy of the following statement: An emphasis on high-technology medical care and lifesaving techniques will not reduce the rate of preterm and low-birth-weight infants in the United States.

3. Propose three changes in health care and its delivery that you believe would improve the health status and well-being of mothers and their infants and reduce the rate of infant and maternal mortality. Support your answer by using the content presented in Chapter 1 and your own experiences with the health care system.

4. Many barriers interfere with a woman's participation in early and ongoing prenatal care. Describe incentives and services that you would offer to pregnant women to encourage their participation in prenatal care. State the rationale for your proposals. Your answer should reflect an understanding of the barriers.

5. You are a nurse at a prenatal clinic. Human immunodeficiency virus (HIV) testing is included in the assessment process for all pregnant women. Your patient expresses reluctance to have the test done, stating, "I can't be positive, and what difference would it make for my baby anyway since there is no cure?" What would you tell your patient?

6. Many patients who come to a prenatal clinic speak English as a second language and often have difficulty speaking fluently. Explain what measures nurses working in this clinic should use to ensure health literacy among their patients.

The Family and Culture $\boxed{2}$

I. REVIEWING KEY CONCEPTS AND CONTENT

MATCHING: Match the family described in Column I with the appropriate family category in Column II.

COLUMN I	COLUMN II
1. _____ Miss M. lives with her 4-year-old adopted Korean daughter, Kim.	a. Binuclear family
2. _____ Anne and Duane are married and live with their daughter, Susan, and Duane's mother, Ruth.	b. Single-parent family
3. _____ Gloria and Andy are a married couple living with their new baby girl, Annie.	c. Homosexual family
4. _____ Carl and Allan are a gay couple living with Carl's daughter, Sally, whom they are raising together.	d. Nuclear family
5. _____ The Smith family consists of Jim; his second wife, Jane; and Jim's two daughters by a previous marriage.	e. Extended family
6. _____ Laurie and John have been divorced for 3 years. They share custody of their four children.	f. Reconstituted (blended) family

MATCHING: Match the description in Column I with the appropriate cultural concept in Column II.

COLUMN I	COLUMN II
7. _____ Mrs. M., a Mexican-American who just gave birth, tells the nurse not to include certain foods on her meal tray because her mother told her to avoid those foods while breastfeeding. The nurse tells her that she doesn't have to avoid any foods and should eat whatever she desires.	a. Cultural relativism
	b. Ethnocentrism
8. _____ Ms. P. an immigrant from Vietnam, has lived in the United States for 1 year. She tells you that she enjoys the comfort of wearing blue jeans and sneakers for casual occasions, like shopping, even though she never would have done so in Vietnam.	c. Assimilation
	d. Subculture
9. _____ A Cambodian family immigrated to the United States and has been living in Denver for over 5 years. The parents express concern about their children ages 10, 13, and 16, stating, "The children act so differently now. They are less respectful to us, want to eat only American food, and go to rock concerts. It's hard to believe they are our children."	e. Acculturation
10. _____ The Amish represent an important ethnic community in Lancaster, Pennsylvania.	
11. _____ The nurse is preparing a healthy diet plan for Mrs. O. In doing so, she takes the time to include the Polish foods that Mrs. O. favors.	

FILL IN THE BLANKS: Insert the cultural concept that corresponds to each of the following definitions.

12. _____ A unified set of values, ideas, beliefs, and standards of behavior shared by a group of people.

13. _____ A group existing within a larger cultural system that retains its own characteristics.

14. _____ Recognizing that people from different cultural backgrounds comprehend the same objects and situations differently; that a culture determines a person's viewpoint.

15. _____ Changes that occur within one group or among several groups when people from different cultures come in contact with one another and exchange and adopt each other's mannerisms, styles, and practices.

16. _____ Process in which one cultural group loses its identity and becomes a part of the dominant culture.

17. _____ A belief that one's cultural way of doing things is the right way, supporting the notion that "My group is the best."

18. _____ Approach that involves the ability to think, feel, and act in ways that acknowledges, respects, and builds upon ethnic, [socio]cultural, and linguistic diversity; to act in ways that meet the needs of the patient and are respectful of ways and traditions that may be different from one's own.

19. _____ Families or people with this type of time orientation maintain a focus on achieving long-term goals; they are more likely to return for follow-up visits related to health care and to participate in primary prevention activities.

20. _____ Families or people with this type of time orientation are more likely to strive to maintain tradition and have little motivation for formulating future goals.

21. _____ Families or people with this type of time orientation may have difficulty adhering to strict schedules and are often described as living for the moment.

22. _____ Cultural concept that reflects dimensions of personal comfort zones. Actions such as touching, placing the woman in proximity to others, taking away personal possessions, and making decisions for the woman can decrease personal security and heighten anxiety.

23. _____ The primary unit of socialization; the basic structural unit within a community and the primary institution in society that preserves and transmits culture.

24. _____ Family category in which male and female partners and their children live as an independent unit, sharing roles, responsibilities, and economic resources.

25. _____ Family category that includes the nuclear family and other people related by blood (kin) such as grandparents, aunts, uncles, and cousins.

26. _____ Family category that refers to the family after divorce, in which the child is a member of both the maternal and paternal nuclear households.

27. _____ Family category in which there is only one parent as head of the household; it is becoming an increasingly recognized structure in our society. These families tend to be vulnerable both _____ and _____.

28. _____ Family category that includes stepparents and stepchildren. It is also called a blended, combined, or remarried family.

29. _____ Family category in which gay or lesbian couples are the parents.

30. _____ Essential family activities that are described as _____, _____, _____, _____, and _____.

31. _____ Family activity that focuses on meeting family members' needs for affection and understanding. It is one of the most vital of family functions.

32. _____ Family activity that refers to the learning experiences provided within the family to teach children their culture and how to function and assume adult social roles. It is a lifelong process that includes internalizing norms and values appropriate for each developmental milestone.

33. _____ Family activity that ensures family continuity over the generations and the survival of society.

34. _____ Family activity that involves the family's provision and allocation of sufficient resources.

35. _____ Family activity that involves the provision of physical necessities such as food, shelter, clothing, and health care.

36. _____ Interactions and communication that allow family members to work cooperatively with each other to accomplish family activities/functions. Family members use _____ to determine roles and responsibilities. _____ are set up by a family between itself and society. A family sets up _____ through which it interacts with society and ensures that its members receive their share of social resources.

37. _____ A family theory that views the family as a unit and focuses on observing the interactions among family members rather than studying family members individually.

38. _____ A family theory that focuses on the family as it moves through stages across time.

39. _____ A family theory concerned with the ways families react to stressful events and suggests factors that promote adaptation to these events.

TRUE OR FALSE: Circle T if true or F if false for each of the following statements. Correct the false statements.

40. T F A subculture's beliefs and practices related to childbearing and parenting must be assessed for each woman and family representing that subculture, because variations in beliefs and practices are possible.

41. T F Women from Southeast Asia often vocalize while experiencing the pain and discomfort associated with the childbirth process.

42. T F African-American women seek prenatal care early because they view pregnancy as a time when women require medical care and supervision.

43. T F Hispanic women appreciate the opportunity to shower or bathe as soon as possible after birth.

44. T F The nurse should recognize that a Vietnamese woman may not wish to breastfeed until her milk comes in because she believes that newborns should not be fed colostrum because it is "filthy" or "spoiled."

45. T F European-American women typically prefer a technology dominated childbirth approach rather than a natural approach.

46. T F Native-American women often use herbal preparations to promote uterine contractions during labor and to stop bleeding in the postpartum period.

47. T F Hispanic-American women often desire and expect reduced activity or even bed rest for as long as 3 days after birth.

48. Discuss why the nurse should take each of the following "products of culture" into considera- tion when providing care within a cultural context:

    a. Communication

    b. Personal space

    c. Time orientation

    d. Family roles

MULTIPLE CHOICE QUESTIONS: Circle the one correct option and state the rationale for the option chosen.

49. A family with open boundaries
    a. uses available support systems to meet its needs.
    b. is more prone to crisis, related to increased exposure to stressors.
    c. discourages family members from setting up channels.
    d. strives to maintain family stability by avoiding outside influences.

50. Families in the launching stage of the family life cycle are involved in accomplishing which of the following developmental tasks?
    a. Establishing financial independence
    b. Realigning relationships with extended family
    c. Renegotiating the marital relationship as a dyad
    d. Maintaining own and/or couple functioning and interests in the face of physiologic decline

51. Which one of the following nursing actions is most likely to reduce a patient's anxiety and enhance the patient's personal security as it relates to the concept of personal space needs?
    a. Touching the patient before and during procedures
    b. Providing explanations when performing tasks
    c. Making eye contact as much as possible
    d. Reducing the need for the patient to make decisions

52. A Native-American woman gave birth to a baby girl 12 hours ago. The nurse notes that the woman keeps her baby in the bassinet except for feeding and states that she will wait until she gets home to begin breastfeeding. The nurse recognizes that this behavior is most likely a reflection of
    a. embarrassment.
    b. delayed attachment.
    c. disappointment that the baby is a girl.
    d. a belief that babies should not be fed colostrum.

II. THINKING CRITICALLY

1. Imagine that you are a nurse working in a clinic that provides prenatal services to a multicultural community predominated by Hispanic, African-American, and Asian families. Describe how you would adapt care measures to reflect the cultural beliefs and practices of pregnant women and their families from each of the following cultural groups.

    a. Hispanic

    b. African-American

    c. Asian-American

2. Pamela is a 20-year-old Native-American woman. She is 3 months pregnant and has come to the prenatal clinic on the reservation where she lives for her first visit to obtain some prenatal vitamins, which her friends at work told her are important.

    a. State the questions the nurse should ask to determine Pamela's cultural expectations about childbearing.

    b. Describe the communication approach you would consider when interviewing Pamela.

    c. Identify the Native-American beliefs and practices regarding childbearing that may influence Pamela's approach to her pregnancy and birth.

3. A nurse has been providing care to Family M, a Hispanic family. This family recently experienced the birth of twin girls at 38 weeks of gestation. It is the first birth experience for both parents and the first grandchildren for the extended family. Both newborns are healthy and living at home.

   a. Identify the family life stage being experienced by this family.

   b. State the developmental tasks that this family needs to accomplish.

   c. Describe the cultural beliefs and practices that the family, as Hispanic, might use as guidelines to provide care to their newborn twin girls.

4. The nurse-midwife at a prenatal clinic has been assigned to care for a Sunni refugee couple from Iraq who recently emigrated to the United States. The woman has just been diagnosed as 2 months pregnant. Neither she nor her husband speaks English. Outline the process that this nurse should use when working with a translator to facilitate communication with this couple to enhance care management.

3 Community and Home Care

I. REVIEWING KEY CONCEPTS AND CONTENT

TRUE OR FALSE: Circle T if true or F if false for each of the following statements. Correct the false statements.

1. T   F   Infant mortality is a statistic widely used to compare the health status of different populations.

2. T   F   Mortality or death rates are calculated on the number of deaths attributed to a particular health problem such as lung cancer per 10,000 population.

3. T   F   Breast self-examination is an example of secondary prevention.

4. T   F   Immunization programs are an example of tertiary prevention.

5. T   F   The majority of homeless families in rural areas are headed by young, single women.

6. T   F   Most migrant laborers value their health and readily seek health promotion and disease prevention services if offered.

7. T   F   Female refugees are often the victims of physical or sexual violence, including rape.

8. T   F   The perinatal continuum of care starts with family planning and ends when the infant is 1 year of age.

9. T   F   An independent proprietary home care perinatal service is considered to be a nonprofit agency.

10. T   F   Women who require intravenous fluids during their pregnancies must be hospitalized and therefore are not candidates for home care.

11. T   F   Infection control measures are less important when care is given in the patient's home.

12. T   F   When documenting a home visit, the nurse should avoid statements such as "no change" or "same as last visit."

FILL IN THE BLANKS: Insert the term that corresponds to each of the following descriptions.

13. Community, in its broadest definition, refers to a _____ area, its _____, their _____, _____, and _____ characteristics and the _____ or _____ through which the needs of the residents are met.

14. A _____ survey is a community assessment technique that involves observing a community by traveling through it.

15. _____ are a useful community assessment method that involves being part of the community you wish to learn about, in order to understand the community more fully and to validate observations.

16. _____ are collected every 10 years by the United States government. Information is gathered regarding _____ size, _____ ranges, _____ and _____ distribution, _____ status, _____ level, _____ and _____ characteristics.

17. _____ is a group of people who have shared characteristics.

18. _____ involves efforts made before the development of illness to promote general health and well-being.

19. _____ involves early detection of health problems with the goal of shortening disease duration and severity, thus enabling an individual to return to normal function as quickly as possible.

20. _____ follows the occurrence of a defect or disability that is permanent and irreversible. Its goal is to provide people who have developed disease with treatment and rehabilitation to prevent complications and further deterioration and to maintain optimal level of function.

10

21. _____ or
_____ are groups of
people who are at higher risk of developing
physical, mental, or social health problems or who
are more likely to have worse outcomes from
these health problems than the population as a
whole. For the perinatal nurse, these groups
include _____ girls,
_____, _____, and
_____ women, and
_____ and _____.

22. A committee of experts from many community
health-related organizations have identified a set
of indicators that can be used to assess the health
status and well-being of a community.

   a. List the indicators of health status outcome.

   b. List the indicators of risk factors.

23. Community health promotion requires the
collaborative efforts of many individuals and
groups within a community. Cite several
programs that could be established to promote
the health of a community's childbearing families.

24. Cite the social and health problems faced by
migrant laborers and their families.

25. State three characteristics of refugees that can
significantly increase the difficulties they
experience as they strive to adapt to a new
language and culture.

26. Describe the ways that nurses can provide care to
perinatal patients using the telephone.

II. THINKING CRITICALLY

1. As a nurse working in home care, it would be helpful for the nurse to become familiar with the neighborhood
and resources with which her/his patients interact.

   a. Describe a walking survey.

   b. Discuss how the nurse could use the findings from this survey to provide health care to the patients who
   reside in the assessed community.

2. Marie is a single parent of 2 young children ages 4 years and 1 year. She and her children have been homeless
for 3 months since her husband abandoned her and she lost her job because she had no one to help her care
for her children.

   a. Discuss the basis for the types of health problems to which Marie and her children are most vulnerable.

b. Research indicates that Marie is at increased risk for becoming pregnant again. State the factors that make Marie more vulnerable.

c. Outline the principles that should guide a nurse in providing care to Marie and her children should they present themselves to the homeless shelter's clinic for health care.

3. Consuelo is the wife of a migrant laborer. She and her husband, along with their two children, have been working on a California farm for 2 weeks. She has arrived at a health center established for migrant laborers. Consuelo states that she is 4 months pregnant. As the woman's health nurse practitioner assigned to care for Consuelo, what approaches would you use to ensure that she obtains quality health care that addresses her unique health risks as a migrant worker?

4. Write a series of questions that you would ask when making a postpartum follow-up call to a woman who gave birth 3 days ago.

5. Eileen gave birth to a son 36 hours ago. A home care nurse has been assigned to visit Eileen and her husband in their home to assess the progress of her recovery after birth, the health status of her newborn son, and the adaptation of family processes to the responsibilities of newborn care.

a. Outline the approach the nurse should take in preparing for this visit.

b. Describe the nurse's actions during the visit using the care management process as a format.

c. Discuss how the nurse should end the visit.

 d. Identify interventions the nurse should implement at the conclusion of the visit with Eileen and her husband.

 e. Specify how the nurse should protect her personal safety both outside and inside Eileen's home.

 f. Cite the infection control measures the nurse should use when conducting the visit and providing care in Eileen's home.

6. Angela has recently been diagnosed with hyperemesis gravidarum and has been hospitalized to stabilize her fluid and electrolyte balance. The hospital-based nurse must evaluate Angela for referral to home care.

 a. State the criteria that this nurse should follow in order to determine Angela's readiness for discharge from hospital to home care.

 b. Angela has been discharged and will be receiving parenteral nutrition in her home. Discuss the additional information required related to high-technology home care.

 c. Identify specific home environment criteria that must be met to ensure the safety and effectiveness of Angela's treatment.

7. A nurse is seeking funding to start a home care agency designed to provide home visits to postpartum women and their families within 1 week of birth and follow-up visits as indicated. State the points the nurse should emphasize as a rationale for the importance of this health care service and the cost-effectiveness of funding such a service.

4 Health Promotion and Prevention

I. REVIEWING KEY CONCEPTS AND CONTENT

TRUE OR FALSE: Circle T for true or F for false for each of the following statements. Correct the false statements.

1. T   F   Most women enter the heath care system for the first time to seek assistance regarding a reproductive system–related situation.

2. T   F   A sexually active teen who does not use contraception has a 50% chance of pregnancy within 2 years.

3. T   F   The rate of teen pregnancies has been steadily increasing since 1991.

4. T   F   A woman's ethnicity often influences her health risks and health behaviors.

5. T   F   Preconception care and counseling is a health care service designed primarily for women of childbearing age who have chronic health problems.

6. T   F   Women older than 35 years of age experience a different physical response to pregnancy than women who are younger.

7. T   F   Smoking increases the risk for osteoporosis after menopause.

8. T   F   Cigarette smoking impairs both male and female fertility.

9. T   F   Women are more likely than men to use primary care services.

10. T   F   High caffeine consumption has been associated with an increased risk for birth defects.

11. T   F   Choice of contraceptive has no impact on the risk for contracting an STD.

12. T   F   In the United States, a major risk factor for cervical cancer is a woman's race.

13. T   F   It is recommended that the first Pap smear take place no later than age 21.

14. T   F   Clinical breast examination by a health care provider is recommended every 1 to 3 years for women starting at the age of 30.

15. T   F   The American Cancer Society recommends an annual mammogram beginning at age 35.

16. T   F   Neural tube defects are more common in infants born of women with a diet poor in folate.

17. T   F   Swimming should be recommended to perimenopausal women as an exercise that can help prevent osteoporosis.

18. T   F   Kegel exercises help strengthen abdominal muscles.

19. T   F   Cigarette smoking during pregnancy causes a decrease in placental perfusion.

20. T   F   Race, religion, social background, age, and educational level are all significant factors in differentiating women at risk for abuse.

21. T   F   The key feature to establish rape is the absence of consent.

22. T   F   Approximately 25% of women are beaten when they are pregnant.

23. T   F   Battering follows a cyclic pattern.

24. T   F   Nurses should assess all women, entering the health care system, for abuse.

25. T   F   Date and acquaintance rape occurs most often to women in their 20s.

FILL IN THE BLANKS: Insert the term that corresponds to each of the following definitions or descriptions.

26. _____ provides women and their partners with information that is needed to make decisions about their reproductive future.

27. _____ involve the use of self-care measures designed to prevent transmission of sexually transmitted diseases.

28. _____, _____, _____, and _____ are the four *A's* of interventions for smoking cessation.

29. _____, _____, _____, and _____ or _____ violence are terms applied to a pattern of assaultive and coercive behaviors inflicted by a male partner in a marriage or other heterosexual, significant, intimate relationship.

30. According to the cycle of violence theory, battering occurs in _____ cycles. The three-phase cyclic pattern that occurs begins with a period of _____ leading to the _____, which is then followed by a period of _____ and _____ known as the _____ phase.

31. _____ or _____ is an act of violence that consists of sexual contact with or without _____ but with _____ or _____. Types of this act of violence include _____, _____, _____, and_____.

32. _____ is the use of power and control tactics to victimize women sexually, particularly in the workplace.

33. _____ is the intentional removal of all or part of the external female genitalia. Complications of this procedure include _____, _____, and _____ complications as well as higher _____ and _____ morbidity and mortality during _____.

34. A nurse involved in the health care of women needs to be alert for factors in a woman's health history that have been associated with an increased risk for specific reproductive tract malignancies.

    a. Identify the factors that would increase a woman's risk for cervical cancer.

    b. Describe several measures that nurses could recommend to women to help them reduce their risk for cervical cancer.

35. A nurse is preparing a pamphlet designed to alert adolescents to the dangers of sexually transmitted infections and what they can do to prevent their transmission.

    a. Describe what the nurse should say about "safer sex."

    b. As an impetus to motivate adolescents to use safer sex measures, the nurse decides to include a section on the consequences of sexually transmitted infections. Discuss the points the nurse should emphasize in this section of the pamphlet.

36. Explain why violent crimes against women are underreported.

37. Describe the characteristics of women who are battered.

MULTIPLE CHOICE QUESTIONS: Circle the one correct option and state the rationale for the option chosen.

38. A 52-year-old woman asks the nurse practitioner about how often she should be assessed for the common health problems women of her age could experience. The nurse would recommend
    a. an endometrial biopsy every 2 to 3 years.
    b. a fecal occult blood test twice a year.
    c. a mammogram every other year.
    d. a blood cholesterol level at least every 5 years.

39. Which of the following statements is most accurate regarding persons who should participate in preconception counseling?
    a. All women and their partners as they make decisions about their reproductive future including becoming parents
    b. All women during their childbearing years
    c. Sexually active women who do not use birth control
    d. Women with chronic illnesses such as diabetes who are planning to get pregnant

40. When teaching a group of young women about contraceptive methods the nurse would state:
    a. Using condoms may prevent the transmission of human immunodeficiency virus (HIV).
    b. Oral contraceptive pills containing estrogen and progesterone provide some protection from developing cervical cancer later in life.
    c. Pelvic inflammatory disease is more likely to occur when barrier methods are used as a method of contraception.
    d. A diaphragm offers the most protection from sexually transmitted infections (STIs).

41. A newly married 25-year-old woman has been smoking since she was a teenager. She has come to the women's health clinic for a checkup before she begins trying to get pregnant. The woman demonstrates a need for further instruction about the effects of smoking on reproduction and health when she states:
    a. "Smoking can interfere with my ability to get pregnant."
    b. "My husband also needs to stop smoking because secondhand smoke can have an adverse effect on my pregnancy and the development of the baby."
    c. "Smoking can make my pregnancy last longer than it should."
    d. "Smoking can reduce the amount of calcium in my bones."

42. When assessing young women who are sexually active, the nurse should be aware that which of the following represents a risk factor for developing cervical cancer?
    a. First sexual intercourse after age 30
    b. Multiple sexual partners
    c. Nulliparity
    d. Early or late menopause

43. A nurse caring for pregnant women needs to be aware that physical abuse during pregnancy can result in
    a. excessive weight gain as a result of the inappropriate intake of food to reduce stress.
    b. use of alcohol or tobacco as a means of coping.
    c. postterm pregnancy.
    d. preeclampsia.

II. THINKING CRITICALLY

1. A nurse is teaching a group of young adult women about health promotion activities. As part of the discussion the nurse identifies preconception care as an important health promotion activity. One woman in the class asks, "I know you need to go for checkups once you are pregnant, but why would you need to see a doctor before you get pregnant? Isn't that a big waste of time and money?" Explain how the nurse should respond to this woman's question.

2. During a routine checkup for her annual Pap smear, Julie, a 26-year-old woman, asks the nurse for advice regarding nutrition and exercise. She is considered to be overweight with a body mass index (BMI) of 27.4 and wants to lose weight sensibly. Discuss the advice the nurse should give to Julie.

3. Alice, a 30-year-old woman comes to the women's health clinic complaining of fatigue, insomnia, and feeling anxious. She works as a stockbroker for a major Wall Street brokerage firm. Alice states that, although she enjoys the challenge of her job, she never can seem to find time for herself or to socialize with her friends. Alice tells the nurse practitioner that she has been drinking more and started to smoke again to help her relax. She is glad that she has lost some weight, attributing this occurrence to her diminished appetite.

   a. State the physical and psychologic manifestations of stress that the nurse should take note of when assessing Alice.

   b. Discuss how the nurse can help Alice cope with stress and its consequences in a healthy manner.

   c. Alice expresses interest in attempting to stop smoking. "I felt so much better when I stopped the first time. That was over 2 years ago and now, here I am back at it again." Describe an approach the nurse could use to help Alice achieve a desired change in health behavior that is long lasting.

4. Laura is a 28-year-old pregnant woman at 8 weeks of gestation. This is her first pregnancy. During the health history interview she reveals that she smokes at least 2 packs of cigarettes each day. When discussing this practice with the nurse, Laura states, "My friends smoked when they were pregnant and their babies are okay. In fact, two of them had pregnancies that were a little shorter than expected and they had nice small babies." Describe how the nurse should respond to Laura's comments.

5. During a routine women's health checkup a woman expresses concern to the nurse practitioner about the increase in violence against women. She states, "One of my friends was raped and a colleague at work was beaten by her boyfriend." Discuss how the nurse practitioner should respond to this woman's concern, including measures she could use to protect herself from violence and injury.

6. Supply the facts to disprove each of the following myths concerning violence against women.

   a. Battering occurs only in "problem" or lower-class families.

   b. Battering occurs in a small percentage of the population.

   c. Battered women like to be beaten and deliberately provoke the attack. They are masochistic.

   d. Being pregnant protects the woman from battering.

7. As a nurse working in a prenatal health clinic you must be alert to cues indicative of battery committed against women when they are pregnant.

   a. Identify the body parts of pregnant women targeted during a battering episode.

   b. Carol, a 24-year-old married woman, comes to the clinic to confirm her belief that she is pregnant. During the assessment phase of the visit, you note cues that lead you to suspect that Carol is being abused by her husband. Discuss the approach you would take to confirm your suspicion that Carol is being abused.

c. Carol admits to you that her husband "beats her sometimes and it has been increasing." Now she is afraid it will get worse since she "was not supposed to get pregnant." Discuss the nursing actions that you could take to help Carol.

d. List the possible reasons why Carol, now that she is pregnant, is experiencing an escalation of battering/abuse from her husband.

e. Discuss how Carol's pregnancy could be adversely affected by the abuse she is experiencing.

5 Health Assessment

I. REVIEWING KEY CONCEPTS AND CONTENT

FILL IN THE BLANKS: Insert the term that corresponds to each of the following definitions related to the female reproductive system and breasts.

1. _____ Fatty pad that lies over the anterior surface of the symphysis pubis.

2. _____ Two rounded folds of fatty tissue covered with skin that extend downward and backward from the mons pubis; their purpose is to protect the inner vulvar structures.

3. _____ Two flat, reddish folds composed of connective tissue and smooth muscle, which are supplied with nerve endings that are extremely sensitive.

4. _____ Hoodlike covering of the clitoris.

5. _____ Fold of tissue under the clitoris.

6. _____ Thin flat tissue formed by the joining of the labia minora; it is underneath the vaginal opening at the midline.

7. _____ Small structure underneath the prepuce composed of erectile tissue with numerous sensory nerve endings; it increases in size during sexual arousal.

8. _____ Almond-shaped area enclosed by the labia minora that contains openings to the urethra, Skene's glands, vagina, and Bartholin's glands.

9. _____ Skin-covered muscular area between the fourchette and the anus that covers the pelvic structures.

10. _____ Fibromuscular, collapsible tubular structure that extends from the vulva to the uterus and lies between the bladder and rectum. Its mucosal lining is arranged in transverse folds called _____.
_____ and _____ glands secrete mucus that lubricates the vagina.

11. _____ Anterior, posterior, and lateral pockets that surround the cervix.

12. _____ Muscular pelvic organ located between the bladder and the rectum and just above the vagina. The _____ is a deep pouch, or recess, posterior to the cervix formed by the posterior ligament.

13. _____ Upper triangular portion of the uterus.

14. _____ Also known as the lower uterine segment, it is the short constricted portion that separates the corpus of the uterus from the cervix.

15. _____ Dome-shaped top of the uterus.

16. _____ Highly vascular lining of the uterus.

17. _____ Layer of the uterus composed of smooth muscles that extend in three different directions.

18. _____ Lower cylindric portion of the uterus composed of fibrous connective tissue and elastic tissue.

19. _____ Canal connecting the uterine cavity to the vagina. The opening between the uterus and this canal is the _____. The opening between the canal and the vagina is the

_____.

20. _____ Location in the cervix where the squamous and columnar epithelium meet; it is also known as the _____ zone; it is the most common site for neoplastic changes; cells from this site are scraped for the Pap smear.

21. _____ Passageways between the ovaries and the uterus; they are attached at each side of the dome-shaped uterine fundus.

22. _____ Almond-shaped organs located on each side of the uterus; their two functions are _____ and the production of the

hormones _____, _____, and _____.

26. _____ Pigmented section of the breast that surrounds the nipple.

23. _____ The paired mammary glands.

27. _____ Sebaceous glands that cause the areola to appear rough.

24. _____ Segment of mammary tissue that extends into the axilla.

28. _____ Breast structures lined with epithelial cells that secrete colostrum and milk.

25. _____ Mammary papilla.

29. _____ Milk reservoirs.

30. A nurse working in the field of women's health must have knowledge of the female reproductive systems, including the internal and external structures, the interrelationship of these structures, and their normal characteristics. Label each of the following illustrations as indicated, using the figures in Chapter 5 and those found in a physical assessment or anatomy textbook to assist you.

    a. External female genitalia

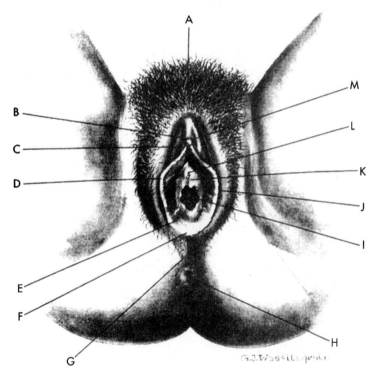

    b. Perineal body with surrounding tissues and organs

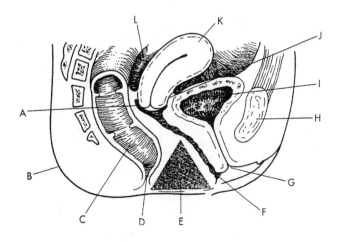

c. Cross section of uterus, adnexa, and upper vagina

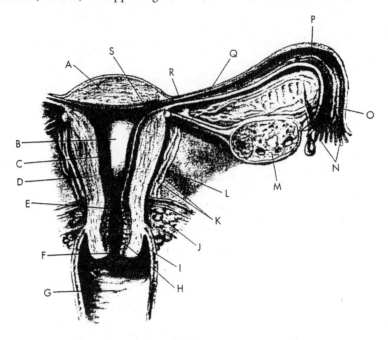

d. Female breast

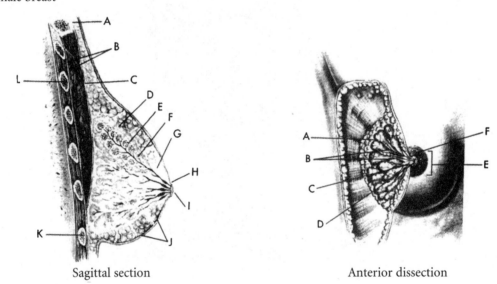

Sagittal section   Anterior dissection

e. Female pelvis

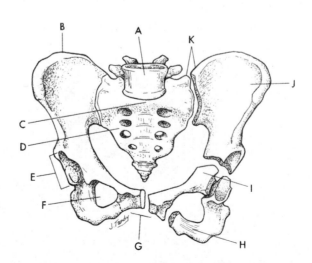

31. The diagram below illustrates the cyclical changes that occur during the menstrual cycle of a woman of childbearing age.

   a. Label the diagram as indicated in terms of hormones, phases and cycles, and specific ovarian structures.

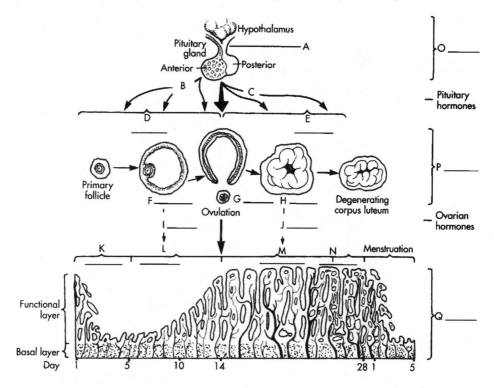

   b. Hormones play an important role in the regulation of the menstrual cycle. Describe how each of the following hormones influences the changes and events that occur during the cycle.

   Gonadotropin-releasing hormone (GnRH)

   Follicle-stimulating hormone (FSH)

   Luteinizing hormone (LH)

   Estrogen

   Progesterone

   Prostaglandins

TRUE OR FALSE: Circle T if true or F if false for each of the following statements. Correct the false statements.

32. T   F   The breasts of a healthy, mature woman should be symmetric.

33. T   F   Progesterone is the hormone responsible for the maturation of mammary gland tissue, specifically the lobules and acinar structures.

34. T   F   The breasts often change in size and nodularity during the menstrual cycle.

35. T F Breast swelling, tenderness, and leakage from the nipple are expected assessment findings during the postmenstrual period.

36. T F In North America, girls experience menarche at approximately 15 years of age.

37. T F Menstruation usually begins at about 14 days after ovulation.

38. T F The last day of bleeding or menses is day one of a new menstrual cycle.

39. T F Pregnancy is possible at any time after menarche occurs.

40. T F Variations in the length of the follicular phase account for almost all variations in ovarian cycle length.

41. T F Implantation (nidation) of a fertilized ovum usually occurs about 14 days after ovulation.

42. T F Mittelschmerz refers to the stretchable quality of cervical mucus that occurs in response to estrogen secretion before ovulation.

43. T F Dysmenorrhea (painful menstruation) is most often associated with the production of estrogen.

44. T F The average age for natural menopause is approximately 60 years.

45. T F Men and women are more alike than different in terms of their physiologic response to sexual excitement and orgasm.

46. T F Sexual arousal is characterized by increased muscular tension called myotonia.

47. T F The acidity of vaginal secretions is an important body defense against infection.

48. T F For many women, modesty, fear, and anxiety can make the health history interview and the physical examination an ordeal.

49. T F Vulvar self-examination (VSE) should be performed at least once a month between menstrual periods.

50. It is essential that guidelines for laboratory and diagnostic procedures be followed exactly in order to ensure the accuracy of the results obtained. Outline the guidelines that should be followed when performing a Papanicolaou smear in terms of each of the following:

a. Patient preparation

b. Timing during examination when the specimen is obtained

c. Sites for specimen collection

d. Handling of specimens

e. Frequency of performance

51. During a clinical examination of a woman's breasts, the nurse identifies a lump in one of the breasts. Cite the characteristics that the nurse should document regarding the palpated lump.

52. Sara, a 20-year-old woman, tells the nurse that she performs breast self-examination (BSE) on a regular basis. The nurse evaluates Sara's understanding of BSE and ability to perform the technique correctly. The nurse's findings are documented below. Indicate with a "+" those findings that reflect accurate knowledge and correct technique and with a "−" those findings that require further instruction and demonstration. State the nursing instruction for those findings requiring further teaching and demonstration.

a. _____ Performs examination every 1 to 2 months.

b. _____ Performs BSE about 2 days after menstruation begins.

c. _____ Stands in front of a mirror and observes characteristics of her breasts with her arms in at least two positions: at rest at her sides and above her head.

d. _____ Observes the size of her breasts, the direction of her nipples, appearance of her skin, and if there are dimples or lumps anywhere when looking at her breasts in the mirror.

e. _____ Lies down on her bed and puts a pillow under the shoulder of the breast she is going to palpate. Then she places the arm on that side under her head.

f. _____ Uses the tips of her four fingers to palpate her breast.

g. _____ Palpates her breast, using an overlapping circular pattern around her entire breast.

h. _____ Gently compresses her nipple between her thumb and forefinger to check for discharge.

i. _____ Palpates her breasts and up into her axilla while taking a shower.

MULTIPLE CHOICE QUESTIONS: Circle the one correct option and state the rationale for the option chosen.

53. When palpating the small breasts of a young slender woman, the nurse should
    a. wear sterile gloves.
    b. lift hands when moving from one segment of the breast to another.
    c. use both hands.
    d. follow a systematic, overlapping pattern.

54. A nurse instructed a female patient regarding vulvar self-examination (VSE). Which of the statements made by the patient will require further instruction?
    a. "I will perform this examination at least once a month, especially if I change sexual partners or am sexually active."
    b. "I will become familiar with how my genitalia look and feel so that I will be able to detect changes."
    c. "I will use the examination to determine when I should get medications at the pharmacy for yeast infections."
    d. "I will wash my hands thoroughly before and after I examine myself."

55. A women's health nurse practitioner is going to perform a pelvic examination on a female patient. Which of the following nursing actions would be least effective in enhancing the patient's comfort and relaxation during the examination?
    a. Encourage the patient to ask questions and express feelings and concerns before and after the examination.
    b. Ask the patient questions as the examination is performed.
    c. Allow the patient to keep her shoes and socks on when placing her feet in the stirrups.
    d. Instruct the patient to place her hands over her diaphragm and take deep, slow breaths.

56. To enhance the accuracy of the Papanicolaou (Pap) smear, the nurse should instruct the patient to do which of the following?
    a. Take a tub bath the morning of the test.
    b. Stop taking birth control pills for 2 days before the test.
    c. Avoid intercourse for 24 hours before the test.
    d. Douche with a specially prepared antiseptic solution the night before the test.

57. When assessing women, it is important for the nurse to keep in mind the possibility that they are victims of violence. The nurse should
    a. use an abuse assessment screen during the assessment of every woman.
    b. recognize that abuse rarely occurs during pregnancy.
    c. assess a woman's legs and back as the most commonly injured areas.
    d. notify the police immediately if abuse is suspected.

II. THINKING CRITICALLY

1. An inner-city women's health clinic serves a diverse population in terms of age, ethnic background, and health problems. Describe how each of the following factors should influence a women's health nurse practitioner's approach when assessing the health of the women who come to the clinic for care.

   a. Culture

   b. Age

   c. Disabilities

   d. Abuse

2. Imagine that you are a nurse working at a clinic that provides health care to women. Describe how you would respond to each of the following concerns or questions of women who have come to the clinic for care.

   a. Jane, a newly married woman, is concerned that she did not bleed during her first coital experience with her husband. She states, "I was a virgin and always thought you had to bleed when you had sex for the first time. Do you think my husband will still believe I was a virgin on our wedding night?"

   b. Serena, a 17-year-old woman, has just been scheduled for her first women's health checkup, which will include a pelvic examination and Pap smear. She nervously asks if there is anything she needs to do to get ready for the examination.

   c. Andrea is trying to get pregnant. She wonders if there are signs she could observe in her body that would indicate that she is ovulating and therefore able to conceive a baby with her partner.

   d. Anne, a 24-year-old woman asks the nurse about a recommended douche to use a couple of times a week to stay "nice and clean down there."

3. Julie, a 21-year-old woman, has come to the women's health clinic for a women's health checkup. During the health history interview she becomes very anxious and states, "I have to tell you this is my first examination. I am very scared; my friends told me that it hurts a lot to have this examination." Describe how the nurse should respond in an effort to reduce Julie's anxiety.

4. As a nurse working in a women's health clinic, you have been assigned to interview Angie, a 25-year-old new patient, to obtain her health history.

   a. List the components that should be emphasized in gathering Angie's history.

   b. Write a series of questions that you would ask to obtain data related to Angie's reproductive and sexual health and practices.

   c. Discuss the therapeutic techniques that you would use to facilitate communication. Give an example of each technique.

5. Self-examination of the breasts and vulva (genitalia) are important assessment techniques to teach a woman. Outline the procedure that you would use to teach each technique to one of your patients. Include the teaching methodologies that you would use to enhance learning.

   a. Breast self-examination

   b. Vulvar (genital) self-examination

6. Lu is a 25-year-old exchange student from China who has been living in the United States for 3 months. This is the first time that she is away from home. She comes to the university women's health clinic for a checkup and to obtain birth control. Describe how the nurse assigned to Lu would approach and communicate with her in a culturally sensitive manner.

7. Nurses working in women's health care must be aware of the growing problem of violence against women. All women should be screened when being assessed during health care for the possibility of abuse.

   a. Describe how you as a nurse would adjust the environment and your communication style when conducting the health history interview and physical examination in order to elicit a woman's confidence and trust.

   b. Identify indicators of possible abuse that you would look for before the appointment and then during the health history interview and physical examination.

   c. State the questions you would ask to screen for abuse.

   d. Discuss the approach you would take if abuse is confirmed during the assessment.

8. When teaching a group of preadolescent girls about menstruation, one student asks the nurse, "What will happen to me when all of this stuff starts?" Describe what the nurse should tell the girls about the changes that they can expect and what is happening to their bodies during each of the following components of the menstrual cycle:

   a. Hypothalamic-pituitary cycle

   b. Ovarian cycle

   c. Endometrial cycle

9. As a student you may be assigned to assist a health care provider during the performance of a pelvic examination for one of your patients.

   a. Describe how you would do each of the following:

   Prepare your patient for the examination

   Support your patient during the examination

   Assist your patient after the examination

   b. Describe how you would assist the health care provider who is performing the examination.

Common Health Problems

6

I. REVIEWING KEY CONCEPTS AND CONTENT

FILL IN THE BLANKS: Insert the term that corresponds to each of the following descriptions related to menstrual problems.

1. _____ refers to the absence or cessation of menstrual flow. It is a clinical sign of a variety of disorders, but it is most commonly associated with _____. It is one of the classic signs of _____. Hypogonadotropic _____ is often related to the suppression of the hypothalamus by _____ or sudden and severe _____, _____ disorders, _____, or _____.

2. Disordered _____, _____, and premature _____ have been described as the female athlete triad.

3. _____ or painful menstruation is one of the most common gynecologic problems for women of all ages. Symptoms usually begin _____ or _____ menstruation. _____ is a type of painful menstruation that occurs as a result of a physiologic alteration in some women. It usually appears within _____ months after menarche when _____ is established since both _____ and _____ are necessary for it to occur. _____ is a type of painful menstruation that occurs later, typically after age 25, and is associated with pelvic abnormality.

4. _____ is a cluster of physical, psychologic, and behavioral symptoms beginning in the luteal phase of the menstrual cycle. A diagnosis is made only if the following three criteria are met: _____, _____, and _____.

5. _____ is a menstrual disorder that is characterized by the presence and growth of endometrial tissue outside of the uterus. This tissue responds to hormonal stimulation by growing during the _____ and _____ phases of the menstrual cycle and bleeding during or immediately after _____ resulting in an _____ response with subsequent _____ and _____ to adjacent organs. The major symptoms of this disorder are _____ and deep pelvic _____. Many women also experience bowel symptoms such as _____, pain with _____, and _____. Impaired _____ may result from adhesions around the uterus and uterine tubes.

6. _____ is any form of uterine bleeding that is irregular in amount, duration, or timing and is not related to regular menstrual bleeding. _____ is a subset of this disorder defined as excessive uterine bleeding with no demonstrable cause. It is most frequently associated with _____ at the extremes of a woman's reproductive years.

TRUE OR FALSE: Circle T if true or F if false for each of the following statements related to menstrual problems. Correct the false statements.

7. T F A pregnancy test is recommended as an important initial step when a woman experiences amenorrhea.

8. T F Premature osteoporosis can occur as a consequence of low levels of progesterone associated with hypogonadotropic amenorrhea.

9. T F A woman being treated for hypogonadotropic amenorrhea requires a daily 800 mg calcium supplement.

10. T F The exact cause of premenstrual syndrome (PMS) is unknown.

11. T F Oral contraceptive pills (OCPs) are the first-line medications for the treatment of primary dysmenorrhea.

12. T F Endometriosis is a menstrual disorder primarily affecting Caucasian women during their late teens to early twenties.

13. T F Nafarelin (Synarel) is a gonadotropin-releasing hormone agonist administered to reduce pain associated with primary dysmenorrhea.

14. T F The only definitive cure for endometriosis is a total abdominal hysterectomy (TAH) with bilateral salpingo-oophorectomy (BSO).

15. T F Primary dysmenorrhea most often is related to excessive prostaglandin secretion during an ovulatory cycle.

16. T F Women often experience a decrease in dysmenorrhea after a full-term pregnancy.

17. T F Women who experience primary dysmenorrhea should avoid physical activity, including exercising for the first few days of menstrual bleeding.

18. T F The pain associated with secondary dysmenorrhea is often sharp, radiating over the abdomen from umbilicus to symphysis pubis.

19. T F Lifestyle changes usually have little effect in the treatment of premenstrual syndrome.

20. T F Evening primrose oil taken daily has been found to be effective in relieving breast symptoms associated with premenstrual syndrome.

21. T F Pregnancy is contraindicated for women who have endometriosis and are being treated with danazol.

FILL IN THE BLANKS: Insert the term that corresponds to each of the following descriptions related to infection.

22. _____ Infections or infectious disease syndromes primarily transmitted by close intimate contact. The most common infections of this type in women are _____, _____, _____, _____, _____, and _____.

23. _____ Precautions used during sexual activity to prevent the transmission of pathogens. These precautions include _____, _____, _____, and _____.

24. _____ The physical barrier promoted for the prevention of sexual transmission of human immunodeficiency virus (HIV) and other sexually transmitted infections (STIs).

25. _____ Bacterial infection that is the most common and fastest spreading STI in American women. This infection is often silent and highly destructive to the female reproductive tract.

26. _____ The oldest communicable disease in the United States. Since it is a reportable communicable disease, health care providers are legally responsible for reporting all cases to health authorities.

27. _____ One of the earliest sexually transmitted diseases (STDs). It is caused by *Treponema pallidum*, a spirochete. _____ is characterized by a lesion or _____ that appears _____ days after infection. _____ occurs ____weeks to _____ months after the appearance of the primary lesion and is characterized by a widespread _____ on the _____ and _____ and generalized _____. The infected individual may experience_____, _____, and _____. _____ may develop on the vulva, perineum, and anus. If left untreated the patient enters a _____ phase that is asymptomatic for most persons. _____ is characterized by neurologic, cardiovascular, musculoskeletal, and multiorgan system complications.

28. _____ Infectious process that most commonly involves the uterine tubes, uterus, and more rarely ovaries and peritoneal surfaces. The ascending spread of microorganisms most commonly happens at the end of or just after _____ or following an _____, _____, or _____.

29. _____ Infection previously named genital or venereal warts. It is now the most common viral STI seen in ambulatory health care settings. The visible lesions caused by the infection are called _____.

30. _____ A viral infection that is transmitted sexually and is characterized by painful recurrent genital ulcers. Patients with an initial or primary genital infection exhibit multiple painful _____, _____, _____, _____, and severe _____ that may last _____ weeks.

31. _____ Viral infection acquired primarily through a fecal-oral route by ingestion of contaminated food, particularly _____, _____, or polluted _____, or _____ contact.

32. _____ Viral infection involving the liver that is transmitted parenterally, perinatally, and through intimate contact. It is 50 to 100 times more contagious than HIV. A vaccine is available to protect infants, children, and adults.

33. _____ The most common blood-borne infection in the United States. It is a disease of the liver that is transmitted parenterally and through intimate contact. No vaccine is available to provide protection against this infection.

34. _____ A retrovirus that is transmitted primarily though exchange of body fluids. Severe depression of the _____ system is associated with this infection.

35. _____ A normal vaginal flora that is present in 9% to 23% of healthy pregnant women. It is associated with poor pregnancy outcomes. Vertical transmission to the newborn during birth has been implicated as an important factor in perinatal and neonatal morbidity and mortality.

36. _____ Vaginal infection formerly called nonspecific vaginitis, _Haemophilus vaginitis_, or _Gardnerella_; it is the most common type of vaginitis and is characterized by a profuse, thin, and white, gray, or milky discharge that has a _____ odor.

37. _____ This yeast infection is the second most common type of vaginal infection in the United States. Common symptoms include _____, _____, and _____. The discharge is _____, _____, _____, and _____. It appears as patches on the _____, _____, and _____.

38. _____ A vaginal infection caused by an anaerobic one-celled protozoan with characteristic flagella. The typically copious discharge is yellowish green, frothy, mucopurulent, and malodorous.

TRUE OR FALSE: Circle T if true or F if false for each of the following statements related to infections. Correct false statements.

39. T F Sexually transmitted infections are among the most common health problems in the United States today.

40. T F Safer sex practices are secondary prevention activities.

41. T F Anal intercourse is a safe alternative to vaginal intercourse if a condom is not available.

42. T F The most common sexually transmitted bacterial pathogen in American women is gonorrhea.

43. T F The majority of women contracting gonorrhea are 30 years of age or older.

44. T F Chlamydia can be transmitted by direct sexual contact or exposure at birth.

45. T F The Centers for Disease Control and Prevention (CDC) recommends that all women between the ages of 18 and 40 be screened for chlamydia every year at the time of the Papanicolaou (Pap) smear.

46. T F Women over age 30 have the lowest rate of infection with chlamydia.

47. T F Gonorrhea can be spread by direct contact with infected lesions and indirectly by transfer from inanimate objects.

48. T F Erythromycin is the preferred drug for the treatment of syphilis.

49. T F _C. trachomatis_ is estimated to cause at least half of all cases of pelvic inflammatory disease (PID).

50. T F Visible warts characterize the types of human papillomavirus (HPV) associated with cervical dysplasia.

51. T F HPV infections are thought to be more common in pregnant women than in nonpregnant women.

52. T F Lesions characteristic of recurrent episodes of herpes simplex virus type 2 (HSV-2) infections are unilateral, beginning as vesicles and progressing rapidly to ulcers.

53. T F Vaginal birth is acceptable if visible HSV-2 lesions are not present at the onset of labor.

54. T F Women who test positive for hepatitis B should not breastfeed their newborn.

55. T F Women are the fastest growing population with HIV infection and AIDS.

56. T F Once HIV enters the body, seroconversion to HIV positivity occurs within 2 to 4 weeks.

57. T F HIV can be transmitted to the newborn via the breast milk of an infected mother.

58. T F Zidovudine (AZT) has been found to be a safe and effective treatment method for women who are HIV positive during pregnancy.

59. T F Vaccination of a woman for hepatitis B during pregnancy can infect the fetus and is therefore contraindicated until after birth.

60. T F The recommended treatment for women in labor who test positive for Group B streptococcus is the intravenous administration of penicillin G.

61. T F Standard Precautions are to be used as soon as a patient is diagnosed with a blood-borne infection.

62. Cite several common risk factors for sexually transmitted diseases.

63. State two specific precautions for each of the following categories:

Standard Precautions

Precautions for invasive procedures

64. Complete the following table related to common reproductive tract infections.

Infection	Clinical Manifestations	Management Guidelines
Chlamydia		
Gonorrhea		
Human papillomavirus		
Herpes simplex virus		
Bacterial vaginosis		
Candidiasis		
Trichomoniasis		

65. Heterosexual transmission is the most common means of infecting women with HIV.

    a. State the mode of transmission for HIV

    b. List the clinical manifestations that may be exhibited during seroconversion to HIV positivity.

    c. Outline the care management approach that should be used by nurses who care for women who test HIV positive.

TRUE OR FALSE: Circle T if true or F if false for each of the following statements related to breast problems. Correct the false statements.

66. T   F   Approximately 50% of fibrocystic conditions of the breast have changes that indicate a risk for cancer.

67. T   F   Typically fibrocystic change is noted as lumpiness in both breasts.

68. T   F   Clinical manifestations associated with fibrocystic change are rarely related to the menstrual cycle.

69. T   F   When a breast lump is palpated, a fine-needle aspirate (FNA) is performed to determine if the lump is fluid filled or solid.

70. T   F   The tenderness associated with fibrocystic breast change is often reduced when caffeine is eliminated from the diet.

71. T   F   The most common benign breast problem is fibroadenoma.

72. T   F   Fibroadenomas tend to increase in size when a woman is pregnant.

73. T   F   Bilateral serous drainage expressed during nipple stimulation requires a microscopic analysis to determine causation.

74. T   F   Risk factors help identify less than 30% of women who will eventually develop breast cancer.

75. T   F   The most important predictor of risk for breast cancer is a family history of breast cancer.

76. T   F   The United States has one of the lowest rates of breast carcinoma in the world.

77. T   F   The risk of an American woman developing breast cancer is 1 in 8.

78. T   F   The mortality rate for breast cancer is higher in Caucasian women.

79. T   F   Ultrasonography can be used to distinguish between cysts and solid tumors found in the breast.

MATCHING: Match the description in Column I with the appropriate breast disorder in Column II.

COLUMN I

80. _____ Lumpiness in both breasts with or without tenderness, usually associated with changes in the menstrual cycle.

81. _____ Fatty breast tumor that is soft, nontender, mobile with discrete borders. It is most often found in women over the age of 45.

82. _____ Unilateral, solid, nontender, discrete breast mass that is unresponsive to dietary changes or hormone therapy.

83. _____ Spontaneous, bilateral milky breast discharge.

84. _____ Inflammatory process in the breast characterized by a thick, sticky, white or colored discharge. Burning pain and itching may be experienced. A mass may be palpated behind the nipple.

COLUMN II

a. Fibroadenoma

b. Fibrocystic change

c. Mammary duct ectasia

d. Lipoma

e. Galactorrhea

85. Breast cancer is a major health problem facing women in the United States. Nurses are often responsible for educating women about breast cancer.

    a. Outline the information the nurse should give women about the risk factors associated with breast cancer.

    b. List the clinical manifestations that are strongly suggestive of breast cancer.

    c. Specify the tests that can be performed to diagnose breast problems.

86. Define each of the following treatment approaches used in the care of women with breast cancer.

    a. Lumpectomy

    b. Modified radical mastectomy

    c. Autologous flap reconstruction

    d. Breast reconstruction using saline implants

    e. Radiation

    f. Adjuvant therapy

    g. Hormonal therapy

    h. Chemotherapy

MULTIPLE CHOICE QUESTIONS: Circle the one correct option and state the rationale for the option chosen.

87. Which of the following women is at greatest risk for developing hypogonadotropic amenorrhea?
    a. 48-year-old woman experiencing perimenopausal changes
    b. 13-year-old figure skater
    c. 18-year-old softball player
    d. 30-year-old (G3 P3003) breastfeeding woman

88. Pharmacologic preparations can be used to treat primary dysmenorrhea. Choose the preparation that would be least effective in relieving the symptoms of primary dysmenorrhea.
    a. Oral contraceptive pill (OCP)
    b. Naproxen sodium (Anaprox)
    c. Acetaminophen (Tylenol)
    d. Ibuprofen (Motrin)

89. Women experiencing primary dysmenorrhea should be advised to avoid which of the following foods?
    a. Red meats
    b. Asparagus
    c. Cranberry juice
    d. Whole grain cereals

90. The nurse counseling a 30-year-old woman regarding effective measures to use to relieve symptoms associated with PMS could suggest:
    a. Decrease intake of fruits especially peaches and watermelon.
    b. Avoid exercise during the luteal phase of the menstrual cycle when symptoms are at their peak.
    c. Take a vitamin supplement containing vitamin B_6 twice a day.
    d. Limit tobacco, alcohol, and caffeine use.

91. A 28-year-old woman has been diagnosed with endometriosis. She has been placed on a course of treatment with danazol (Danocrine). The woman exhibits understanding of this treatment when she says:
    a. "Since this medication stops ovulation I do not need to use birth control."
    b. "I will experience more frequent and heavier menstrual periods when I take this medication."
    c. "I can experience a decrease in my breast size, oily skin, and hair growth on my face as a result of taking this medication."
    d. "I will need to spray this medication into my nose twice a day."

92. A 55-year-old woman tells the nurse that she has started to experience pain when she and her husband have intercourse. The nurse would record that this woman is experiencing:
    a. dyspareunia.
    b. dysmenorrhea.
    c. dysuria.
    d. dyspnea.

93. Infections of the female midreproductive tract, such as chlamydia, are dangerous primarily because these infections:
    a. are asymptomatic.
    b. cause infertility.
    c. lead to PID.
    d. are difficult to treat effectively.

94. A finding associated with HPV infection would include which of the following?
    a. White, curdlike, adherent discharge
    b. Soft papillary swelling occurring singly or in clusters
    c. Vesicles progressing to pustules and then to ulcers
    d. Yellow to green frothy malodorous discharge

95. A recommended medication effective in the treatment of vulvovaginal candidiases would be
    a. Metronidazole (Flagyl).
    b. Miconazole (Monistat).
    c. Erythromycin.
    d. Acyclovir.

96. A woman is determined to be Group B streptococcus (GBS) positive at the onset of her labor. The nurse should prepare this woman for
    a. cesarean birth.
    b. intravenous administration of penicillin during labor.
    c. isolation of her newborn after birth.
    d. application of acyclovir to her labial lesions.

97. When providing a woman recovering from primary herpes with information regarding the recurrence of herpes infection of the genital tract, the nurse would tell her:
    a. Fever and flulike symptoms will precede a recurrent infection.
    b. Little can be done to control the recurrence of infection.
    c. Transmission of the virus is possible only when lesions are open and draining.
    d. Itching and tingling often occur before the appearance of vesicles.

98. When teaching women about breast cancer the nurse should emphasize which of the following statements?
    a. The incidence of breast cancer is highest among African-American women.
    b. Breast cancer is most prevalent among women in their thirties and forties.
    c. Most women diagnosed with breast cancer exhibited clear and identifiable risk factors.
    d. Lowering fat intake and maintaining a normal weight could have an effect on reducing a woman's chances of developing breast cancer.

99. When providing discharge instructions to a woman who had a modified right radical mastectomy, the nurse should emphasize the importance of
    a. reporting any tingling or numbness in her incisional site or right arm immediately.
    b. telling health care providers not to take a blood pressure or draw blood from her right arm.
    c. learning how to use her left arm to write and accomplish the activities of daily living such as combing her hair.
    d. wearing clothing that snugly supports her right arm.

100. A 26-year-old woman has just been diagnosed with fibrocystic change in her breasts. Which of the following nursing diagnoses would be a priority for this woman?
    a. Pain related to cyclical enlargement of breast cysts or lumps
    b. Risk for infection related to altered integrity of the areola associated with leakage from the nipples
    c. Anxiety related to anticipated surgery to remove the cysts in her breasts
    d. Fear related to high risk for breast cancer

101. When assessing a woman with a diagnosis of fibroadenoma, the nurse would expect to find which of the following characteristics?
    a. Bilateral tender lumps behind the nipple
    b. Milky discharge from one or both nipples
    c. Soft and nonmoveable lumps
    d. Small, well-delineated lump in the upper outer quadrant of one breast

II. THINKING CRITICALLY

1. Marie is a 16-year-old gymnast who has been training vigorously for a placement on the U.S. Olympic team. She has been experiencing amenorrhea, and the development of her secondary sexual characteristics has been limited. Marie expresses concern because her nonathletic friends have all been menstruating for at least 1 year and have well-developed breasts. After a health assessment, Marie was diagnosed with hypogonadotropic amenorrhea.

   a. State the risk factors for this disorder that Marie most likely exhibited during the assessment process.

   b. State one nursing diagnosis reflective of Marie's concern.

   c. Write two expected outcomes for a plan of care for Marie.

   d. Outline a typical care management plan for Marie that will address the issues associated with hypogonadotropic amenorrhea.

2. Mary, a 17-year-old who experienced menarche at age 16, comes to the women's health clinic for a routine checkup. She complains to the nurse that her last few periods have been very painful. "I have missed a few days of school because of it. What can I do to reduce the pain that I feel during my periods?" Physical examination and testing reveal normal structure and function of Mary's reproductive system. A medical diagnosis of primary dysmenorrhea is made.

   a. Compare and contrast the medical diagnoses of primary and secondary dysmenorrhea in terms of etiology and characteristics of the pain and discomfort experienced.

   b. State the priority nursing diagnosis appropriate for Mary.

   c. Identify appropriate relief measures for primary dysmenorrhea that the nurse could suggest to Mary.

3. Susan experiences physical and psychologic signs and symptoms associated with PMS during every ovulatory menstrual cycle.

   a. List the signs and symptoms most likely described by Susan that led to the diagnosis of PMS.

   b. Identify one nursing diagnosis that may be appropriate for Susan when she is experiencing the signs and symptoms of PMS.

   c. Describe the approach the nurse would use in helping Susan deal with this menstrual disorder.

4. Lisa is 26 years old and has been diagnosed recently with endometriosis.

   a. List the signs and symptoms Lisa most likely exhibited to lead to this medical diagnosis.

   b. Lisa asks, "What is happening to my body as a result of this disease?" Describe the nurse's response.

   c. Lisa asks about her treatment options. "Are there medications I can take to make me feel better?" Describe the action/effect and potential side effects for each of the following pharmacologic approaches to treatment.

      Oral contraceptive pills

      Gonadotropin-releasing hormone agonists

      Androgenic synthetic steroids

   d. Identify support measures the nurse can suggest to assist Lisa to cope with the effects of endometriosis.

5. Terry, a 20-year-old woman, comes to a women's health clinic for her first visit.

   a. During the health history interview, it is imperative that the nurse practitioner determine Terry's risk for contracting an STI, including HIV. Write one question for each of the following risk categories.

      Sexual risk

      Drug use–related risk

      Blood-related risk

      HIV concerns

   b. Terry asks the nurse about measures she could use to protect herself from STIs. Cite the major points that the nurse practitioner should emphasize when teaching Terry about prevention measures.

c. Terry tells the nurse that she does not know if she could ever tell a partner that he must wear a condom. Describe the approach the nurse can take to enhance Terry's assertiveness and communication skills.

6. Martha is 4 weeks pregnant. As part of her prenatal assessment, it was discovered that she was HIV positive. Identify the measures that can be used to reduce the risk of transmission of HIV from Martha to her baby.

7. Suzanne, a 20-year-old woman, is admitted for suspected severe, acute PID.

a. Identify the risk factors for PID that the nurse would be looking for in Suzanne's health history.

b. A complete physical examination is performed to determine if the criteria for PID are met. Specify the criteria that Suzanne's health care provider would be alert for during the examination.

c. Suzanne is hospitalized when the diagnosis of PID secondary to chlamydial infection is confirmed. Intravenous antibiotics will be used as the primary medical treatment followed by oral antibiotics at the time of discharge. State three priority nursing diagnoses that are likely to be present during the acute stage of Suzanne's infection and treatment.

d. Outline a nursing management plan for Suzanne in terms of each of the following:

Position and activity

Comfort measures

Support measures

Health education in preparation for discharge

e. List the recommendations for Suzanne's self-care during the recovery phase.

f. Identify the reproductive health risks that Suzanne may face as a result of the pelvic infection she experienced.

8. Laura has just been diagnosed with gonorrhea, a sexually transmitted disease.

   a. Laura, who is very upset by the diagnosis, states, "This is just awful. What kind of sex life can I have now?" Cite a nursing diagnosis that reflects Laura's concern.

   b. Outline a management plan that will assist Laura to take control of her self-care and prevent future infections.

9. Cheryl, a 27-year-old woman, is being treated for HPV. A primary diagnosis identified for Cheryl is "pain related to lesions on the vulva and around the anus secondary to HPV infection." State the measures the nurse could suggest to Cheryl to reduce the pain from the condylomata and enhance their healing.

10. Mary, a 20-year-old woman, has just been diagnosed with a primary herpes simplex 2 infection. In addition to the typical systemic symptoms, Mary exhibits multiple, painful genital lesions.

    a. Relief of pain and healing without the development of a secondary infection are two expected outcomes for care. Identify several measures that the nurse can suggest to Mary in an effort to help her achieve the expected outcomes of care.

    b. Mary asks the nurse if there is anything she can do so that this infection does not return. Discuss what the nurse should tell Mary about the recurrence of HSV-2 infection and the influence of self-care measures.

11. Sonya is concerned that she has been exposed to HIV and has come to the women's health clinic for testing.

    a. During the health history the nurse questions Sonya about behaviors that could have placed her at risk for HIV transmission. Cite the behaviors that the nurse would be looking for.

    b. Explain the testing procedure that will most likely be followed to determine Sonya's HIV status.

    c. Outline the counseling protocol that should guide the nurse when caring for Sonya before and after the test.

    d. Sonya's test result is negative. Discuss the instructions the nurse should give Sonya regarding guidelines she should follow to reduce her risk for the transmission of HIV with future sexual partners.

12. Mary Anne comes to the women's health clinic complaining that her breasts feel lumpy.

    a. Outline the assessment process that should be used to determine the basis for Mary Anne's complaint.

    b. A diagnosis of fibrocystic breast changes is made. Describe the signs and symptoms Mary Anne most likely exhibited to support this diagnosis.

    c. State one nursing diagnosis that the nurse would identify as a priority when preparing a plan of care for Mary Anne.

    d. Identify measures the nurse could suggest to Mary Anne for lessening the symptoms she experiences related to fibrocystic changes.

13. Molly, a 50-year-old woman, found a lump in her left breast during a breast self-examination. She comes to the women's health clinic for help.

    a. Describe the diagnostic protocol that should be followed to determine the basis for the lump Molly found in her breast.

    b. Molly elects to have a simple mastectomy based on the information provided by her health care providers and in consultation with her husband. Identify two priority postoperative nursing diagnoses and outline the nursing care management for the postoperative phase of Molly's treatment.

    Nursing diagnoses

    Postoperative phase care measures

    c. Molly will be discharged within 48 hours after her surgery. Describe the instructions that the nurse should give Molly to prepare her for self-care at home.

    d. Discuss support measures the nurse should use to address the concerns that Molly and her husband will most likely experience and express.

Infertility, Contraception, and Abortion

7

I. REVIEWING KEY CONCEPTS AND CONTENT

TRUE OR FALSE: Circle T if true or F if false for each of the following statements regarding infertility. Correct the false statements.

1. T F Infertility is a problem for 25% of reproductive age couples in the United States.

2. T F Infertility that is solely a result of female factors is responsible for approximately 70% of infertility cases.

3. T F A combination of male and female factors and unexplained and unusual problems account for approximately one third of infertility.

4. T F Emotional stresses can influence a woman's fertility.

5. T F Clinical tests for the detection of ovulation such as basal body temperature (BBT) and secretory endometrial changes are based on the secretion of large amounts of estrogen.

6. T F An increase in scrotal temperature when using hot tubs and saunas may lessen fertility by interfering with spermatogenesis.

7. T F Hysterosalpingography is scheduled for day 7 to 10 of the menstrual cycle.

8. T F An endometrial biopsy is typically performed in the proliferative phase of the menstrual cycle before ovulation.

9. T F The use of condoms during genital intercourse for 2 months will reduce the female antibody production in most women who have elevated antisperm antibody titers.

10. T F The multifetal pregnancy rate with the use of medications that stimulate or enhance ovulation can be as high as 25% or greater.

11. T F Herbal preparations that promote fertility include licorice root and passion flower.

FILL IN THE BLANKS: Insert the term that corresponds to each of the following descriptions of reproductive alternatives.

12. _____
A woman's eggs are collected, fertilized in the laboratory with sperm, and transferred into her uterus after normal embryo development has occurred.

13. _____
Selection of one sperm cell that is injected directly into the egg to achieve fertilization; it is used with in vitro fertilization (IVF).

14. _____
Oocytes are retrieved from the ovary, placed in a catheter with sperm, and immediately transferred into the fimbriated end of the uterine tube.

15. _____
After IVF the ova are placed in one uterine tube during the zygote stage.

16. _____
Sperm from a person other than the male partner are used to inseminate the female partner.

17. _____ Embryo(s) from one couple are transferred into the uterus of another woman who has contracted with the couple to carry the baby to term. This woman has no genetic connection with the child.

18. _____ Process by which a woman is inseminated with the semen from the infertile woman's partner and then carries the baby until birth.

19. _____ The zona pellucida is penetrated chemically or manually to create an opening for the dividing embryo to hatch and to implant into the uterine wall.

MATCHING: Match the description in Column I with the appropriate test in Column II.

<table>
<tr><td align="center">COLUMN I</td><td align="center">COLUMN II</td></tr>
</table>

20. _____ Immunologic test to determine sperm and cervical mucus interaction and compatibility

a. Laparoscopy

21. _____ Basic test for male infertility

b. Postcoital test (Sims-Huhner)

22. _____ Examination of the lining of the uterus to detect secretory changes and receptivity to implantation

c. Endometrial biopsy

d. Hysterosalpingography

23. _____ Test for adequacy of coital technique, cervical mucus, sperm, and degree of sperm penetration through cervical mucus.

e. Sperm immobilization antigen-antibody reaction

24. _____ Examination of uterine cavity and tubes using radiopaque contrast material instilled through the cervix. It is often used to determine tubal patency and to release a blockage if present.

f. Semen analysis

25. _____ Examination of pelvic structures by inserting a small endoscope through an incision in the anterior abdominal wall.

26. Mary and Jim have come for their first visit to the fertility clinic. The nurse needs to instruct them about the interrelated structures, functions, and processes essential for conception, emphasizing that they are a biologic unit of reproduction.

    a. Identify and describe each component required for normal fertility.

    b. Support the statement, "Assessment of infertility must involve both partners."

27. Cite several surgical procedures that could be helpful in treating the causes of infertility.

TRUE OR FALSE: Circle T if true or F if false for each of the following statements regarding contraception and abortion. Correct the false statements.

28. T F Despite the large number of persons who use contraception, almost one third of pregnancies in the United States are unintended.

29. T F Contraception failure rate refers to the percentage of contraceptive users expected to have an accidental pregnancy during the first year of use, even when they use the method consistently and correctly.

30. T F The fertile period extends from 4 days before to 3 to 4 days after ovulation.

31. T F Coitus interruptus is similar to barrier methods with regard to effectiveness.

32. T F The typical failure rate for all fertility awareness methods is about 25% during the first year of use.

33. T F When preparing to use the calendar rhythm method, a woman needs to accurately record the lengths of the previous two menstrual cycles.

34. T F The luteinizing hormone (LH) surge in urine just before ovulation can be affected if the woman is ill at the time of the test.

35. T F Research has demonstrated that polyurethane condoms are highly effective in protecting against sexually transmitted diseases and human immunodeficiency virus (HIV) infections.

36. T F The female condom can be inserted up to 8 hours before intercourse.

37. T F Use of a diaphragm can increase the risk for urethritis and recurrent cystitis.

38. T F An advantage of using a cervical cap is that it can be left in place longer than a diaphragm.

39. T F When using a cervical cap, the woman must apply spermicide before each act of intercourse.

40. T F A new contraceptive sponge needs to be inserted for each act of sexual intercourse.

41. T F Broad-spectrum antibiotics can decrease the effectiveness of the oral contraceptive pill.

42. T F. The mini-pill contains both estrogen and progesterone.

43. T F The patch used in the transdermal contraceptive system should be changed twice a week.

44. T F After injecting Depo-Provera intramuscularly the nurse should massage the injection site to fully distribute the progestin.

45. T F Depo-Provera injections must be repeated every 12 weeks.

46. T F An antiemetic taken 1 hour before each oral dose of estrogen and progesterone used for emergency contraception will help minimize nausea.

47. T F There is an increased risk of pelvic inflammatory disease (PID) during the first 20 days after insertion of an intrauterine device (IUD).

48. T F Female sterilization, by occluding both fallopian tubes, has a 100% success rate for preventing pregnancy.

49. T F Most abortions are performed during the second trimester.

50. T F Mifepristone (RU 486) can be taken up to 9 weeks after conception to terminate a pregnancy.

FILL IN THE BLANKS: Insert the term that corresponds to each of the following descriptions of contraceptive methods.

51. _____ Method that requires the male partner to withdraw his penis from the woman's vagina before ejaculation.

52. _____ Group of contraceptive methods that rely on avoidance of intercourse during fertile days.

53. _____ Method that combines the charting of signs and symptoms of the menstrual cycle with the use of abstinence or other contraceptive methods during fertile periods.

54. _____ Method based on the number of days in each cycle counting from the first day of menses. The fertile period is determined after accurately recording lengths of menstrual cycles for 6 months.

55. _____ Method based on variations in a woman's lowest body temperature, which is determined after waking and before getting out of bed.

56. _____ Term used to refer to the stretchiness of cervical mucus.

57. _____ Method that uses the physiologic and psychologic changes that occur during each phase of the menstrual cycle to determine the occurrence of ovulation and the fertile period.

58. _____ Chemical that destroys sperm. When inserted into the vagina it acts as both a chemical and physical barrier to sperm. It is also an effective lubricant.

59. _____ Thin, stretchable sheath that covers the penis or is inserted into the vagina.

60. _____ Shallow, dome-shaped rubber device with a flexible rim that covers the cervix.

61. _____ A soft natural rubber dome with a firm but pliable rim that fits snugly around the base of the cervix close to the junction of the cervix and vaginal fornices.

62. _____ A small round polyurethane device that contains a spermicide. It fits over the cervix and has a woven polyester loop to facilitate its removal.

63. _____ Form of hormonal contraception in which six Silastic capsules containing progestin are implanted subdermally into the inner aspect of the upper arm.

64. _____ Progesterone antagonist that prevents the implantation of a fertilized ovum. It can be used up to 9 weeks after conception with effectiveness being enhanced when a _____ is administered 36 to 48 hours later.

65. _____ Small, T-shaped object inserted into the uterine cavity. It can be loaded with copper or a progestational agent.

66. _____ Surgical procedures intended to render the person infertile. Method used to render a female infertile is termed tubal _____ and can be accomplished by _____, _____, or the application of _____ or _____. _____ is the easiest and most commonly used method for males. It involves ligating and then severing the _____ of each testicle.

67. _____ Purposeful interruption of a pregnancy before 20 weeks of gestation. If it is performed at the woman's request it is termed an _____. If it is performed for reasons of maternal or fetal health or disease it is termed a _____.

68. A nurse is working with a couple to help them choose a method of contraception that is right for them. List the factors that should be considered when helping this couple choose their contraceptive method.

69. A woman is a little uncomfortable about checking her cervical mucus and asks the nurse what she could possibly find out about doing this assessment. State the useful purpose of self-evaluation of cervical mucus.

70. June's religious and cultural beliefs prohibit her from using any artificial method of birth control. She is interested in learning about fertility awareness and natural family planning methods. Fill in the blanks in each of the following statements concerning this method.

   a. The two principal problems with fertility awareness methods are that the _____ and it is often difficult to _____. Women with _____ have the greatest risk for failure.

   b. Using the calendar method, June and her husband would abstain from day _____ to _____ of her menstrual cycle because her shortest cycle was 23 days and the longest cycle was 33 days.

   c. Basal body temperature (BBT) may _____ about _____ ° C around the time of ovulation. After ovulation, because of increasing levels of _____, the BBT will _____ about _____ ° C. This change in BBT will last until _____ before menstruation. This change in temperature is termed the _____.

   d. The _____ method would require June to recognize and interpret the cyclical changes in the characteristics of her _____ such as _____ and _____.

   e. The symptothermal method combines _____ and _____ methods with awareness of secondary cycle phase–related symptoms such as _____, _____, _____, _____, or _____, and _____. The woman is taught to palpate her _____ to assess for changes indicating ovulation such as _____, _____, and _____ in the vagina.

   f. The predictor test for ovulation detects the sudden surge of _____ in the urine that occurs approximately _____ hours before ovulation.

71. Joyce has chosen the diaphragm as her method of contraception. Label each of the following actions with *C* if correct or *I* if incorrect. Indicate how the action should be changed for those actions labeled *I*.

   a. _____ Joyce came to be refitted after healing was complete following the term vaginal birth of her son.

   b. _____ Joyce applies a spermicide only to the rim of the diaphragm just before insertion because she dislikes the stickiness of the spermicide.

c. _____ Joyce empties her bladder before inserting the diaphragm.

d. _____ Joyce inserts the diaphragm about 3 to 4 hours before intercourse to increase spontaneity.

e. _____ Joyce applies more spermicide for each act of intercourse.

f. _____ Joyce removes the diaphragm within 1 hour of intercourse.

g. _____ After removal, Joyce washes the diaphragm with warm water and an antiseptic-type soap, dries it, and then applies baby powder.

h. _____ Joyce always uses the diaphragm during her menstrual periods.

72. Cite four factors that can contribute to a woman's decision to seek an induced abortion.

MULTIPLE CHOICE QUESTIONS: Circle the one correct option and state the rationale for the option chosen.

73. A woman must assess herself for signs that ovulation is occurring. Which of the following is a sign associated with ovulation?
    a. Reduction in level of LH in the urine 12 to 24 hours before ovulation
    b. Spinnbarkeit
    c. Drop in BBT, following ovulation
    d. Increase in amount and thickness of cervical mucus

74. A couple is to undergo a postcoital (Huhner) test. The nurse should tell the couple that
    a. intercourse should occur daily for 3 days before the test.
    b. the test will be used to determine how sperm penetrate and survive in cervical mucus.
    c. the test will be scheduled for the day after menstruation ceases.
    d. the examination of cervical mucus must be performed within 30 minutes of intercourse.

75. A single, young adult woman received instructions from the nurse regarding the use of an oral contraceptive. The woman would demonstrate a need for further instruction if she
    a. stops asking her sexual partners to use condoms with spermicide.
    b. enrolls in a smoking cessation program.
    c. takes a pill every morning.
    d. uses a barrier method of birth control if she misses two or more pills.

76. The most common, and for some women the most distressing, side effect of progestin-only contraceptives, is
    a. irregular menstrual bleeding.
    b. headache.
    c. nervousness.
    d. nausea.

77. A woman with an IUD should confirm its placement by checking the IUD's string
    a. before each menstrual period.
    b. after intercourse.
    c. at the time of ovulation.
    d. during menstrual bleeding.

78. When using a cervical cap, the woman should
    a. apply spermicide inside the cap and around the rim.
    b. leave it in place for a minimum of 8 hours and maximum of 48 hours after the last act of coitus.
    c. continue to use the cap during menstrual periods.
    d. check the position of the cap and insert additional spermicide before each act of coitus.

II. THINKING CRITICALLY

1. Mark and his wife, Mary, are undergoing testing for impaired fertility.

   a. Describe the nursing support measures that should be used when working with this couple.

   b. Mark must provide a specimen of semen for analysis. Describe the procedure he should follow to ensure accuracy of the test.

   c. State the semen characteristics that will be assessed.

   d. A postcoital test will be part of the diagnostic process for Mary and Mark. Describe the instructions you would give them to maximize the effectiveness and accuracy of the test.

2. Alternative birth technologies are being developed and perfected, creating a variety of ethical, legal, financial, and psychosocial concerns. Discuss the issues and concerns engendered by these alternative technologies.

3. Kathy, an 18-year-old, has come to Planned Parenthood for information on birth control methods and assistance with making her choice. She tells the nurse that she is planning to become sexually active with her boyfriend of 6 months and is worried about getting pregnant. "I know I should know more about all of this, but I just don't."

   a. State the nursing diagnosis that reflects Kathy's concern.

   b. Outline the approach the nurse should use to help Kathy make an informed decision in choosing contraception that is right for her.

4. June plans to use a combination estrogen-progestin oral contraceptive.

   a. Describe the action for this type of contraception.

   b. List the advantages of using oral contraception.

   c. Using the acronym ACHES, identify the signs and symptoms that would require June to stop taking the pill and notify her health care provider.

A

C

H

E

S

d. Specify the instructions the nurse should give June about taking the pill to ensure maximum effectiveness.

5. Beth has decided to try the cervical cap as her method of contraception.

   a. Identify factors that if present in Beth's health history would make her a poor candidate for this contraceptive method.

   b. Following assessment, Beth is determined to be a good candidate for using the cervical cap. Describe the principles that the nurse should teach Beth to guide her in the safe and effective use of this method.

6. Anita has just had a Copper-T 380 A IUD inserted. Specify the instructions that the nurse should give Anita before she leaves the women's health clinic after the insertion.

7. Judy (6-4-0-2-4) and Allen, both age 36, are contemplating sterilization now that their family is complete. They are seeking counseling regarding this decision.

   a. Describe the approach a nurse should use in helping Judy and Allen make the right decision for them.

   b. They decide that Allen will have a vasectomy. Discuss the preoperative and postoperative care and instructions required by Allen.

8. Anne and her husband, Ian, will be using the symptothermal method of fertility awareness.

   a. List the assessment components of this method.

b. Outline the points the nurse should emphasize when teaching Anne and Ian to ensure that they will accurately:

Measure BBT

Evaluate cervical mucus characteristics

c. State the effectiveness of the symptothermal fertility awareness method of contraception.

9. Edna is a 20-year-old unmarried woman. She is 9 weeks pregnant and is unsure about what to do. She comes to the women's health clinic and asks for the nurse's help in making her decision, stating, "I just cannot support a baby right now. I am alone and trying to finish my education. What can I do?"

a. Cite the nursing diagnosis reflective of Edna's current dilemma.

b. Describe the approach the nurse should take in helping Edna make a decision that is right for her.

c. Edna elects to have an abortion. A vacuum aspiration will be performed in the morning. *Laminaria* will be used in preparation for the procedure. Edna asks what will happen to her as part of the abortion procedure. Describe how the nurse should respond to Edna's question.

d. Identify three nursing diagnoses related to Edna's decision and the procedure she is facing.

e. Describe the nursing measures related to the physical care and emotional support that Edna will require as part of this procedure.

f. Outline the discharge instructions that Edna should receive.

10. Marlee comes to the women's health clinic to report that she had unprotected intercourse last night. She is worried about getting pregnant since she is at midcycle and has already noticed signs of ovulation. Marlee tells the nurse that she hardly knows her partner and that her emotions just got the best of her. She is very anxious and asks the nurse what her options are. Describe the approach this nurse should use to assist Marlee with her concerns.

Genetics, Conception, and Fetal Development 8

I. REVIEWING KEY CONCEPTS AND CONTENT

FILL IN THE BLANKS: Insert the term that corresponds to each of the following descriptions related to conception and fetal development.

1. _____ Union of a single egg and sperm. It marks the beginning of a pregnancy.

2. _____ Male and female germ cell. The male germ cell is a _____ and the female germ cell is an _____.

3. _____ Process whereby gametes are formed and mature. For the male, the process is called _____ and for the female, the process is called _____.

4. _____ Process of penetration of the membrane surrounding the ovum by a sperm. It takes place in the _____ of the uterine tube. The membrane becomes impenetrable to other sperm, a process termed _____. The _____ number of chromosomes is restored when this union of sperm and ovum occurs.

5. _____ The first cell of the new individual. Within 3 days it becomes a 16-cell solid ball of cells called a _____. This developing structure becomes known as the _____ when a cavity becomes recognizable within it. The outer layer of cells surrounding this cavity is called the _____.

6. _____ Attachment process whereby the blastocyst burrows into the _____. _____ or fingerlike projections develop out of the _____ and extend into the blood filled spaces of the uterine lining. The uterine lining is now called the _____. The portion of this lining directly under the blastocyst is called the _____ and the portion of this lining that covers the blastocyst is called the _____.

7. _____ The term used to refer to the developing baby from day 15 until about 8 weeks after conception.

8. _____ The term used to refer to the developing baby from 9 weeks of gestation to the end of pregnancy.

9. _____ Membranes that surround the developing baby and the fluid. The _____ is the outer layer of these membranes and becomes the covering of the fetal side of the placenta. The _____ is the inner layer.

10. _____ Fluid that surrounds the developing baby in utero.

11. _____ Structure that connects the developing baby to the placenta. It contains three vessels, namely two _____ and one _____. _____ is the connective tissue that prevents compression of the blood vessels to ensure continued nourishment of the developing baby.

12. _____ Structure composed of 15 to 20 lobes called _____. It produces _____ essential to maintain the pregnancy, supplies the _____ and _____ needed by the developing baby for survival and growth, and removes _____ and _____.

13. _____ Capability of fetus to survive outside the uterus.

14. _____ Surface-active phospholipid that needs to be present in fetal/newborn lungs to facilitate breathing after birth. A _____ ratio can be performed using amniotic fluid as one means of determining the degree to which this phospholipid is present in fetal lungs.

15. _____ Special circulatory pathway that allows fetal blood to bypass the lungs.

16. _____ Shunt that allows most of fetal blood to bypass the liver and pass into the inferior vena cava.

17. _____ Opening between the fetal atria.

18. _____ Formation of blood.

19. _____ Maternal perception of fetal movement that occurs sometime between _____ and _____ weeks of gestation.

20. _____ Dark green to black tarry substance that contains fetal waste products. It accumulates in the fetal intestines.

21. _____ Twins that are formed from two zygotes. They are also called _____ twins.

22. _____ Twins that are formed from one fertilized ovum that then divides. They are also called _____ twins.

MATCHING: Match the description in Column I with the appropriate genetic concept in Column II.

COLUMN I	COLUMN II

23. _____ Environmental substances or exposures that result in functional or structural disability of the embryo/fetus.

24. _____ The process by which germ cells divide, producing gametes that each contain 23 chromosomes.

25. _____ Failure of a pair of chromosomes to separate.

26. _____ Small segments of DNA.

27. _____ Abnormalities in chromosome number.

28. _____ Cells that contain half of the genetic material of a normal somatic cell.

29. _____ Union of a normal gamete with a gamete containing an extra chromosome resulting in a cell with 47 chromosomes.

30. _____ X, Y

31. _____ Combination of genetic and environmental factors to result in congenital malformations.

32. _____ Process whereby body (somatic) cells replicate to yield two cells with the same genetic makeup as the parent cell.

33. _____ Single gene controls a particular trait, disorder, or defect.

34. _____ The copy of the genetic material in humans.

35. _____ Disorder reflecting absent or defective enzymes.

36. _____ Genetic material is transferred from one chromosome to another different chromosome.

37. _____ Threadlike strands formed of DNA.

38. _____ Both genes of a pair must be abnormal for disorder to be expressed.

39. _____ Somatic cell containing the full number of 46 chromosomes.

a. Mitosis

b. Meiosis

c. Haploid

d. Diploid

e. Teratogen

f. Human genome

g. Chromosome

h. Gene

i. Sex chromosomes

j. Karyotype

k. Aneuploidy

l. Trisomy

m. Nondisjunction

n. Monosomy

o. Translocation

p. Mutation

q. Unifactorial inheritance

r. Multifactorial inheritance

s. Autosomal dominant inheritance

t. Autosomal recessive inheritance

u. Inborn error of metabolism

40. _____ Union of a normal gamete with a gamete missing a chromosome resulting in a cell with only 45 chromosomes.

41. _____ A spontaneous and permanent change in normal gene structure.

42. _____ Abnormal gene for a trait is expressed even when the other member of the pair is normal.

43. _____ Pictorial analysis of the number, form, and size of an individual's chromosomes.

44. Each of the following structures plays a critical role in fetal growth and development. List the functions of each of the structures listed below.

    a. Yolk sac

    b. Amniotic membranes and fluid

    c. Umbilical cord

    d. Placenta

TRUE OR FALSE: Circle T if true or F if false for each of the following statements. Correct the false statements.

45. T   F   Normal human somatic (body) cells contain 23 pairs of chromosomes.

46. T   F   Hemophilia is an example of X-linked dominant inheritance.

47. T   F   Neural tube defects result from a combination of genetic and environmental factors.

48. T   F   In order for a recessive trait to be expressed in their offspring, both parents must contribute the abnormal gene.

49. T   F   In autosomal dominant inheritance, if one parent is affected by the disorder, there is a 100% chance of passing the abnormal gene to an offspring during each pregnancy.

50. T   F   Cystic fibrosis is an example of an inborn error of metabolism.

51. T   F   The stage of the fetus lasts from 9 weeks of gestation until the end of pregnancy, at about 40 weeks of gestation.

52. T   F   The umbilical cord is composed of two veins, one artery, Wharton's jelly, ligaments, and nerves.

53. T   F   Human chorionic gonadotropin (hCG) is first detected in maternal blood 3 weeks after conception.

54. T   F   The corpus luteum produces estrogen and progesterone to maintain the pregnancy until the placenta is mature enough to take over as an endocrine gland.

55. T   F   The placenta functions as an effective barrier to substances such as viruses and drugs, thereby protecting the fetus from their potentially harmful effects.

56. T   F   Oligohydramnios often indicates fetal renal dysfunction.

57. T   F   Meconium, waste products in the fetal intestine, may be passed into the amniotic fluid if fetal hypoxia occurs.

58. T   F   If a couple give birth to a child with an autosomal dominant disorder, there is a 50% reduction in risk that the next pregnancy will result in an affected child.

59. T   F   Fetal viability is first reached at 30 weeks of gestation.

60. T   F   A human pregnancy reaches term by 40 weeks or 280 days.

61. T   F   The occurrence of multifetal pregnancies with three or more fetuses has steadily decreased as a result of increased maternal exposure to teratogens.

62. T   F   Inborn errors of metabolism are an example of autosomal dominant inheritance.

63. Complete the following table by naming the three primary germ layers and identifying the tissues or organs that develop from each layer.

Primary Germ Layer	Tissue/Organ Formation

64. Angela has come for her first prenatal visit. Identify the questions the nurse should ask during the health history interview to determine if factors are present that would place Angela at risk for giving birth to a baby with an inheritable disorder.

65. Explain each of the following types of inheritance and give an example of each.

   a. Unifactorial inheritance

   b. Multifactorial inheritance

   c. X-Linked inheritance

MULTIPLE CHOICE QUESTIONS: Circle the one correct option and state the rationale for the option chosen.

66. An expectant woman, 40-years-old, undergoes an amniocentesis to detect the presence of Down syndrome. The fetal chromosomes are arranged and photographed to facilitate diagnosis. The term used for this picture is
   a. genotype.
   b. phenotype.
   c. chromosome type.
   d. karyotype.

67. Based on genetic testing of a newborn, a diagnosis of dwarfism was made. The parents ask the nurse if this could happen to future children. Since this is an example of autosomal dominant inheritance, the nurse would tell the parents:
   a. "For each pregnancy, there is a 50–50 chance the child will be affected by dwarfism."
   b. "This will not happen again since the dwarfism was caused by the harmful genetic effects of the infection you had during pregnancy."
   c. "For each pregnancy there is a 25% chance the child will be a carrier of the defective gene but unaffected by the disorder."
   d. "Since you already have had an affected child there is a decreased chance for this to happen in future pregnancies."

68. A female carries the gene for hemophilia on one of her X chromosomes. Now that she is pregnant she asks the nurse how this might affect her baby. The nurse should tell her:
   a. "A female baby has a 50% chance of also being a carrier."
   b. "Hemophilia is always expressed if a male inherits the defective gene."
   c. "Female babies are never affected by this disorder."
   d. "A male baby can be a carrier or have hemophilia."

69. A pregnant woman carries a single gene for cystic fibrosis. The father of her baby does not. Which of the following is true concerning the genetic pattern of cystic fibrosis as it applies to this family?
    a. The pregnant woman has cystic fibrosis herself.
    b. There is a 50% chance her baby will have the disorder.
    c. There is a 25% chance her baby will be a carrier.
    d. There is no chance her baby will be affected by the disorder.

70. When teaching a class of pregnant women about fetal development, the nurse would include which of the following statements?
    a. "The sex of your baby is determined by the ninth week of pregnancy."
    b. "The baby's heart begins to pump blood during the tenth week of pregnancy."
    c. "You should be able to feel your baby move by week 16 to 20 of pregnancy."
    d. "The baby's heart beat will be audible using a special ultrasound stethoscope as early as the eighteenth week of pregnancy."

II. THINKING CRITICALLY

1. Imagine that you are a nurse-midwife working in partnership with an obstetrician. Formulate a response to each of the following concerns or questions directed to you from some of your prenatal patients.

   a. June (2 months pregnant), Mary (5 months pregnant), and Alice (7 months pregnant) each ask for a description of their fetus at the present time.

   June

   Mary

   Alice

   b. Jessica states that a friend told her that babies born after about 35 weeks have a better chance to survive because they can breathe easier. She asks if this is true.

   c. Beth, who is 1 month pregnant, states that she heard that women who are pregnant experience quickening. She wants to know what that could mean and if it hurts.

   d. Susan, who is 6 months pregnant, states that she read in a magazine that a fetus can actually hear and see. She feels that this is totally unbelievable.

e. Alexa is 2 months pregnant. She asks how the sex of her baby was determined and if a sonogram could tell if she were having a boy or a girl.

f. Karen is pregnant for the first time. She reveals that she has a history of twins in her family. She wants to know what causes twin pregnancies to occur and what the difference is between identical and fraternal twins.

2. Mr. and Mrs. G., a Jewish couple, are newly married and are planning for pregnancy. They express to the nurse their concern that Mrs. G. has a history of Tay-Sachs disease in her family. Mr. G. has never investigated his family history.

a. Describe the nurse's role in the process of assisting Mr. and Mrs. G. to determine their genetic risk.

b. Both Mr. and Mrs. G. are found to be carriers of the disorder. Discuss the estimation of risk and interpretation of risk as it applies to the couple for giving birth to a child who is normal, is a carrier, or is affected by the disorder.

c. Outline the nurse's role in the education and emotional support of the couple now that a diagnosis and estimation of risk have been made.

Assessment for Risk Factors

9

I. REVIEWING KEY CONCEPTS AND CONTENT

TRUE OR FALSE: Circle T if true or F if false for each of the following statements. Correct the false statements.

1. T F More than one million births that occur in the United States each year are categorized as high risk.

2. T F According to the latest recorded statistics, the maternal mortality rate in the United Sates is approximately 5.4 per 100,000 live births.

3. T F The three major causes for maternal mortality are hypertensive disorders, infection, and hemorrhage.

4. T F Maternal mortality remains a significant problem because a high proportion of deaths are preventable.

5. T F African-American women have a maternal mortality rate that is twice as high as that of Caucasian women.

6. T F Respiratory distress syndrome continues as the leading cause of neonatal mortality.

7. T F The major expected outcome of antepartum testing is the detection of potential fetal compromise.

8. T F Serial measurement of the fetal biparietal diameter (BPD) and limb length by means of ultrasonography can differentiate between size discrepancies resulting from inaccurate dates and true intrauterine growth restriction (IUGR).

9. T F Hydramnios, or an increase in amniotic fluid amount, has been associated with neural tube defects.

10. T F The presence of meconium in amniotic fluid antepartally is usually associated with adverse fetal outcome.

11. T F After amniocentesis or chorionic villi sampling (CVS), an Rh-negative woman should receive RhoGAM.

12. T F The major disadvantage of a nonstress test relates to its high rate of false-negative results.

13. T F A lower than normal alpha-fetoprotein level in the maternal serum and in the amniotic fluid has been associated with Down syndrome.

14. T F In order to accurately assess results of a contraction stress test, four uterine contractions in a 15-minute period are required.

15. T F Higher than normal levels of alpha-fetoprotein in maternal serum are diagnostic of a fetal neural tube defect.

16. T F A hyperstimulation result on a contraction stress test refers to late deceleration fetal heart rate (FHR) patterns occurring as a result of excessive uterine activity or a persistent increase in uterine tone.

17. T F When performing a daily fetal movement count, a pregnant woman should call her health care provider if she notes 5 or fewer fetal movements in 1 hour.

18. Identify factors that would place the pregnant woman and fetus/neonate at risk, for each of the following categories.

Biophysical:

Psychosocial:

Sociodemographic:

Environmental:

19. Discuss the role of the nurse when caring for high-risk pregnant women who are required to undergo antepartal assessment testing to determine fetal well-being.

20. Annie is a primigravida who is at 10 weeks of gestation. Her prenatal history reveals that she was treated for pelvic inflammatory disease 2 years ago. She describes irregular menstrual cycles and is therefore unsure about the first day of her last menstrual period. Annie is scheduled for a vaginal ultrasound.

    a. Cite the likely reasons for the performance of this test.

    b. Describe how the nurse should prepare Annie for this test.

21. Ally, a pregnant woman at 20 weeks of gestation, is scheduled for a series of abdominal ultrasound tests to monitor the growth of her fetus. Describe the nursing role as it applies to Ally and ultrasound examinations.

22. State two risk factors for each of the following pregnancy problems.

    Preterm labor

    Polyhydramnios

    Intrauterine growth restriction

    Oligohydramnios

    Postterm pregnancy

    Chromosomal abnormalities

FILL-IN-THE-BLANKS: Insert the term that corresponds to each of the following descriptions.

23. A _____ is a pregnancy in which the life or health of the mother or her fetus is jeopardized by a disorder coincidental with or unique to pregnancy.

24. The major expected outcome of antepartum testing is the detecting of potential _____ ideally before intrauterine _____ of the fetus occurs so that the health care provider can take measures to prevent or minimize adverse perinatal outcomes. First and second trimester testing is directed primarily at the diagnosis of _____, whereas the goal of third trimester testing is to determine if the _____ continues to be supportive to the fetus.

25. _____ is the assessment of fetal activity by the mother. It is a simple yet valuable method for monitoring the condition of the fetus. The fetal alarm signal refers to the cessation of fetal movements entirely for _____. A count of fewer than _____ warrants further evaluation by _____ or _____, _____, or a combination of these. Fetal movements are usually not present during the fetal _____; they may be temporarily reduced if the woman is taking _____ medications, drinking _____, or _____; they do not usually _____ as the woman nears term.

26. _____ is the use of sound having a frequency higher than that detectable by humans to examine structures inside the body. It can be done _____ or _____ during pregnancy. _____ is more useful after the first trimester when the pregnant uterus rises out of the pelvis. _____, in which the probe is inserted into the _____, allows _____ anatomy to be evaluated in greater detail and _____ to be diagnosed earlier. It is optimally used in the first trimester to detect _____ pregnancies, monitor the developing _____, help identify _____, and help establish _____.

27. _____ is the noninvasive study of blood flow in the fetus and placenta. It is a helpful adjunct in the management of pregnancies at risk because of _____, _____, _____, _____, or _____.

28. _____ is a noninvasive dynamic assessment of the fetus and its environment by _____ and external _____. This test includes assessment of five variables namely _____, _____, _____, _____, and _____. The presence of normal fetal _____ activities indicates that the _____ is fully functional and the fetus is therefore not _____.

29. _____ is a noninvasive technique used for obstetric and gynecologic diagnosis by providing excellent pictures of soft tissue.

30. _____ is performed to obtain amniotic fluid that contains fetal cells. A needle is inserted _____ into the uterus, _____ is withdrawn, and various assessments are performed. Indications for this procedure are prenatal diagnosis of _____ disorders or _____ anomalies, assessment of _____ maturity, and diagnosis of fetal _____ disease.

31. Direct access to the fetal circulation during the second and third trimesters is possible through _____ or _____, which is the most widely used method for fetal _____ and _____. It involves the insertion of a needle directly into the fetal _____ under ultrasound guidance.

32. _____ is a procedure that involves the removal of a small tissue specimen from the fetal portion of the placenta. Since this tissue originates from the zygote, it reflects the _____ of the fetus. It is performed between _____ and _____ weeks of gestation.

33. Determination of the _____ level is used as a screening tool for neural tube defects in pregnancy. The test is usually performed between _____ and _____ weeks of gestation.

34. The _____ test is a screening test for Down syndrome. It is performed between _____ and _____ weeks of gestation. The levels of three markers namely _____, _____, and _____, in combination with maternal _____ are used to determine risk.

35. A _____ test or _____ determination is based on the fact that the heart rate of a healthy fetus with an intact central nervous system will usually _____ in response to fetal movement.

36. The purpose of a _____ test is to identify the jeopardized fetus who is stable at rest but shows evidence of compromise when exposed to the stress of uterine contractions. If the resultant hypoxia of the fetus is sufficient a _____ of the FHR will result. Two methods used for this test are the _____ _____ test and the _____ test.

MULTIPLE CHOICE QUESTIONS: Circle the one correct option and state the rationale for the option chosen.

37. A 34-year-old woman at 36 weeks of gestation has been scheduled for a biophysical profile. She asks the nurse why the test needs to be performed. The nurse would tell her that the test
    a. determines how well her baby will breathe after it is born.
    b. evaluates the response of her baby's heart to uterine contractions.
    c. measures her baby's head and length.
    d. observes her baby's activities in utero to ensure that her baby is getting enough oxygen.

38. As part of preparing a 24-year-old woman at 42 weeks of gestation for a nonstress test, the nurse would
    a. tell the woman to fast for 8 hours before the test.
    b. explain that the test will evaluate how well her baby is moving inside her uterus.
    c. show her how to indicate when her baby moves.
    d. attach a spiral electrode to the presenting part to determine FHR patterns.

39. A 40-year-old woman at 18 weeks of gestation is having a triple marker test performed. She is obese, and her health history reveals that she is Rh negative. The primary purpose of this test is to screen for
    a. spina bifida.
    b. Down syndrome.
    c. gestational diabetes.
    d. Rh antibodies.

40. During a contraction stress test, 4 contractions lasting 45 to 55 seconds were recorded in a 10-minute period. A late deceleration was noted during the third contraction. The nurse conducting the test would document that the result is
    a. negative.
    b. positive.
    c. suspicious.
    d. unsatisfactory.

41. A pregnant woman is scheduled for a transvaginal ultrasound test to establish gestational age. In preparing this woman for the test the nurse would
    a. place the woman in a supine position with her hips elevated on a folded pillow.
    b. instruct her to come for the test with a full bladder.
    c. administer an analgesic 30 minutes before the test.
    d. lubricate the vaginal probe with transmission gel.

II. THINKING CRITICALLY

1. Mary is at 42 weeks of gestation. Her physician has ordered a biophysical profile (BPP). She is very upset and tells the nurse, "All my doctor told me is that this test will see if my baby is okay. I do not know what is going to happen and if it will be painful to me or harmful for my baby."

   a. State a nursing diagnosis that reflects this situation.

   b. Describe how the nurse should respond to Mary's concerns.

   c. Mary receives a score of 8 for the BPP. List the factors that were evaluated to obtain this score and specify the meaning of Mary's test result of 8.

2. Jan, age 42, is 18 weeks pregnant. Because of her age, Jan's fetus is at risk for genetic anomalies. Jan's blood type is A negative and her partner's, the father of her baby, is B positive. Her primary health care provider has suggested an amniocentesis. Describe the nurse's role in terms of each of the following:

   a. Preparing Jan for the amniocentesis

   b. Supporting Jan during the procedure

   c. Providing Jan with postprocedure care and instructions

3. Susan, who has diabetes and is in week 36 of pregnancy, has been scheduled for a nonstress test.

   a. Discuss what you would tell Susan about the purpose of this test and what will be learned about her baby's well-being.

   b. Describe how you would prepare Susan for this test.

   c. Discuss how you would conduct the test.

   d. Indicate the criteria you would use to determine if the result of the test was:

   Reactive

   Nonreactive

   Unsatisfactory

4. Beth is scheduled for a contraction stress test following a nonreactive result on a nonstress test. Nipple stimulation will be used to stimulate the required contractions.

   a. Discuss what you would tell Beth about the purpose of this test and what will be learned about the well-being of her fetus.

   b. Describe how you would prepare Beth for the test.

   c. Indicate how you would conduct the test.

   d. State how you would conduct the test differently if exogenous oxytocin (Pitocin) is used instead of nipple stimulation.

e. Indicate the criteria you would use to determine if the result of the test was:

Negative

Positive

Suspicious

Hyperstimulation

Unsatisfactory

Anatomy and Physiology of Pregnancy 10

I. REVIEWING KEY CONCEPTS AND CONTENT

FILL IN THE BLANKS: Insert the term that corresponds to each of the following descriptions related to pregnancy.

1. _____ Pregnancy.

2. _____ The number of pregnancies in which the fetus or fetuses have reached viability, not the number of fetuses (e.g., twins) born. Whether the fetus is born alive or is stillborn (i.e., fetus showing no signs of life at birth) after viability is reached does not affect the numeric designation.

3. _____ A woman who is pregnant.

4. _____ A woman who has never been pregnant.

5. _____ A woman who has not completed a pregnancy with a fetus or fetuses who have reached the stage of fetal viability.

6. _____ A woman who is pregnant for the first time.

7. _____ A woman who has completed one pregnancy with a fetus or fetuses who have reached the stage of fetal viability.

8. _____ A woman who has had two or more pregnancies.

9. _____ A woman who has completed two or more pregnancies to the stage of fetal viability.

10. _____ Capacity to live outside the uterus, occurring about 20 to 24 weeks since the last menstrual period, or when the weight of the fetus is greater than 500 g.

11. _____ Designation given to a pregnancy that has reached 20 weeks of gestation but before completion of 37 weeks of gestation.

12. _____ Designation given to a pregnancy from the beginning of the thirty-eighth week of gestation to the end of the forty-second week of gestation.

13. _____ Designation given to a pregnancy that goes beyond 42 weeks of gestation. The designation _____ may also be given to refer to this pregnancy.

14. _____ The biologic marker on which pregnancy tests are based. Its presence in urine or serum results in a positive pregnancy test result.

MATCHING: Match the assessment finding in Column I with the appropriate descriptive term in Column II.

COLUMN I | COLUMN II

15. _____ Menstrual bleeding no longer occurs

16. _____ Fundal height decreased, fetal head in pelvic inlet

17. _____ Cervix and vagina violet-bluish in color

18. _____ Swelling of ankles and feet at the end of the day

19. _____ Cervical tip softened

20. _____ Lower uterine segment is soft and compressible

21. _____ Fetal head rebounds with gentle, upward tapping through the vagina

22. _____ White or slightly gray mucoid vaginal discharge with faint, musty odor

23. _____ Enlarged sebaceous glands in areola on both breasts

24. _____ Plug of mucus fills endocervical canal

25. _____ Pink stretch marks or depressed streaks on breasts and abdomen

26. _____ Thick, creamy fluid expressed from nipples

27. _____ Cheeks, nose, and forehead blotchy, brownish hyperpigmentation

28. _____ Pigmented line extending up abdominal midline

29. _____ Varicosities around the anus

30. _____ Heartburn experienced after supper

31. _____ Lumbosacral curve increased

32. _____ Paresthesia and pain in right hand radiating to elbow

33. _____ Spotting following cervical palpation or intercourse

34. _____ Hematocrit decreased to 36% and hemoglobin to 11 g/dl

35. _____ Vascular spiders on neck and thorax

36. _____ Palms pinkish red, mottled

37. _____ Abdominal wall muscles separated

a. Colostrum

b. Operculum

c. Amenorrhea

d. Angiomas

e. Pyrosis

f. Friability

g. Striae gravidarum

h. Physiologic anemia

i. Linea nigra

j. Ballottement

k. Chadwick's sign

l. Diastasis recti abdominis

m. Lordosis

n. Leukorrhea

o. Chloasma (mask of pregnancy)

p. Lightening

q. Hemorrhoids

r. Palmar erythema

s. Goodell's sign

t. Physiologic/dependent edema

u. Hegar's sign

v. Montgomery's tubercles

w. Carpal tunnel syndrome

38. Complete the following table related to the three categories of signs and symptoms of pregnancy by filling in the blanks and listing the appropriate signs and symptoms for each category.

_____, those changes felt by the woman.	_____, those changes observed by an examiner.	_____, those signs attributed only to the presence of the fetus.

39. Describe the obstetric history for each of the following women, using the 4-digit and 5-digit system.

    a. Nancy is pregnant. Her first pregnancy resulted in a stillbirth at 36 weeks of gestation and her second pregnancy resulted in the birth of her daughter at 42 weeks of gestation.

       4-digit

       5-digit

    b. Marsha is 6 weeks pregnant. Her previous pregnancies resulted in the live birth of a daughter at 40 weeks of gestation, the live birth of a son at 38 weeks of gestation, and a spontaneous abortion at 10 weeks of gestation.

       4-digit

       5-digit

    c. Linda is experiencing her fourth pregnancy. Her first pregnancy ended in a spontaneous abortion at 12 weeks, the second resulted in the live birth of twin boys at 32 weeks, and the third resulted in the live birth of a daughter at 39 weeks.

       4-digit

       5-digit

TRUE OR FALSE: Circle T if true or F if false for each of the following statements. Correct the false statements.

40. T F Pregnancy tests are based on the biologic marker of human chorionic gonadotropin (hCG) found in the urine and serum of pregnant women.

41. T F Most home pregnancy tests are based on ELISA technology.

42. T F Diuretics can contribute to a false-positive pregnancy test result.

43. T F Fetal movements palpated by an examiner are an example of a positive sign of pregnancy.

44. T F The uterine fundus should be above the level of the symphysis pubis by the eighth week of gestation.

45. T F Cervical mucus present during pregnancy does not exhibit ferning.

46. T F During pregnancy, a woman's vulnerability for yeast infections increases.

47. T F Lactation does not occur during pregnancy as a result of the inhibiting effect of high prolactin levels.

48. T F Physiologic anemia is diagnosed in a pregnant woman when the hemoglobin value falls to 10 g/dl or less or if the hematocrit value falls to 35% or less.

49. T F A woman is more vulnerable to thrombus formation during pregnancy as a result of increases in certain clotting factors and depression of fibrinolytic activity.

50. T F A pregnant woman is more likely to experience epistaxis as a result of increased vascularity and congestion of the upper respiratory tract.

51. T F A supine position with head elevated is the best maternal position to facilitate renal perfusion.

52. T F A proteinuria of 1+ or less is acceptable during pregnancy.

53. T F Hypercalcemia is common during pregnancy and can result in muscle cramps or tetany.

54. T F Perspiration is increased during pregnancy as a result of increased peripheral circulation and increased sweat gland activity.

55. T F Carpal tunnel syndrome can occur during the third trimester of pregnancy as a result of edema compressing the median nerve beneath the carpal ligament in the wrist.

56. T F Increased triglyceride levels as a result of higher estrogen secretion may account for the tendency to develop gallstones during pregnancy.

57. T F During the second half of pregnancy, the woman's ability to use her own insulin is decreased to ensure an ample supply of glucose for the developing fetus.

58. T F Glycosuria can be exhibited in a normal pregnancy.

59. When assessing the pregnant woman, the nurse should keep in mind that baseline vital sign values will change as she progresses through her pregnancy. Describe how each of the following would change:

a. Blood pressure (BP)

b. Heart rate and patterns

c. Respiratory rate and patterns

d. Body temperature

60. Calculate the mean arterial pressure (MAP) for each of the following BP readings:

a. 120/76

b. 114/64

c. 110/80

d. 150/90

61. Specify the expected changes that occur in the following laboratory tests as a result of physiologic adaptations to pregnancy:

    a. CBC: hematocrit, hemoglobin, white blood cell count

    b. Clotting activity

    c. Acid/base balance

    d. Urinalysis

62. Explain the expected adaptations in elimination that occur during pregnancy. Include in your answer the basis for the changes that occur.

    RENAL

    BOWEL

63. Discuss how and why the levels of each of the following substances change during pregnancy.

    a. Parathyroid hormone

    b. Estrogen

    c. Progesterone

    d. Thyroid hormones

    e. hCG

MULTIPLE CHOICE QUESTIONS: Circle the one correct option and state the rationale for the option chosen.

64. A pregnant woman at 10 weeks of gestation exhibits the following signs of pregnancy during a routine prenatal checkup. Which one would be categorized as a probable sign of pregnancy?
    a. hCG in the urine
    b. Breast tenderness
    c. Morning sickness
    d. Fetal heart sounds

65. A pregnant woman with 4 children reports the following obstetric history: a stillbirth at 32 weeks of gestation, triplets (2 sons and a daughter) born via cesarean section at 30 weeks of gestation, a spontaneous abortion at 8 weeks of gestation, and a daughter born vaginally at 39 weeks of gestation. Which of the following accurately expresses this woman's current obstetric history using the 5-digit system?
    a. 5-1-4-1-4
    b. 4-1-3-1-4
    c. 5-2-2-0-3
    d. 5-1-2-1-4

66. An essential component of prenatal health assessment of pregnant women is the determination of vital signs. Which of the following would be an expected change in vital sign findings as a result of pregnancy?
    a. Increase in systolic blood pressure by 30 mm Hg or more after assuming a supine position
    b. Increase in diastolic BP by 5 to 10 mm Hg beginning in the first trimester
    c. Increased awareness of the need to breathe as pregnancy progresses
    d. Gradual decrease in baseline pulse rate of approximately 20 beats per minute

67. A woman exhibits understanding of instructions for performing a home pregnancy test to maximize accuracy if she
    a. uses urine collected at the end of the day, just before going to bed.
    b. avoids using Tylenol or aspirin for a headache for about 1 week before performing the test.
    c. performs the test on the day after she misses her first menstrual period.
    d. records the day of her last normal menstrual period and her usual cycle length.

68. During an examination of a pregnant woman the nurse notes that her cervix is soft on its tip. The nurse would document this finding as
    a. friability.
    b. Goodell's sign.
    c. Chadwick's sign.
    d. Hegar's sign.

II. THINKING CRITICALLY

1. Describe how the nurse should respond to each of the following patient concerns and questions.

    a. Tina is 14 weeks pregnant. She calls the prenatal clinic to report that she noticed slight, painless spotting this morning. She reveals that she did have intercourse with her partner the night before.

    b. Lisa suspects she is pregnant because her menstrual period is already 3 weeks late. She asks her friend, who is a nurse, how to use the pregnancy test that she just bought so that she obtains the best results.

    c. Joan is 3 months pregnant. She tells the nurse that she is worried because a friend told her that vaginal and bladder infections are more common during pregnancy. She wants to know if this could be true and if so, why.

    d. Tammy, who is 20 weeks pregnant, tells the nurse that she has noted some "problems" with her breasts: there are "little pimples" near her nipples and her breasts feel "lumpy and bumpy" and "leak a little" when she performs a breast self-examination (BSE).

    e. Tamara is concerned since she read in a book about pregnancy that a pregnant woman's position could affect her circulation, especially to the baby. She asks what positions are good for her circulation now that she is pregnant.

f. Beth, a pregnant woman, calls to tell the nurse that she had a nosebleed this morning and has noticed occasional feelings of fullness in her ears. She asks if these occurrences are anything to worry about.

g. Karen is 7 months pregnant and works as a secretary full time. She asks the nurse if she should take a "water pill" that a friend gave her because she has noticed that her ankles "swell up" at the end of the day.

h. Jan is in her third trimester of pregnancy. She tells the nurse that her posture seems to have changed and that she occasionally experiences low back pain.

i. Monica, who is 36 weeks pregnant with her first baby, calls the clinic stating that she knows the baby is coming because she felt some uterine contractions before getting out of bed in the morning. Monica confirms that they seem to have decreased in intensity and frequency since she has gotten out of bed and walked around.

j. Nina is a primigravida who is at 32 weeks of gestation. When she comes for a prenatal visit she reports that she has been experiencing occasional periods of shortness of breath during the day and sometimes has to use an extra pillow to sleep comfortably. Nina expresses concern that she is developing a breathing problem.

2. Accurate blood pressure readings are critical, if significant changes in the cardiovascular system are to be detected as a woman adapts to pregnancy during the prenatal period. Write a protocol for blood pressure assessment that can be used by nurses working in a prenatal clinic to ensure accuracy of the results obtained during blood pressure assessment.

11 Nursing Care during Pregnancy

I. REVIEWING KEY CONCEPTS AND CONTENT

FILL IN THE BLANKS: Insert the term that corresponds to each of the following descriptions.

1. _____ rule is used to determine the _____ by subtracting _____ from and adding _____ and _____ to the first day of the _____. Alternatively, add _____ to the _____ and count forward _____. Pregnancy is divided into three 3-month periods called _____.

2. _____ can occur when a woman lies on her back for an examination of her abdomen. The _____ and the _____ are compressed by the weight of the abdominal contents, including the uterus. Signs and symptoms that this has occurred would include: _____, _____, _____ and _____, _____, _____, _____, and _____.

3. A variety of assessment methods are used to evaluate the progress of pregnancy. _____is measured beginning in the second trimester as one indicator of the progress of fetal growth. The _____ test determines whether the nipple is everted or inverted, by placing thumb and forefinger on the areola and pressing inward gently.

4. Assessment of fetal health status includes evaluating _____, _____, and _____. The fetal _____ is estimated after determining the duration of pregnancy and the estimated date of birth.

5. Maternal and paternal adaptation during pregnancy includes mastery of certain _____ tasks that include _____, _____, _____, _____, and _____.

6. As a pregnant woman establishes a relationship with her fetus she progresses through three phases. In phase one, she accepts the _____ and needs to be able to state, _____. In phase two, the woman accepts the _____ and a _____. She can now say, _____. Finally, in phase three, the woman prepares realistically for the _____ and _____. She expresses the thought, _____.

7. _____ refers to rapid unpredictable changes in mood.

8. _____ refers to having conflicting feelings about the pregnancy at the same time.

9. _____ refers to the rituals and taboos that a culture expects the male to follow when his partner is pregnant.

10. Certain cultural practices are expected by women of all cultures to ensure a good outcome to their pregnancy. Cultural _____ are directives that tell a woman what to do during pregnancy. Cultural _____ are directives that tell a woman what not to do during pregnancy; they establish _____.

11. The multiple marker or _____ test is used to detect _____. It is done between _____ to _____ weeks of gestation and measures maternal serum levels of _____, _____, and _____.

12. Calculate the expected date of birth (EDB) for each of the following pregnant women using Nägele's rule.

    a. Diane's last menses began on May 5, 2005, and its last day occurred on May 10, 2005.

    b. Sara had intercourse on February 21, 2005. She has not had a menstrual period since the one that began on January 14, 2005, and ended 5 days later.

    c. Beth's last period began on July 4, 2005, and ended on July 10, 2005. She noted that her basal body temperature (BBT) began to rise on July 28, 2005.

13. Cultural beliefs and practices are important influencing factors during the prenatal period.

    a. Describe how cultural beliefs can affect a woman's participation in prenatal care as it is defined by the Western biomedical model of care.

b. Identify one prescription and one proscription for each of the following areas:

Emotional responses

Clothing

Physical activity and rest

Sexual activity

Diet

14. Complete the following table by identifying data to be collected for each component of maternal assessment during the initial visit and follow-up visits during pregnancy.

Component	Initial Visit	Follow-up Visits
Health History Interview		
Physical Examination		
Laboratory and Diagnostic Testing		

15. During a prenatal visit, Marie asks the nurse what can be done to make sure that her baby is healthy and doing well. Identify and describe what the nurse could tell Marie about the components of fetal assessment that will determine her baby's health status.

16. Nurses responsible for the care management of pregnant women must be alert for warning signs of potential complications that women could develop as pregnancy progresses from trimester to trimester.

    a. List the signs of potential complications (warning signs) for each trimester of pregnancy. Indicate possible cause(s) for each sign listed.

    First Trimester

    Second/Third Trimester

b. Describe the approach a nurse should take when discussing potential complications with a pregnant woman and her family.

TRUE OR FALSE: Circle T if true or F if false for each of the following statements. Correct the false statements.

17. T F   Walking and non–weight-bearing exercises such as swimming should be encouraged during pregnancy.

18. T F   If a woman's pulse rises above 100 beats per minute during exercise, she should slow down until it reaches a maximum of 70 beats per minute.

19. T F   The use of a condom is necessary during pregnancy if the woman is at risk for acquiring or transmitting a sexually transmitted disease (STD).

20. T F   Intercourse is safe during a normal pregnancy as long as it is not uncomfortable.

21. T   F   Exposure to second-hand smoke is associated with fetal growth restriction and an increase in perinatal and infant morbidity and mortality.

22. T   F   It is not necessary to screen pregnant women for HIV because there is no effective measure to reduce transmission to the fetus.

23. T   F   Women who are at low risk for complications should be scheduled for prenatal visits every 2 to 3 weeks throughout pregnancy.

24. T   F   An absolute systolic BP of 130 mm Hg or more and a diastolic BP of 80 mm Hg or more suggests hypertension in pregnancy.

25. T   F   A rise in systolic blood pressure of 15 mm Hg or more and/or in diastolic blood pressure of 10 mm Hg or more above baseline should be viewed as an indicator of risk for pregnancy-induced hypertension.

26. T   F   From weeks 18 to 30 the height of the fundus in centimeters is approximately the same as the weeks of gestation if the woman's bladder is empty.

27. T   F   Quickening usually occurs between weeks 16 to 20 of gestation.

28. T   F   A woman should avoid tub bathing and shower instead once she reaches the midpoint of her pregnancy.

29. T   F   The side-lying position promotes uteroplacental perfusion and fetal oxygenation.

30. T   F   Once the uterus enlarges, the pregnant woman should use only the lap belt and avoid using a shoulder harness while in a car.

31. T   F   A woman with inverted nipples should perform nipple rolling and tugging exercises during the third trimester in order to break adhesions.

32. T   F   Hepatitis B vaccination can be administered during pregnancy.

33. T   F   A sign of preterm labor would be uterine contractions occurring every 10 minutes or more often (6 or more per hour) for 1 hour.

34. T   F   Wearing breast shells for 1 to 2 hours each day during the third trimester can help inverted or flat nipples evert or become erect, thereby facilitating the newborn's ability to latch on once breastfeeding begins.

35. T   F   Women who are positive for hepatitis B should not breastfeed.

36. T   F   Women often react to the confirmation of pregnancy with mixed feelings or ambivalence.

37. T   F   Emotional lability (mood swings) may be related to profound hormonal changes that are part of the maternal response to pregnancy.

38. T   F   Children typically respond to their mother's pregnancy in terms of their age and dependency needs.

39. T   F   The reaction of a mother to her daughter's pregnancy can influence her daughter's self-confidence about her pregnancy.

40. T   F   Loss of calcium from teeth during pregnancy increases a woman's risk for dental caries and tooth loss.

41. T   F   No amount of alcohol is considered safe during pregnancy.

42. Create a protocol for fundal measurement that will facilitate accuracy.

43. Identify four factors that can be used to estimate the gestational age of the fetus.

44. Prevention of injury is an important goal for nurses as they teach pregnant women about how to care for themselves during pregnancy.

    a. Describe three principles of body mechanics that a pregnant woman should be taught to prevent injury.

    b. Identify five safety guidelines that the nurse should include in a pamphlet titled "Safety During Pregnancy" that will be distributed to pregnant women during a prenatal visit.

45. During the third trimester, parents often make a decision concerning the method they will use to feed their newborn. List the contraindications for breastfeeding.

46. Men experience pregnancy in many different ways. Three styles of involvement have been exhibited by men during their partners' first pregnancy (May, 1980, 1982). Describe the typical behaviors the nurse would expect to observe in fathers representing each of the following styles of involvement.

    Observer

    Expressive

    Instrumental

MULTIPLE CHOICE QUESTIONS: Circle the one correct option and state the rationale for the option chosen.

47. A nurse is assessing a pregnant woman during a prenatal visit. Several presumptive indicators of pregnancy are documented. Which one of the following is a presumptive indicator?
    a. Uterine enlargement
    b. Quickening
    c. Ballottement
    d. Palpation of fetal movement by the nurse

48. A woman's last menstrual period (LMP) began on September 10, 2005, and it ended on September 15, 2005. Using Nägele's rule, the estimated date of birth would be:
    a. June 17, 2006.
    b. June 22, 2006.
    c. August 17, 2006.
    d. December 3, 2006.

49. A woman at 30 weeks of gestation assumes a supine position for a fundal measurement and Leopold's maneuvers. She begins to complain about feeling dizzy and nauseated. Her skin feels damp and cool. The nurse's first action would be to

a. assess the woman's respiratory rate and effort.
b. provide the woman with an emesis basin.
c. elevate the woman's legs 20 degrees from her hips.
d. turn the woman on her side.

50. During an early bird prenatal class a nurse teaches a group of newly diagnosed pregnant women about their emotional reactions during pregnancy. Which of the following should the nurse discuss with the women?
    a. Sexual desire (libido) is decreased throughout pregnancy.
    b. A referral for counseling should be sought if a woman experiences conflicting feelings about her pregnancy especially in the first trimester.
    c. A quiet period of introspection is often experienced around the time a woman feels her baby move for the first time.
    d. The need to seek safe passage and prepare for birth begins early in the second trimester.

51. The nurse evaluates a pregnant woman's knowledge about prevention of urinary tract infections at the prenatal visit following a class on infection prevention that the woman attended. The nurse would recognize that the woman needs further instruction, when she tells the nurse about which one of the following measures that she now uses to prevent urinary tract infections?
    a. "I drink about 1 quart of fluid a day."
    b. "I have stopped using bubble baths and bath oils."
    c. "I have started wearing panty hose and underpants with a cotton crotch."
    d. "I have yogurt for lunch or as an evening snack."

52. Doulas are becoming important members of a laboring woman's health care team. Which of the following activities should be expected as part of the doula's role responsibilities?
    a. Monitoring hydration of the laboring woman, including adjusting IV flow rates
    b. Interpreting electronic fetal monitoring tracings to determine the well-being of the maternal-fetal unit
    c. Eliminating the need for the husband/partner to be present during labor and birth
    d. Providing continuous support throughout labor and birth, including explanations of labor progress

II. THINKING CRITICALLY

1. A health history interview of the pregnant woman by the nurse is included as part of the initial prenatal visit.

   a. State the purpose of the health history interview.

   b. Write two questions for each component that is included in the initial health history interview. Questions should be clear, concise, and understandable. Most of the questions should be open ended in order to elicit the most complete response from the patient.

   c. Write four questions that should be included in the interview when updating the health history during follow-up visits.

2. Imagine that you are a nurse working in a prenatal clinic. You have been assigned to be the primary nurse for Martha, an 18 year old, who has come to the clinic for confirmation of pregnancy. She tells you that she knows she is pregnant because she has already missed 3 periods and a home pregnancy test that she did last week was positive. Martha states that she has had very little contact with the health care system, and the only reason she came today is because her boyfriend insisted that she "make sure" she is really pregnant. Describe the approach that you would take regarding data collection and nursing interventions appropriate for this woman.

3. Terry is a primigravida in her first trimester of pregnancy. She is accompanied by her husband, Tim, to her second prenatal visit. Answer each of the following questions asked by Terry and Tim:

   a. "At the last visit I was told that my estimated date of birth is December 25, 2005. Can I really count on my baby being born on Christmas Day?"

   b. "Before I became pregnant my friend told me I should be doing Kegel exercises. I was too embarrassed to ask her about them. What are they and is it safe for me to do them while I am pregnant?"

   c. "What effect will pregnancy have on our sex life? We are willing to abstain during pregnancy if we have to keep our baby safe."

   d. "This morning sickness I am experiencing is driving my crazy. I become nauseated in the morning and again late in the afternoon. Occasionally I vomit or have the dry heaves. Will this last for my entire pregnancy? Is there anything I can do to feel better?"

4. Tara is 2 months pregnant. She tells the nurse, at the prenatal clinic, that she is used to being active and exercises every day. Now that she is pregnant she wonders if she should reduce or stop her exercise routine. Discuss the nurse's response to Tara.

5. Write one nursing diagnosis for each of the following situations. State one expected outcome, and list appropriate nursing measures for the nursing diagnosis you identified.

  a. Beth is 6 weeks pregnant. During the health history interview, she tells you that she has limited her intake of fluids and tries to hold her urine as long as she can because, "I just hate having to go to the bathroom so frequently."

Nursing diagnosis	Expected outcome	Nursing measures

  b. Doris, who is 23 weeks pregnant, tells you that she is beginning to experience more frequent lower back pain. You note that when she walked into the examining room her posture exhibited a moderate degree of lordosis and neck flexion. She was wearing shoes with 2-inch narrow heels.

Nursing diagnosis	Expected outcome	Nursing measures

  c. Lisa, a primigravida at 32 weeks of gestation, comes for a prenatal visit accompanied by her partner, the father of the baby. They both express anxiety about the impending birth of the baby and how they will handle the experience of labor. Lisa is especially concerned about how she will survive the pain and her partner is primarily concerned about how he will help Lisa cope with labor and make sure she and the baby are safe.

Nursing diagnosis	Expected outcome	Nursing measures

6. Jane is a primigravida in her second trimester of pregnancy. Answer each of the following questions asked by Jane during a prenatal visit.

  a. "Why do you measure my abdomen every time I come in for a checkup?"

  b. "How can you tell if my baby is doing okay?"

  c. "I am going to start changing the way that I dress now that I am beginning to show. Do you have any suggestions I could follow, especially since I have a limited amount of money to spend?"

  d. "What can I do about gas and constipation? I never had much of a problem before I was pregnant."

e. "Since yesterday I have started to feel itchy all over. Do you think I am coming down with some sort of infection?"

f. "I will be flying out to Chicago to visit my father in 1 month. Is airline travel safe for me when I am 5 months pregnant?"

7. While a nurse is measuring a pregnant woman's fundus, the woman becomes pale and diaphoretic. The woman, who is at 23 weeks of gestation, states that she feels dizzy and lightheaded.

a. State the most likely explanation for the assessment findings exhibited by this woman.

b. Describe the nurse's immediate action.

8. Kelly is a primigravida in her third trimester of pregnancy. Answer each of the following questions asked by Kelly during a prenatal visit.

a. "My husband and I have decided to breastfeed our baby but friends told me it is very difficult if my nipples do not come out. Is there any way I can tell now if my nipples are okay for breastfeeding?"

b. "My ankles are swollen by the time I get home from work late in the afternoon [Kelly teaches second grade]. I have been trying to drink about 3 liters of fluid every day. Should I reduce the amount of liquid I am drinking or ask my doctor for a water pill?"

c. "I woke up last night with a terrible cramp in my leg. It finally went away but my husband and I just did not know what to do. What if this happens again tonight?"

9. Marge, a pregnant woman (2-0-0-1-0) beginning her third trimester, expresses concern about preterm birth. "I already had one miscarriage and my sister's baby died after being born too early. I am so worried that this will happen to me."

a. Identify one nursing diagnosis with an expected outcome that reflects Marge's concern.

b. Indicate what the nurse can teach Marge about the signs of preterm labor.

c. Describe the actions Marge should take if she experiences signs of preterm labor.

10. Carol is 4 months pregnant and beginning to "show." She asks the nurse what she should expect as a reaction from her 13-year-old daughter and 3-year-old son. Describe the response the nurse would make.

11. Your neighbor, Jane, is in her second month of pregnancy. Knowing that you are a nurse, her husband, Tom, confides to you, "I just can't figure out Jane. One minute she is happy and the next minute she is crying for no reason at all! I do not know how I will be able to cope with this for 7 more months."

    a. Write a nursing diagnosis and expected outcome that reflects Tom's concern.

    b. Discuss how you would respond to his concern.

12. Jennifer (2-1-0-0-1) and her husband, Dan, are beginning their third trimester of a low risk pregnancy. As you work with them on their birth plan, they tell you that they are having trouble making a decision about their choice of a birth setting. They experienced a delivery room birth with their first child. Jennifer states, "My first pregnancy was perfectly normal just like this one, but the birth was disappointing, so medically focused with monitors, IVs, and staying in bed." They ask you for your advice about the different birth settings they have heard and read about, namely labor, delivery, recovery, and postpartum (LDRP) rooms at their local hospital, the birthing center a few miles from their home, and even their own home. Describe the approach that you would take to guide Jennifer and Dan in their decision regarding a birth setting.

13. Nancy, a pregnant woman (3-2-0-0-2) at 26 weeks of gestation, asks the nurse about doulas. "My friend had a doula and she said that she was amazing. My first two birth experiences were difficult—my husband and I really needed someone to help us. Do you think a doula could be that person?"

    a. Explain the role of the doula so that Nancy will have the information she will need to make an informed decision.

    b. Nancy decides to try a doula for her upcoming labor. Identify what you would tell Nancy about finding a doula.

    c. Specify questions that Nancy should ask when she is making a choice about the doula she will hire for her labor.

14. Tony and Andrea are considering the possibility of giving birth to their second baby at home. They have been receiving prenatal care from a certified nurse-midwife who has experience with home birth. Their 5-year-old son and both sets of grandparents want to be present for the birth.

   a. Discuss the decision-making process that Tony and Andrea should follow to ensure that they make an informed decision that is right for them and their family.

   b. Tony and Andrea decide that home birth is an ideal choice for them. Outline the preparation measures you would recommend to Tony and Andrea to ensure a safe and positive experience for everyone.

12 Maternal and Fetal Nutrition

I. REVIEWING KEY CONCEPTS AND CONTENT

FILL IN THE BLANKS: Insert the term that corresponds to each of the following descriptions.

1. A _____ is the best way to ensure that adequate nutrients are available for the developing fetus. Adequate intake of _____ is important for decreasing risk for _____ or failures in the closure of the neural tube. An intake of _____ daily is recommended for all women capable of becoming pregnant.

2. Inadequate maternal nutrition and inadequate weight gain may impair fetal growth and development resulting in _____. _____ is defined as a birth weight of 2500 g (5½ pounds) or less. Infants born at this weight may be _____ and/or _____.

3. Obesity, either preexisting or developed during pregnancy, increases the likelihood of
   _____,
   _____,
   _____,
   _____,
   _____,
   _____, and
   _____.

4. When individualizing the recommended daily allowances (RDAs) for pregnant and lactating women, nurses need to consider variations in a pregnant woman's situation, including such factors as _____, _____, _____, _____, and stage of _____. _____ needs are met by carbohydrates, fats, and protein in the diet and should be increased _____ above prepregnancy needs during the second and third trimesters.

5. Women at greatest risk for inadequate protein intake would include
   _____,

_____, and
_____.

6. Inadequate intake of iron can lead to the development of _____ during pregnancy, a nutritional health problem that is more common among _____ and _____ than among adult Caucasian women.

7. _____ is the inability to digest milk sugar because of the absence of the lactase enzyme in the small intestine.

8. _____ is the practice of consuming nonfood substances such as _____, _____, and _____ or excessive amounts of food stuffs low in nutritional value such as _____, _____, _____, and _____. _____ is the urge to consume specific types of foods such as ice cream, pickles, and pizza and are thought to be caused by an innate drive to consume _____ missing from the diet.

9. Assessment of nutritional status begins with a diet history that should include
   _____,
   _____, and
   _____. Physical examination includes _____ measurement such as _____ and _____. Calculation of the _____ is a method of evaluating the appropriateness of weight for height and is used to guide a woman's weight gain during pregnancy.

10. Vegetarian diets can vary in terms of the foods allowed. Basic to almost all vegetarian diets are
    _____, _____,
    _____, _____,
    _____, and _____.
    _____ eat fish, poultry, eggs, and dairy products, but they do not eat beef or pork. _____ also consume dairy products and eggs. Strict _____ or _____ consume only plant products.

11. Complete the following table by stating the importance of each of the following nutrients for healthy maternal adaptation to pregnancy and optimum fetal growth and development. Indicate the major food sources for each nutrient.

Nutrient	Importance for Pregnancy	Major Food Sources
Protein		
Iron		
Calcium		
Zinc		
Fat-soluble Vitamins (A, D)		
Water-soluble Vitamins (folic acid, B_6, C)		

12. When assessing pregnant women, it is critical that nurses are alert for factors that could place women at nutritional risk so that early intervention can be implemented. Name five such indicators or risk factors of which the nurse should be aware.

13. At her first prenatal visit, Marie, a 20-year-old primigravida, reports that she has been a strict vegetarian for the past 3 years. Identify two major guidelines that the nurse should follow when planning menus with Marie.

14. Evaluation of nutritional status is an essential part of a thorough physical assessment of pregnant women. Cite four signs of good nutrition and four signs of inadequate nutrition that the nurse should observe for during the assessment of a pregnant woman.

15. Identify three nursing measures appropriate for each of the following nursing diagnoses:

    a. Imbalanced nutrition: less than body requirements related to inadequate intake associated with moderate nausea and vomiting (morning sickness).

b. Constipation related to decreased intestinal motility associated with increased progesterone levels during pregnancy.

c. Pain related to reflux of gastric contents into esophagus following dinner.

16. Determine the recommended weight gain and pattern for each woman based on her BMI.

Woman	BMI	Weight Gain
a. June: 5 feet 3 inches, 120 pounds		
b. Alice: 5 feet 6 inches, 180 pounds		
c. Ann: 5 feet 5 inches, 95 pounds		

TRUE OR FALSE: Circle T if true or F if false for each of the following statements. Correct the false statements.

17. T   F   Good maternal nutrition before and during pregnancy is considered to be one of the most important preventive measures for low birth weight (LBW).

18. T   F   A series of 24-hour diet recalls is the best way to determine the appropriateness of a woman's caloric intake.

19. T   F   An overweight woman whose BMI is 28 should gain approximately 0.3 kg/per week during the second and third trimesters of pregnancy.

20. T   F   During pregnancy, women should drink at least 2 liters of fluid each day.

21. T   F   A caloric increase of 600 kcal per day is recommended for pregnant women beginning in the first trimester.

22. T   F   A weight gain of more than 2 kg in a month after the twentieth week of gestation is strongly suggestive of gestational hypertension.

23. T   F   Iron deficiency anemia increases the risk for postpartum infection and/or poor wound healing.

24. T   F   Pregnant women should avoid caffeine because an intake of more than 300 mg daily increases the risk for miscarriage and intrauterine growth restriction (IUGR).

25. T   F   Women should begin taking an iron supplement starting at 12 weeks of gestation.

26. T   F   All pregnant women require a supplement of 60 mg of ferrous iron daily.

27. T   F   If moderate peripheral edema occurs during pregnancy, the woman's sodium intake should be reduced.

28. T   F   Excessive intake of vitamin A, a fat-soluble vitamin, during pregnancy can cause congenital malformations of the fetus.

29. T   F   Development of neural tube defects appears to be more common in the fetuses of pregnant women whose diets are low in vitamin B_6.

30. T   F   Dehydration may increase the risk for contractions of the uterus and preterm labor.

31. T   F   Lactating women need to consume at least 2500 kcal/day.

32. T   F   Lactating women should be told that loss of the weight gained during pregnancy will begin after they stop breastfeeding.

33. T   F   The most common nutrition-related laboratory test for a pregnant woman is a hematocrit and hemoglobin measurement.

34. T   F   A 1200 mg calcium supplement daily may be required if the lactating woman consumes a diet that is low in calcium.

35. Jean intends to breastfeed her infant until she returns to work in 6 months. State three guidelines the nurse should teach Jean to follow to ensure adequate nutrition during lactation.

36. Mary asks the nurse why her nutrient needs increase during pregnancy. State four factors that the nurse should explain to Mary as reasons why her needs increase.

MULTIPLE CHOICE QUESTIONS: Circle the one correct option and state the rationale for the option chosen.

37. A nurse teaching a pregnant woman about the importance of iron in her diet would tell her to avoid consuming which of the following foods at the same time as her iron supplement because it will decrease iron absorption?
    a. Tomatoes
    b. Strawberries
    c. Meat
    d. Eggs

38. A 25-year-old pregnant woman is at 10 weeks of gestation. Her BMI is calculated to be 24. Which one of the following is recommended in terms of weight gain during pregnancy?
    a. Total weight gain of 18 kg
    b. First trimester weight gain of 1 to 2.5 kg
    c. Weight gain of 0.4 kg each week for 40 weeks
    d. Weight gain of 3.0 kg per month during the second and third trimesters

39. A pregnant woman at 6 weeks of gestation tells her nurse midwife that she has been experiencing nausea with occasional vomiting every day. The nurse could recommend which of the following as an effective relief measure?
    a. Eat starchy foods such as buttered popcorn or peanut butter with crackers in the morning before getting out of bed.
    b. Avoid eating before going to bed at night.
    c. Alter eating patterns to small meals every 2 to 3 hours.
    d. Skip a meal if nausea is experienced.

40. A woman demonstrates an understanding of the importance of increasing her intake of foods high in folic acid when she includes which of the following foods in her diet?
    a. Seafood
    b. Legumes
    c. Eggs
    d. Cheese

41. A 30-year-old woman at 16 weeks of gestation comes for a routine prenatal visit. Her 24-hour dietary recall is evaluated by the nurse. Which of the following entries would indicate that this woman needs further instructions regarding nutrient needs during pregnancy?
    a. Six servings (total of 8 ounces) from the meat, poultry, fish, dry beans, eggs, and nuts group
    b. Total kcal intake is 300 kcal above her calculated prepregnancy needs
    c. Daily iron supplement taken at bedtime with a glass of orange juice
    d. Three servings from the milk and milk products group

II. THINKING CRITICALLY

1. Nutrition and weight gain are important areas of consideration for nurses who care for pregnant women. In addition, weight gain is often a source of stress and body image alteration for the pregnant woman. Discuss the approach you would use in each of the following situations.

   a. Kelly (5' 8" and 120 pounds) complains to you that her physician recommended a weight gain of approximately 30 pounds during her pregnancy. She states, "Babies only weigh about 7 pounds when they are born. Why do I have to gain much more than that?"

   b. Kate (5' 4" and 125 pounds) has just found out that she is pregnant. She states, "I am so glad to be pregnant. I love to eat, and now I can start eating for two. It will be great not to have to watch the scale or what I eat."

c. June tells you that she does not have to worry about her nutrient intake during her pregnancy. "I take plenty of vitamins—everything from A to Z."

d. Erin is 7 months pregnant. She asks you what she can do to relieve the heartburn she experiences after meals, especially dinner.

e. Sara (BMI = 28.7) is 1 month pregnant. She asks you for dietary guidance, including a weight reduction diet because she does not want to gain too much weight with this pregnancy.

f. Beth is 2 months pregnant. She states, "I have cut down on my water intake. I do get a little thirsty, but it's worth it since I don't have to urinate so often."

g. Hedy is 2 months pregnant and has come for her second prenatal visit. During a discussion about nutritional needs during pregnancy she states, "I know I will never get enough calcium because I get sick when I drink milk."

h. Lara is 36 weeks pregnant. She states that she would like to breastfeed her baby but is concerned about getting back into shape and losing weight after the baby is born. "My friends told me that I will lose weight more slowly since I will not be able to start on a weight reduction diet as long as I am breastfeeding."

2. Yvonne's hemoglobin is 13 g/dl and her hematocrit is 37% at the onset of her pregnancy. She asks the nurse if she will have to take iron during her pregnancy if she tries to follow a good diet. "My friend took iron when she was pregnant and it made her sick to her stomach." Discuss the appropriate response by the nurse.

3. Gloria is an 18-year-old Native-American woman (5′ 6″ and 98 pounds) who has just been diagnosed as 8 weeks pregnant. In her discussions with you at her first prenatal visit, she expresses a lack of knowledge regarding the nutritional requirements of pregnancy and an interest in learning about what to eat because she wants to have a healthy baby.

a. Outline the approach that you would use to help Gloria learn about and meet the nutritional requirements of her pregnancy.

b. Plan a 1-day menu that incorporates Gloria's nutritional needs and reflects the traditions of her culture.

Pregnancy at Risk: Preexisting Conditions

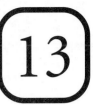

I. REVIEWING KEY CONCEPTS AND CONTENT

1. Explain the interrelationship of each of the following clinical manifestations associated with diabetes mellitus.

   Hyperglycemia

   Polyuria

   Glycosuria

   Polydipsia

   Weight loss

   Polyphagia

FILL IN THE BLANKS: Insert the term that corresponds to each of the following descriptions related to diabetes mellitus.

2. Diabetes mellitus is a group of metabolic diseases characterized by _____ resulting from defects in _____, _____, or both.

3. _____ refers to excretion of large volumes of urine. _____ refers to excessive thirst and _____ refers to excessive eating. Excretion of unusable glucose results in _____.

4. _____ is the label given to type 1 or type 2 diabetes that existed before pregnancy.

5. _____ is any degree of glucose intolerance with its onset or first recognition occurring during pregnancy. Diagnosis of this form of diabetes is usually made during the _____ of pregnancy.

6. The key to optimal outcome of a diabetic pregnancy is strict maternal _____ control before _____ and throughout the _____.

7. During the first trimester, insulin dosage needs to be decreased to avoid _____.

8. During the second and third trimester the dosage of insulin must be increased to avoid _____ and _____.

9. Glycemic control over the previous 4 to 6 weeks can be evaluated based on the determination of the level of _____ in the blood. Acceptable fasting blood glucose levels should be between _____ and _____. The 1-hour postprandial glucose should be between _____ and the 2-hour postprandial should be between _____. The goal of treatment is to maintain a state of _____ or normal blood glucose within a range of _____ and _____.

10. Dietary management during a diabetic pregnancy must be based on _____ levels. Energy needs are usually based on _____ calories/kg of ideal body weight. _____ of total calories should be from carbohydrates. _____ carbohydrates should be limited, whereas _____ carbohydrates high in _____ content should be emphasized when food choices are made. _____ of total calories should be from protein and _____ should be from fat with no more than _____ from saturated fat. Weight gain should be approximately _____ during pregnancy.

11. Blood glucose levels are measured throughout each day: before _____, _____, and _____, _____, at _____, and in the _____. _____measurements are performed 2 hours after meals and are most likely to identify _____. More frequent testing may be done during the _____ and _____trimesters when insulin needs are _____. In addition, glucose levels should be checked at any sign of _____ or _____; when there is a readjustment of _____ or _____; when _____, _____, or _____ occurs or when _____ is present.

12. Urine testing for _____ is still recommended because it may provide information related to the onset of _____.

13. Typically _____ of the daily insulin dose is given in the morning before _____using a combination of _____ and _____ insulin. The remaining _____ may be administered in the evening before _____. To reduce the risk of _____ during the night, separate injections often are given with _____ insulin before _____ followed by _____ insulin at _____. Another insulin regimen would be to administer _____ insulin before each meal and _____ insulin at bedtime.

14. Complete the following table by identifying the major maternal and fetal/neonatal risks and complications associated with diabetic pregnancies.

Maternal Risks/Complications	Fetal and Neonatal Risks/Complications

15. Complete the following table by identifying the metabolic changes that occur during pregnancy and indicating how these changes affect the woman with pregestational diabetes during the first trimester, the second and third trimesters, and the postpartum period.

Stage of Pregnancy	Metabolic Changes of Pregnancy	Impact on Diabetes
First Trimester		
Second/Third Trimesters		
Postpartum Period		

16. Explain the current recommendations for screening for and diagnosing gestational diabetes mellitus developed by the Expert Committee on the Diagnosis and Classification of Diabetes Mellitus.

17. State how hyperthyroidism and hypothyroidism can affect reproductive well-being and pregnancy.

TRUE OR FALSE: Circle T if true or F if false for each of the following statements related to preexisting conditions during pregnancy. Correct the false statements.

18. T   F   Preconception counseling is a critical factor in the care management of the pregnancy of a woman with pregestational diabetes mellitus.

19. T   F   Insulin requirements may decrease during the first trimester but need to increase during the second and third trimesters.

20. T   F   Women with type 2 diabetes can continue to use an oral hypoglycemic agent to maintain glycemic control during pregnancy.

21. T   F   Strict metabolic control before conception and in the early weeks of pregnancy is an essential factor in reducing the risk of congenital anomalies.

22. T   F   Even mild to moderate hypoglycemic episodes can have significant harmful effects on the fetus including macrosomia.

23. T   F   The most important cause of perinatal deaths in diabetic pregnancy is intrauterine growth restriction (IUGR).

24. T   F   Fasting blood glucose (FBS) levels should fall between 40 and 75 mg/dl.

25. T   F   Multiple injections of insulin daily are usually required to maintain glucose control for the pregestational diabetic woman, especially during the second half of pregnancy.

26. T   F   Ketoacidosis occurring at any time during pregnancy can lead to intrauterine fetal death.

27. T   F   Cardiac defects are the most common congenital anomalies associated with pregestational diabetes.

28. T   F   A glycosylated hemoglobin level of 13% to 20% indicates good diabetic control.

29. T   F   Diabetic women should avoid a bedtime snack when they are pregnant.

30. T   F   It is recommended that the 2-hour postmeal (postprandial) blood glucose level be less than 130 mg/dl.

31. T   F   During labor a woman's blood glucose level should be maintained between 60 and 100 mg/dl to prevent neonatal hypoglycemia.

32. T   F   Insulin requirements decrease substantially during the postpartum period with loss of placental-induced insulin resistance.

33. T   F   Many women diagnosed with gestational diabetes may require insulin at some point during their pregnancy to maintain glycemic control.

34. T   F   The majority of women with gestational diabetes convert to type 2 diabetes mellitus within 1 year after pregnancy.

35. T   F   Gestational diabetes is primarily a condition complicating the pregnancies of Caucasian women.

36. T   F   The incidence of congenital anomalies among infants of gestational diabetic mothers is nearly the same as for the general population.

37. T   F   A 1-hour 50 g glucose tolerance test result that is greater than 140 mg/dl confirms the diagnosis of gestational diabetes.

38. T   F   The urine of diabetic pregnant women is tested periodically for the presence of acetone, which could signal the onset of ketoacidosis.

39. T   F   To avoid the risk of fetal intrauterine death, labor should be induced for the diabetic woman as soon as the fetal lungs are mature, usually at approximately 36 weeks of gestation.

40. T   F   The primary treatment of hyperthyroidism during pregnancy is drug therapy with propylthiouracil (PTU).

41. T   F   Effectiveness of treatment for hyperthyroidism involves the monitoring of free T_3 levels on a weekly basis.

42. T   F   Infants of women with hypothyroidism often exhibit thyroid dysfunction for several months after birth.

43. T   F   Women should take L-thyroxine (Synthroid) with their iron supplement to facilitate absorption of the Synthroid.

44. T   F   Phenylketonuria (PKU) is an inborn error of metabolism that causes mental retardation if left untreated.

45. T   F   A pregnant woman with a cardiac problem may be experiencing cardiovascular decompensation if she notices a sudden limitation of her ability to perform her usual activities.

46. T   F   Pregnant women with cardiac problems may require a diet low in salt.

47. T   F   Women using heparin during pregnancy should increase their intake of foods high in vitamin K to enhance the anticoagulant effects of the drug.

48. T   F   Epidural anesthesia is recommended as an effective method of pain relief for the labor of a woman with cardiac problems.

49. T   F   Anemia is the most common medical disorder of pregnancy.

50. T   F   Folic acid deficiency anemia is the most common type of anemia in pregnancy.

51. T   F   A pregnant woman in the first trimester is considered anemic when her hemoglobin level is less than 10 g/dl or her hematocrit is less than 33%.

52. T   F   Iron deficiency anemia increases the incidence of cleft lip and cleft palate.

53. T   F   A well-balanced diet alone is unable to prevent an iron deficit in pregnancy.

54. T   F   For the pregnant woman with iron-deficiency anemia, oral iron supplementation should be taken in a dose of 30 mg daily.

55. T   F   Exacerbations of sickle cell crises are diminished with pregnancy.

56. T   F   Preeclampsia is more common in pregnancies complicated by thalassemia major.

57. T   F   The physiologic alterations induced by pregnancy increase the risk for asthmatic attacks.

58. T F Fentanyl should be avoided for laboring women with asthma because it may precipitate an asthmatic attack.

59. T F In the management of care for a laboring woman with cystic fibrosis, close monitoring of serum sodium and fluid balance is critical.

60. T F The pregnant woman is more vulnerable to cholelithiasis than the nonpregnant woman.

61. T F Preeclampsia and the HELLP syndrome are more common among pregnant women with systemic lupus erythematosus (SLE).

62. T F Therapeutic abortion is recommended when a woman has multiple sclerosis because pregnancy can cause irreversible worsening of the condition.

63. T F In the United States, about 78% of HIV-infected women are African American or Hispanic.

64. T F About 50% of all pediatric AIDS cases are due to transmission of the virus from mother to child during the perinatal period.

65. Identify the maternal and fetal complications that are more common among pregnant women who have cardiac problems.

66. Explain the modifications that should be made in the protocol used for cardiopulmonary resuscitation (CPR) and the Heimlich maneuver when a woman is pregnant.

FILL IN THE BLANKS: Insert the term that corresponds to each of the following descriptions related to selected preexisting medical disorders during pregnancy.

67. _____ is the inability of the heart to maintain a sufficient cardiac output. Physiologic stress on the heart is greatest between the _____ and _____ weeks of gestation because the cardiac output is at its peak. Risk for this complication is also higher during _____ and the first _____ to _____ hours after birth.

68. _____ is a classification system for cardiovascular disorders developed by the New York Heart Association. Class I implies _____. Class II implies _____. Class III implies _____. Class IV implies _____.

69. _____ refers to the damage of the heart valves and the chordae tendineae cordis as a result of an infection originating from an inadequately treated group A β-hemolytic streptococcal infection of the throat. The American Heart Association recommends lifelong prophylaxis with _____ even during pregnancy.

70. _____ is a narrowing of an opening of the valve between the left atrium and the left ventricle of the heart by stiffening of the valve leaflets, which obstructs blood flow from the atrium to the ventricles.

71. _____ is an inflammation of the innermost lining of the heart caused by invasion of microorganisms.

72. _____ is a common, usually benign, cardiac condition that involves the protrusion of the leaflets of the mitral valve back into the left atrium during ventricular systole, allowing some backflow of blood.

73. _____ is a disease caused by the presence of abnormal hemoglobin in the blood. It is a recessive, hereditary, familial hemolytic _____ that affects those of _____ or _____ ancestry.

74. _____ is a relatively common anemia in which an insufficient amount of globin is produced to fill red blood cells.

75. _____ is an acute respiratory illness caused by allergens, a marked change in ambient temperature, or emotional tension. In response to stimuli, there is widespread but reversible narrowing of the _____ making it difficult to _____. The clinical manifestations are expiratory _____, productive _____, thick _____, and _____.

76. _____ is a common autosomal recessive genetic disorder in which the exocrine glands produce excessive viscous secretions, causing problems with both respiratory and digestive functions.

77. _____ is a disorder of the brain causing recurrent seizures; it is the most common neurologic disorder accompanying pregnancy.

78. _____ is a chronic, multisystem, inflammatory disease characterized by autoimmune antibody production that affects the skin, joints, kidneys, lungs, central nervous system (CNS), liver, and other body organs.

79. _____ refers to presence of gallstones in the gallbladder.

80. _____ refers to inflammation of the gallbladder.

81. The T-ACE test and the TWEAK test are important assessment tools.

   a. State the purpose of each of these assessment tools.

   T-ACE test

   TWEAK test

   b. Indicate the question represented by each letter

   T

   A

   C

   E

   T

   W

   E

   A

   K

   c. Specify how the answers should be interpreted or scored for each of these assessment tools.

82. Explain why women who abuse substances may delay seeking prenatal care.

MULTIPLE CHOICE QUESTIONS: Circle the one correct option and state the rationale for the option chosen.

83. A pregestational diabetic woman at 20 weeks of gestation exhibits the following: thirst, nausea and vomiting, abdominal pain, drowsiness, and increased urination. Her skin is flushed and dry and her breathing is rapid with a fruity odor. A priority nursing action when caring for this woman would be to
   a. provide the woman with a simple carbohydrate immediately.
   b. request an order for an antiemetic.
   c. assist the woman into a lateral position to rest.
   d. administer insulin according to the woman's blood glucose level.

84. During her pregnancy, a woman with pregestational diabetes has been monitoring her blood glucose level several times a day. Which of the following levels would require further assessment?
   a. 85 mg/dl—before breakfast
   b. 90 mg/dl—before lunch
   c. 135 mg/dl—2 hours after supper
   d. 100 mg/dl—at bedtime

85. Specific guidelines should be followed when planning a diet with a pregestational diabetic woman to ensure a euglycemic state. An appropriate diet would reflect
   a. 40 calories per kg of prepregnancy weight daily.
   b. a caloric distribution among three meals and one or two snacks.
   c. a minimum of 350 g of carbohydrate daily.
   d. a protein intake of at least 30% of the total kcalories in a day.

86. An obese pregnant woman with gestational diabetes is learning self-injection of insulin. While evaluating the woman's technique for self-injection, the nurse would recognize that the woman understood the instructions when she
    a. washes her hands and puts on a pair of clean gloves.
    b. shakes the NPH insulin vial vigorously to fully mix the insulin.
    c. draws the NPH insulin into her syringe first.
    d. spreads her skin taut and punctures the skin at a 90° angle.

87. When assessing a pregnant woman at 28 weeks of gestation who is diagnosed with mitral valve stenosis, the nurse must be alert for signs indicating cardiac decompensation. A sign of cardiac decompensation is:
    a. a dry, hacking cough.
    b. supine hypotension.
    c. wheezing with inspiration and expiration.
    d. rapid pulse that is irregular and weak.

88. A woman at 30 weeks of gestation with a Class II cardiac disorder calls her primary health care provider's office and speaks to the nurse practitioner. She tells the nurse that she has been experiencing a frequent, moist cough for the past few days. In addition, she has been feeling more tired and is having difficulty completing her routine activities as a result of some difficulty with breathing. The nurse's best response would be
    a. "Have someone bring you to the office so we can assess your cardiac status."
    b. "Try to get more rest during the day because this is a difficult time for your heart."
    c. "Take an extra diuretic tonight before you go to bed, since you may be developing some fluid in your lungs."
    d. "Ask your family to come over and do your housework for the next few days so you can rest."

89. A pregnant woman with a cardiac disorder will begin anticoagulant therapy to prevent clot formation. In preparing this woman for this treatment measure, the nurse would expect to teach the woman about self-administration of which of the following medications?
    a. Furosemide
    b. Propranolol
    c. Heparin
    d. Warfarin

90. At a previous antepartal visit, the nurse taught a pregnant woman diagnosed with a Class II cardiac disorder about measures to use to lower her risk for cardiac decompensation. This woman would demonstrate need for further instruction if she
    a. increases roughage in her diet.
    b. remains on bed rest getting out of bed only to go to the bathroom.
    c. sleeps 10 hours every night and rests after meals.
    d. states she will call the nurse immediately if she experiences any pain or swelling in her legs.

II. THINKING CRITICALLY

1. Mary is a 24-year-old woman with diabetes. When Mary informed her gynecologist that she and her husband are trying to get pregnant, she was referred to an endocrinologist for preconception counseling. Mary tells the nurse that she just cannot understand why this is necessary. "I have had diabetes since I was 12 years old, and I have not had many problems. All I want to do is get pregnant!" Discuss how the nurse should respond to Mary's comments.

2. Luann is a 25-year-old nulliparous woman in her first trimester of pregnancy (sixth week of gestation). She has had type 1 diabetes since she was 15 years old. Recently, she has been experiencing some nausea and is eating less as a result. She took her usual dose of regular and NPH insulin before eating a very light breakfast of tea and a piece of toast. Just before her midmorning snack at work she began to experience nervousness and weakness. She felt dizzy and became diaphoretic and pale.

   a. Identify the problem that Luann is experiencing. Indicate the basis for her symptoms.

   b. State the action that Luann should take.

3. Judy's pregnancy has just been confirmed. She also has type 1 diabetes.

   a. As a result of her high risk status a variety of additional assessment measures are emphasized during her prenatal period to evaluate the status of her fetus. Identify these additional assessment measures and their relevance in a diabetic pregnancy.

   b. Discuss the stressors that might confront Judy and her family as a result of her status as a diabetic woman who is pregnant.

   c. Write two nursing diagnoses that reflect Judy's current health status.

   d. Indicate the activity and exercise recommendations that Judy should be given.

   e. Complete the following table by describing the focus, nursing interventions, and health teaching for the major components of health care required at each stage of Judy's pregnancy.

Care Component	Antepartum	Intrapartum	Postpartum
Diet			
Glucose Monitoring			
Insulin Requirements			

f. After birth, Judy, who will be bottle-feeding, asks the nurse about birth control. Discuss the birth control options that would be best for Judy and her partner.

4. Elena (2-1-0-0-1) is a 32-year-old Hispanic-American woman in week 28 of her pregnancy. She is obese. Her mother, who is 59, was recently diagnosed with type 2 diabetes. Elena's first pregnancy resulted in the birth of a 10 pound 6 ounce daughter who is now 2 years old. A 1-hour, 50 g glucose tolerance test last week revealed a glucose level of 152 mg/dl. A 3-hour glucose tolerance test was done yesterday with the following results: Fasting—108 mg/dl, 1 hr—195 mg/dl, 2 hr—170 mg/dl, 3 hr—140 mg/dl.

a. Identify the complication of pregnancy Elena is exhibiting. State the rationale for your answer.

b. List the risk factors for this health problem that are present in Elena's assessment data.

c. Describe the pathophysiology involved in creating Elena's problem.

d. Identify the maternal and fetal/neonatal risks and complications that are possible in this situation.

e. Outline the ongoing assessment measures necessitated by Elena's health problem.

f. State two nursing diagnoses for Elena and her fetus

g. State the dietary changes Elena will have to make to maintain glycemic control during the rest of her pregnancy.

h. Before discharge after the birth of her second daughter, Elena asks the nurse if the health problem she experienced during this pregnancy will continue now that she has had her baby. She also wonders if it will happen with her next pregnancy because she wants to get pregnant again soon so she can "try for a son." Discuss the response the nurse should give to Elena's concerns.

5. Jennifer's pregnancy has just been confirmed. She has type 2 diabetes and is told that she now must learn how to give herself insulin. Jennifer becomes very upset and states, "I cannot possibly give myself a shot. Why not let me continue to take my pills since they have been working fine so far?" Describe how you would respond to Jennifer.

6. Linda, age 26, had rheumatic fever as a child and subsequently developed mitral valve stenosis. She is presently 6 weeks pregnant. She is classified as Class II according to the New York Heart Association functional classification of heart disease. This is the first pregnancy for Linda and her husband, Sam.

a. Identify two nursing diagnoses appropriate for Linda related to her cardiac status and her anticipated care management. State an expected outcome for each nursing diagnosis identified.

b. Discuss a recommended therapeutic plan for Linda that will reduce her risk for cardiac decompensation in terms of each of the following:

Rest/sleep/activity patterns

Prevention of infection

Nutrition

Bowel elimination

c. Identify physiologic and psychosocial factors that could increase the stress placed on Linda's heart during her pregnancy.

Physiologic Factors   Psychosocial Factors

d. List the subjective symptoms that the nurse should teach Linda and her family to look for as indicators of possible cardiac decompensation.

e. List the objective signs that could indicate that Linda is experiencing signs of cardiac decompensation and heart failure.

f. Linda is admitted to the labor unit. Her cardiac condition is still classified as Class II. Outline the nursing measures designed to assess Linda and promote optimum cardiac function during labor and birth.

g. Linda should be observed carefully during the postpartum period because cardiac risk continues. Indicate the physiologic events after birth that place Linda at risk for cardiac decompensation.

h. Identify two nursing diagnoses that would be appropriate for the first 24 to 48 hours of Linda's postpartum period.

i. Discuss the measures the nurse can use to reduce the stress placed on Linda's heart during the postpartum period.

j. Linda indicates that she wishes to breastfeed her infant. Describe the nurse's response.

k. Identify the important factors to be considered when preparing Linda's discharge plan.

7. Allison is a pregnant woman with a cardiac disorder. As part of her medical regimen, her primary health care provider substituted subcutaneous heparin for the oral warfarin sodium (Coumadin) she had been taking before pregnancy.

a. Allison states, "I cannot give myself a shot! Why can't I just take the medication orally?" Discuss how you would respond as to the purpose of heparin and why it must be used instead of the Coumadin she is used to taking.

b. Indicate the information that the nurse should give Allison to ensure safe use of the heparin.

8. Jean is a primigravida at 4 weeks of gestation. She has been an epileptic for several years and her seizures have been controlled with phenytoin (Dilantin). Jean expresses concern regarding how her medication use will affect her pregnancy and her baby. She wants to stop taking the Dilantin. Describe the approach you would take in addressing Jean's concern and the course of action she is contemplating.

9. Lorraine is a 26-year-old pregnant woman. During her first prenatal visit she is tested for HIV and is found to be positive. Describe the care management of Lorraine during each period of pregnancy.

a. Antepartum

b. Intrapartum

c. Postpartum

10. Imagine that you are an advanced practice nurse who specializes in the treatment of men and women who are alcohol and drug dependent. You have been asked to establish a treatment program specifically designed for pregnant women. Outline the approach you would take to ensure that the program you establish takes into consideration the unique characteristics and needs of women in general and pregnant women in particular who abuse alcohol and drugs.

14 Pregnancy at Risk: Gestational Conditions

I. REVIEWING KEY CONCEPTS AND CONTENT

FILL IN THE BLANKS: Insert the term that corresponds to each of the following descriptions of hypertensive disorders during pregnancy and hyperemesis gravidarum.

1. The two basic types of hypertension during pregnancy are _____ and _____. _____ is hypertension that is present and observable before pregnancy or is diagnosed before week 20 of gestation. _____ is the onset of hypertension without proteinuria after the twentieth week of pregnancy.

2. _____ is a pregnancy-specific condition in which hypertension develops after _____ weeks in a previously normotensive woman. It is a multisystem, vasospastic disease process characterized by the presence of _____ and _____; it is usually categorized as _____ or _____ in terms of management.

3. _____ is defined as a systolic blood pressure (BP) greater than _____ or a diastolic blood pressure greater than _____ or a mean arterial pressure (MAP) greater than _____. Diagnosis is based on at least _____ measurements more than _____ hours apart.

4. _____ is defined as a protein concentration of _____ or more in at least _____ random urine specimens collected at least _____ hours apart.

5. _____ is clinically evident, generalized accumulation of fluid in the face, hands, or abdomen that is not responsive to _____ hours of bed rest. It may also be manifested as a rapid weight gain of more than _____ in 1 week.

6. _____ is the presence of any one of the following in women diagnosed with preeclampsia: systolic BP of at least _____ or a diastolic pressure of at least _____; protein concentration in the urine greater than _____ on dipstick measurement; _____, less than 400 to 500 ml of urine output over 24 hours; _____ or _____ disturbances; _____ involvement; _____ with a platelet count less than _____; _____ or _____ involvement; development of _____; development of _____ syndrome; increased serum _____; and certain cases of severe fetal _____.

7. _____ is the onset of seizure activity or coma in the woman diagnosed with preeclampsia, with no history of preexisting pathology that can result in seizure activity.

8. _____ syndrome is a laboratory diagnosis for a variant of severe preeclampsia that involves hepatic dysfunction; it is characterized by _____, _____, and _____.

9. _____ is gestational hypertension with no signs of preeclampsia present at the time of birth. Hypertension resolves by _____ weeks postpartum.

10. Arteriolar _____ diminishes the diameter of blood vessels, which impedes blood flow to all organs and raises BP. Impaired _____ leads to degenerative aging of the placenta and possible fetal _____. Reduced kidney perfusion leads to _____.

11. A diagnosis of _____ is made when vomiting becomes excessive enough to cause weight loss of at least _____ of prepregnancy weight and is accompanied by _____, _____, _____, and _____. Women with this disorder tend to be _____, _____, and have a _____ gestation.

12. State the principles you would follow to ensure the accuracy of BP measurement during pregnancy.

TRUE OR FALSE: Circle T if true or F if false for each of the following statements related to hypertensive disorders during pregnancy. Correct the false statements.

13. T   F   Preeclampsia complicates less than 10% of all pregnancies that progress beyond the first trimester.

14. T   F   The rate for preeclampsia has risen since the early 1990s.

15. T   F   The major maternal hazard of preeclampsia is liver failure.

16. T   F   A genetic disposition may be partly responsible for the development of preeclampsia in some women.

17. T   F   HELLP syndrome appears in approximately 2% to 12% of women with severe preeclampsia.

18. T   F   HELLP syndrome occurs most often in young, nulliparous African-American women.

19. T   F   Calcium gluconate is the antidote for magnesium sulfate toxicity.

20. T   F   The therapeutic serum magnesium level for the treatment of severe preeclampsia would be 10 to 12 mg/dl.

21. T   F   Pregnant women with chronic renal disease are at increased risk for developing preeclampsia.

22. T   F   Research studies have confirmed that a daily dose of low-dose aspirin is effective in preventing preeclampsia.

23. T   F   When on bed rest, the woman with preeclampsia should maintain a dorsal recumbent position.

24. T   F   Sodium should be restricted to a minimal level when a woman has preeclampsia.

25. T   F   Administration of magnesium sulfate to a woman with severe preeclampsia may precipitate labor by stimulating the uterus to contract.

26. T   F   An expected outcome for the use of magnesium sulfate is the prevention of progress from preeclampsia to eclampsia.

27. T   F   Hydralazine (Apresoline) may be used to lower the BP of a woman with preeclampsia.

28. T   F   Severe epigastric or right upper quadrant pain is one sign of impending eclampsia.

29. T   F   Protein restriction in the diet of a woman with preeclampsia can reduce BP and edema.

30. T   F   Prompt treatment of a woman using appropriate medications, bed rest, and diet can cure preeclampsia.

31. T   F   Methergine is the oxytocic of choice to prevent or treat postpartum hemorrhage for women with preeclampsia.

32. Preeclampsia is a serious complication of pregnancy. State the risk factors associated with preeclampsia for which the nurse should be alert when doing the health history interview at the first prenatal visit.

33. Describe the assessment technique used to determine if the following findings are present in women with preeclampsia. (Note: You may wish to review this information in a physical assessment textbook for a complete explanation of each technique.)

   a.   Hyperreflexia and ankle clonus

   b.   Proteinuria

   c.   Pitting edema

MATCHING: Match the client description in Column I with the appropriate diagnosis from Column II.

<table>
<tr><td>COLUMN I</td><td>COLUMN II</td></tr>
</table>

34. _____ At 30 weeks of gestation, Angela's MAP was 108 mm Hg; her urinalysis indicated a protein level of 2+; her weight increased 2 kg in 1 week; she exhibited dependent and upper body edema.

a. Eclampsia

b. Chronic hypertension

35. _____ At 24 weeks of gestation, Mary's BP rose from a prepregnant baseline of 120/70 to 150/92. No other problematic signs and symptoms were noted.

c. Gestational hypertension

d. HELLP syndrome

36. _____ Susan, a 34-year-old pregnant woman, has had a consistently high BP ranging from 148/92 to 160/98 since she was 28 years old. Her weight gain has followed normal patterns, and urinalysis remains normal as well.

e. Preeclampsia

37. _____ At 32 weeks of gestation, Maria, with hypertension since 28 weeks, generalized edema, and proteinuria of 4+, has a convulsion.

38. _____ Dawn has been hypertensive since her twenty-fourth week of pregnancy. Urinalysis indicates a protein content of 3+. Further testing reveals a platelet count of 95,000 and elevated AST and ALT levels; in addition, her hematocrit is decreased and burr cells appear on a peripheral smear.

39. Preeclampsia and eclampsia affect both maternal and fetal well-being.

    a. Describe how preeclampsia and eclampsia can adversely affect the health and well-being of the fetus.

    b. Indicate the fetal surveillance measures recommended for women experiencing preeclampsia.

TRUE OR FALSE: Circle T if true or F if false for each of the following statements related to hemorrhagic disorders during pregnancy. Correct the false statements.

40. T   F   Miscarriages are often related to maternal behavior.

41. T   F   There is little that nurses can do to reduce the incidence of miscarriages.

42. T   F   A missed miscarriage refers to a pregnancy in which the fetus has died but the products of conception are retained in the uterus for up to several weeks.

43. T   F   An etiologic factor for recurrent premature dilation of the cervix (incompetent cervix) is the use of diethylstilbestrol by the woman's mother during pregnancy with the woman.

44. T   F   Ectopic pregnancy accounts for 30% of all maternal deaths.

45. T   F   Ectopic pregnancy is the leading pregnancy-related cause of first trimester maternal mortality.

46. T   F   Ectopic pregnancy is a leading cause of infertility.

47. T   F   The incidence of ectopic pregnancy is decreasing in part because of more effective treatment for pelvic inflammatory disease.

48. T   F   Complete molar pregnancies contain embryonic or fetal parts and an amniotic sac.

49. T   F   There is a lower rate of malignant transformation with a partial molar pregnancy.

50. T   F   Multiple gestation and closely spaced pregnancies increase the risk for placenta previa.

51. T   F   The standard for the diagnosis of placenta previa is transabdominal ultrasound examination.

52. T   F   The greatest fetal risk related to placenta previa is malpresentation.

53. T   F   Maternal mortality is approximately 5% with placenta previa.

54. T   F   A vaginal examination performed when a woman is exhibiting signs of placenta previa can result in profound hemorrhage.

55. T   F   Premature separation of the placenta accounts for 15% to 30% of all perinatal deaths.

56. T   F   Cesarean birth is recommended for women experiencing signs of abruptio placentae.

57. T   F   Abdominal trauma is the most consistently identified risk factor for abruptio placentae.

58. T   F   Use of cocaine can precipitate a premature separation of the placenta partly because of cocaine-induced hypertension.

59. T   F   It is safe to manage a woman with a Grade I premature separation of the placenta at home.

60. T   F   The urinary output of women diagnosed with disseminated intravascular coagulation should be carefully monitored since renal failure is a potential complication.

FILL IN THE BLANKS: Insert the appropriate term for each description of antepartal bleeding.

61. In the first trimester, most bleeding is the result of _____ and _____.

62. Approximately 50% of bleeding in the third trimester is caused by _____ and _____.

63. _____ is defined as the termination of pregnancy that occurs before the fetus has reached the point of _____ and is capable of surviving in an _____ environment. In the United States this point is before _____ weeks of gestation. A fetal weight of less than _____ may also be used to define this type of pregnancy loss. A _____ results from natural causes. There are five types of this form of pregnancy termination, namely _____, _____, _____, _____, and _____.

64. Evaluation of the serum level of the placental hormone _____ and determination of the presence of a viable _____ using _____ are two diagnostic tests that can be used when a pregnant woman is exhibiting signs of threatened abortion.

65. Incompetent cervix or _____ is a cause of late miscarriage or preterm birth. Current research contends that cervical incompetence is variable and exists as a continuum that is determined in part by cervical _____. Other factors include _____ of the cervical tissue and the individual circumstances associated with the pregnancy in terms of maternal _____ and _____. Short _____ and _____ of the pregnancy at a progressively earlier gestational age are characteristics of this cervical disorder.

66. _____ pregnancy is one in which the _____ is implanted outside the uterine cavity, usually in the _____ of the uterine _____. An ecchymotic blueness around the umbilicus called _____ sign indicates _____ as a result of an undiagnosed ruptured intraabdominal pregnancy.

67. _____ or _____ is a gestational trophoblastic disease. There are two distinct types: _____, resulting from fertilization of an egg whose nucleus has been lost or inactivated and _____, resulting from two sperm fertilizing an apparently normal ovum.

68. _____ is the implantation of the placenta in the lower uterine segment, and as a result, it covers the _____ in the third trimester. It is termed _____ when the distance of the placenta is 2 to 3 cm from the _____ and does not cover it. The term _____ is used when the exact relationship of the os to the placenta has not been determined. Risk for postpartum hemorrhage is increased because the _____ is unable to _____ around the open blood vessels of the placental site. The most important risks factors for this placental disorder are previous _____, previous _____, and treatment of miscarriage or induced abortion with _____.

69. _____ or abruptio placentae is the _____ of part or all of the placenta from its _____ site. A woman who experienced abruptio placentae is at higher risk for postpartum hemorrhage as a result of _____ uterus, _____, or both. Risks for abruptio placentae include maternal _____, _____ use, _____ trauma, maternal _____, and poor _____.

70. _____ is a placental anomaly in which the cord vessels begin to branch at the membranes and then course into the placenta. Rupture of the _____ or traction on the _____ may tear one or more of the fetal vessels leading to fetal hemorrhage. _____ placenta is the term used for a marginal insertion of the cord into the placenta which also increases the risk for fetal hemorrhage. _____ placenta refers to a condition in which the placenta is divided into two or more separate lobes.

71. _____ is a pathologic form of clotting that is diffuse and consumes large amounts of clotting factors, causing widespread external and internal _____. It is an overactivation of the clotting cascade and the fibrinolytic system that results in the depletion of _____ and _____.

72. Disseminated intravascular coagulation (DIC) can result from a number of obstetric problems.

   a. Identify three predisposing conditions for DIC.

   b. Describe the pathophysiology that leads to DIC.

   c. Indicate the clinical manifestations of DIC that would be noted during physical examination and with laboratory testing.

   d. Describe four priority nursing measures that should be used when caring for a woman experiencing DIC.

73. TORCH infections can have serious consequences.

   a. TORCH infections are a group of organisms capable of _____ the placenta and adversely affecting the _____ of the fetus. Generally, TORCH infections produce _____ symptoms in the mother, but fetal and neonatal effects are more serious.

b. Complete the following table by indicating the infections represented by each letter of the acronym TORCH and identifying their mode of transmission, prevention measures, and treatment.

Infection	Mode of Prevention	Treatment
T		
O		
R		
C		
H		

74. At times pregnant women require abdominal surgery.

   a. Identify the factors that can complicate diagnosis of and surgical treatment for abdominal problems during pregnancy.

   b. List the most common conditions necessitating surgery during pregnancy.

   c. Cite the major fear most often expressed by the pregnant woman undergoing surgery.

   d. Preoperative care for a pregnant woman differs from that for a nonpregnant woman in one significant aspect, namely the presence of the _____. General preoperative observations and ongoing care are the same as for any surgery, with the addition of continuous _____ and _____ monitoring if the fetus is considered to be viable. Intraoperatively fetal oxygenation is improved by placing the woman on an operating table with a _____ to avoid maternal _____.

Continuous _____ and _____ monitoring must take place during the surgical procedures and in the postoperative period if intrauterine pregnancy continues. There is an increase for the onset of _____. _____ may be required to suppress uterine contractions.

   e. Identify the nursing considerations and topics for teaching related to the discharge planning process of the pregnant woman who experienced abdominal surgery.

MULTIPLE CHOICE QUESTIONS: Circle the one correct option and state the rationale for the option chosen.

75. When measuring the BP to ensure consistency and to facilitate early detection of BP changes consistent with gestational hypertension, the nurse should
   a. place the woman in a supine position.
   b. allow the woman to rest for at least 15 minutes before measuring her BP.
   c. use the same arm for each BP measurement.
   d. use a proper sized cuff that covers at least 50% of her upper arm.

76. When caring for a woman with mild preeclampsia, it is critical that during assessment the nurse is alert for signs of progress to severe preeclampsia. Progress to severe preeclampsia would be indicated by which one of the following assessment findings?
    a. Proteinuria of 2+ or greater
    b. Platelet level of 200,000/mm³
    c. Deep tendon reflexes 2+, ankle clonus is absent
    d. BP of 154/94 and 156/100, 6 hours apart

77. A woman's preeclampsia has advanced to the severe stage. She is admitted to the hospital and her primary health care provider has ordered an infusion of magnesium sulfate be started. In implementing this order the nurse would
    a. prepare a loading dose of 20 g of magnesium sulfate in 100 ml of 5% glucose in water.
    b. monitor maternal vital signs, fetal heart rate (FHR) patterns, and uterine contractions every 2 hours.
    c. expect the maintenance dose to be approximately 4 g/hour.
    d. report a respiratory rate of 12 breaths or less per minute to the primary health care provider immediately.

78. The primary expected outcome for care associated with the administration of magnesium sulfate would be met if the woman
    a. exhibits a decrease in both systolic and diastolic BP.
    b. experiences no seizures.
    c. states that she feels more relaxed and calm.
    d. urinates more frequently, resulting in a decrease in pathologic edema.

79. A woman has been diagnosed with mild preeclampsia and will be treated at home. The nurse, in teaching this woman about her treatment regimen for mild preeclampsia would tell her to
    a. weigh herself daily after dinner or just before going to bed.
    b. place a dipstick into her urine stream as she begins to urinate to check for protein in the urine.
    c. reduce her fluid intake to four to five 8 ounce glasses each day.
    d. Do gentle exercises such as hand and feet circles and gently tensing and relaxing arm and leg muscles.

80. A woman has just been admitted with a diagnosis of hyperemesis gravidarum. She has been unable to retain any oral intake and as a result has lost weight and is exhibiting signs of dehydration with electrolyte imbalance and acetonuria. The care management of this woman would include which of the following?
    a. Administering diphenhydramine (Benadryl) to control nausea and vomiting
    b. Keeping the woman NPO for at least 24 hours after vomiting has stopped
    c. Avoiding oral hygiene until the woman is able to tolerate oral fluids
    d. Providing small frequent meals consisting of bland foods and warm fluids once the woman begins to respond to treatment

81. A primigravida at 10 weeks of gestation reports slight vaginal spotting without passage of tissue and mild uterine cramping. When examined, no cervical dilation is noted. The nurse caring for this woman would
    a. anticipate that the woman will be sent home and placed on bed rest with instructions to avoid stress and orgasm.
    b. prepare the woman for a dilation and curettage.
    c. notify a grief counselor to assist the woman with the imminent loss of her fetus
    d. tell the woman that the doctor will most likely perform a cerclage to help her maintain her pregnancy.

82. A woman is admitted through the emergency room with a medical diagnosis of ruptured ectopic pregnancy. The primary nursing diagnosis at this time would be
    a. acute pain related to irritation of the peritoneum with blood.
    b. risk for infection related to tissue trauma.
    c. deficient fluid volume related to blood loss associated with rupture of the uterine tube.
    d. anticipatory grieving related to unexpected pregnancy outcome.

83. A woman diagnosed with an ectopic pregnancy is given an intramuscular injection of methotrexate. The nurse would tell the woman which of the following?
    a. Methotrexate is an analgesic that will relieve the dull abdominal pain she is experiencing.
    b. She should avoid alcohol until her primary care provider tells her the treatment is complete.
    c. Follow-up blood tests will be required for at least 6 months after the injection of the methotrexate.
    d. She should continue to take her prenatal vitamin to enhance healing.

84. A pregnant woman at 32 weeks of gestation comes to the emergency room because she has begun to experience bright red vaginal bleeding. She reports that she is experiencing no pain. The admission nurse suspects
    a. abruptio placentae.
    b. disseminated intravascular coagulation.
    c. placenta previa.
    d. preterm labor.

85. A pregnant woman, at 38 weeks of gestation diagnosed with marginal placenta previa, has just given birth to a healthy newborn male. The nurse recognizes that the immediate focus for the care of this woman would be:
    a. preventing hemorrhage.
    b. relieving pain.
    c. preventing infection.
    d. fostering attachment of the woman with her new son.

II. THINKING CRITICALLY

1. Jean (2-1-0-0-1) is at 30 weeks of gestation and has been diagnosed with mild preeclampsia. The treatment plan includes home care with limited activity consisting of bed rest with bathroom privileges and out of bed twice a day for meals, appropriate nutrition, and stress reduction. She and her husband are very anxious about the diagnosis and are also concerned about how they will manage the care of their active 3-year-old daughter, Anne.

    a. Indicate the clinical manifestations that would have been present to indicate this diagnosis.

    b. List three priority nursing diagnoses for Jean and her family.

    c. Describe how you would help this couple organize their home care routine.

    d. Specify what you would teach them with regard to assessment of Jean's status in terms of each of the following:

       BP

       Weight

       Protein in urine

       Fetal well-being

       Signs of a worsening condition

    e. Describe the instructions you would give Jean regarding her nutrient and fluid intake.

   f. Discuss the measures Jean can use to cope with the boredom and alteration in circulation and muscle tone that accompany bed rest.

   g. Limited activity can lead to a nursing diagnosis of constipation related to changes in bowel function associated with pregnancy and limited activity. Cite two measures that Jean can use to enhance bowel elimination and prevent constipation.

2. Ellen, a pregnant woman at 37 weeks of gestation, is admitted to the hospital with a diagnosis of severe preeclampsia.

   a. Indicate the signs and symptoms that would have been present to indicate this diagnosis.

   b. List three priority nursing diagnoses for Ellen.

   c. Specify the precautionary measures that should be taken to protect Ellen and her fetus from injury.

   d. Ellen's physician orders magnesium sulfate to be infused at 4 g in 20 minutes as a loading dose then a maintenance intravenous infusion of 2 g/hr.

   • Identify the guidelines that must be followed when administering the magnesium sulfate infusion.

   • Write one nursing diagnosis related to the treatment with magnesium sulfate.

   • Explain the expected therapeutic effect of magnesium sulfate to Ellen and her family.

   e. List the maternal-fetal assessments that should be accomplished on a regular basis during the infusion of magnesium sulfate.

   • Identify the progressive signs of magnesium sulfate toxicity.

   • State the interventions that must be instituted immediately if magnesium sulfate toxicity occurs.

   f. Despite all prevention efforts, Ellen has a convulsion.

     • Specify the nursing measures that should be implemented at the onset of the convulsion and immediately afterward.

     • List the problems that can occur as a result of the convulsion that Ellen experienced.

   g. Ellen successfully gave birth vaginally despite her high risk status. Describe Ellen's care management during the first 48 hours of her postpartum recovery period.

3. Marie, an 18-year-old obese primigravida at 9 weeks of gestation, is diagnosed with hyperemesis gravidarum. She is unmarried and lives at home with her parents. Marie is admitted to the high risk antepartal unit. During the admission interview, Marie confides to the nurse that her parents have been very unhappy about her pregnancy. She now is worried that she may have made the wrong decision to continue with her pregnancy and raise her baby as a single parent.

   a. Identify the etiologic factors that may have contributed to Marie's current health problem.

   b. List the physiologic and psychologic factors that the nurse should be alert for when assessing Marie upon her admission.

   c. State two nursing diagnoses related to Marie's current health status.

   d. Outline the nursing care measures appropriate for Marie while hospitalized.

   e. Once stabilized, Marie is discharged to home care. She is able to tolerate oral food and fluid intake. Explain the important care measures that the nurse should discuss with Marie and her family before she goes home.

4. Andrea is admitted to the hospital, where a diagnosis of acute ruptured ectopic pregnancy in her fallopian tube is made.

   a. State the risk factors associated with ectopic pregnancy.

   b. Describe the findings that were most likely experienced and exhibited by Andrea as her ectopic pregnancy progressed and then ruptured.

   c. Identify the other health care problems that share the same or similar clinical manifestations as ectopic pregnancy.

   d. State the major care management problem at this time. Support your answer.

   e. Identify two priority nursing diagnoses appropriate for Andrea.

   f. Outline the nursing measures Andrea will require during the preoperative and postoperative period.

5. Janet is 10 weeks pregnant. She comes to the clinic and states that she has been experiencing slight bleeding with mild cramping for about 4 hours. No tissue has been passed and pelvic examination reveals that the cervical os is closed.

   a. Indicate the most likely basis for Janet's signs and symptoms.

   b. Outline the expected care management of Janet's problem.

6. Denise, a primigravida, calls the clinic. She is crying while she tells the nurse that she has noted "a lot of bleeding" and that she is sure she is losing her baby.

   a. Write several questions the nurse should ask Denise to obtain a more definitive picture of the bleeding she is experiencing.

   b. Based on the data collected Denise is admitted to the hospital for further evaluation. A medical diagnosis of incomplete abortion is made. Describe the assessment findings that would indicate the diagnosis of incomplete abortion.

   c. State the nursing diagnosis that would take priority at this time.

   d. Outline the nursing measures that would be appropriate for the priority nursing diagnosis you identified and for the expected medical management of Denise's health problem.

   e. Specify the instructions that Denise should receive before her discharge from the hospital.

f. List the nursing measures appropriate for the nursing diagnosis: anticipatory grieving related to unexpected outcome of pregnancy.

7. Mary has been diagnosed with hydatidiform mole (complete).

a. Identify the typical signs and symptoms Mary would most likely exhibit to establish this diagnosis.

b. Specify the post-treatment instructions that the nurse must stress when discussing follow-up management with Mary.

c. A major concern, associated with hydatidiform mole, is the development of _____ which is indicated by a rising _____ titer and enlarging _____ .

8. Two pregnant women are admitted to the labor unit with vaginal bleeding. Sara is at 29 weeks of gestation and is diagnosed with marginal placenta previa. Jane is at 34 weeks of gestation and is diagnosed with a moderate (grade II) premature separation of the placenta (abruptio placentae).

a. Compare the clinical picture each of these women is likely to exhibit during assessment.

   Sara   **Jane**

b. Identify two priority nursing diagnoses for both Sara and Jane.

c. Contrast the care management approach required by each of the women as it relates to their diagnosis and the typical medical management.

   Sara   **Jane**

d. Indicate the considerations that must be given top priority following birth for each of these women.

   Sara   **Jane**

9. Trauma continues to be a common complication during pregnancy that may require obstetric critical care.

   a. Discuss the significance of this complication using statistical data to describe the scope of the problem in terms of incidence, timing during pregnancy, and forms of trauma.

   b. Indicate the effects trauma can have on pregnancy.

   c. Describe the potential impact of trauma on the fetus.

   d. Priorities of care for the pregnant woman following trauma must be to _____ the woman and _____ her condition first and then consider _____ needs. This method of approach in care management is important because _____ survival is dependent on _____ survival. The ABCs of resuscitation are _____, _____, and _____.

   e. Outline the major components of the assessment and care of a pregnant woman who has experienced trauma.

   Primary survey

   Secondary survey

   f. Explain the critical components of discharge planning as it applies to a pregnant woman who has experienced trauma.

Labor and Birth Processes

I. REVIEWING KEY CONCEPTS AND CONTENT

FILL IN THE BLANKS: Insert the term that corresponds to each of the following descriptions.

1. The five factors of labor are
_____,
_____, _____,
_____, and _____.

2. _____are membrane-filled spaces that are located where _____in the fetal/neonatal skull intersect.

3. _____ is the slight overlapping of the bones of the fetal skull that occurs during childbirth.

4. _____ refers to the part of the fetus that enters the pelvic inlet first. The three main types are_____ (head first), _____ (buttocks first), and _____.

5. The _____ refers to the part of the fetal body first felt by the examining finger during a vaginal examination. The four types are _____, _____, _____, and _____.

6. The _____ occurs when the fetal head is fully flexed, making the _____ the fetal part first felt by the examining finger.

7. Fetal _____ is the relationship of the long axis (spine) of the fetus to the long axis (spine) of the mother. There are two types: _____ when the spines are parallel to each other and _____ when the spines are at right angles or diagonal to each other.

8. _____ is the relationship of the fetal body parts to each other. The most common type is one of general _____.

9. The _____ diameter is the largest transverse diameter of the fetal skull. The _____ diameter is the smallest anteroposterior diameter of the fetal skull to enter the maternal pelvis when the fetal head is in complete _____.

10. Fetal _____ refers to the relationship of the fetal presenting part to the four quadrants of the maternal pelvis.

11. _____ occurs when the largest transverse diameter of the presenting part has passed through the maternal pelvic brim or inlet into the true pelvis reaching the level of the _____ or _____ station.

12. Station is the relationship of the _____ of the fetus to an imaginary line drawn between the _____. It is measured in terms of _____ above or below the _____, thereby serving as a method of determining the progress of fetal _____.

13. _____ refers to the shortening and thinning of the cervix during the _____ stage of labor. Degree of effacement is expressed as a _____.

14. _____ is the enlargement or widening of the cervical opening (os) and the cervical canal, which occurs once labor has begun. Degree of progress is expressed in _____from _____ to _____.

15. _____ occurs when the fetus's presenting part descends into the true pelvis approximately _____ weeks before term in the primigravida. For the multiparous woman, this event may not occur until after _____ are established and _____ is in progress.

16. The primary powers of labor are _____ and the secondary powers are the woman's _____ efforts or _____.

17. _____ is discharge of brownish or blood-tinged cervical mucus representing the passage of the _____ as the cervix _____ in preparation for labor.

18. The _____ refers to the turns and adjustments of the fetal head, to facilitate passage through the birth canal. They are also known as the _____ of labor, they include: _____, _____, _____, _____, _____, _____ and _____, and finally birth by _____.

19. _____ maneuver is a pushing method during the second stage of labor characterized by a closed _____ with _____ holding and prolonged _____. It is not recommended because it has been associated with fetal _____ and _____. _____ have been associated with directed pushing.

20. The first stage of labor is considered to last from the _____ to full _____ of the cervix. It is divided into three phases, namely _____, _____, and _____.

21. The second stage of labor lasts from the time the cervix is fully _____ to the _____ of the fetus.

22. The third stage of labor lasts from the _____ until the _____ is delivered.

23. The fourth stage of labor is the period of immediate _____ when _____ is reestablished. It lasts approximately _____.

24. The four factors that affect fetal circulation during labor are maternal _____, _____, _____, and _____.

25. Describe how the five factors (the five *Ps*) affect the process of labor and birth.

26. Explain how the cardinal movements of labor facilitate the birth of the fetus.

27. Label the following illustrations of the fetal skull and the maternal pelvis with the appropriate landmarks and diameters.

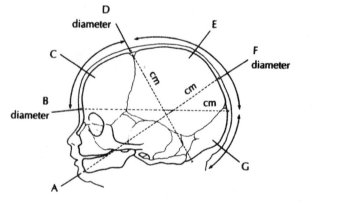

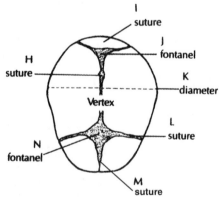

Fetal Skull

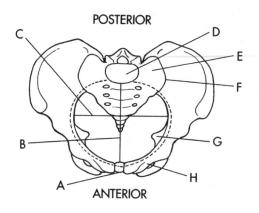

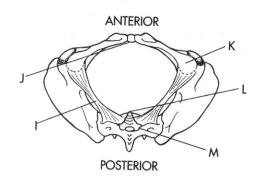

Pelvic Brim from Above

Pelvic Outlet from Above

Maternal Pelvis

28. Indicate the presentation, presenting part, position, lie and attitude of the fetus, for each of the following illustrations.

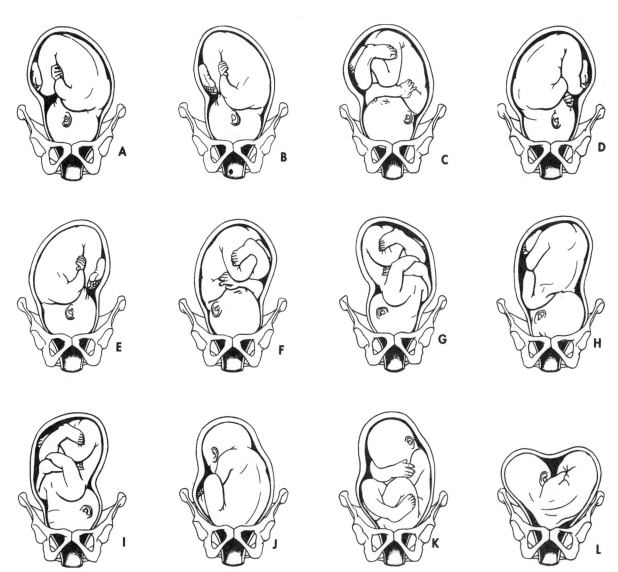

TRUE OR FALSE: Circle T if true or F if false for each of the following statements. Correct the false statements.

29. T   F   The most common fetal attitude is one of full extension of body parts.

30. T   F   A longitudinal lie results in either a cephalic or a breech presentation.

31. T   F   Fetal position is unlikely to change once labor begins.

32. T   F   A woman must have a gynecoid pelvis in order to experience a spontaneous vaginal birth.

33. T   F   Effacement usually precedes dilation for a nulliparous woman.

34. T   F   Women with a history of sexually transmitted infections or surgery may experience slowed or ineffective progress of cervical dilation as a result of scarring.

35. T   F   The hands and knees position is most helpful when the fetal presentation is breech.

36. T   F   Women often experience decreased dyspnea but increased urinary frequency after lightening occurs.

37. T   F   The expected range of the fetal heart rate of a full-term fetus is 100 to 140 beats/min.

38. T   F   An increase in fetal P_{O_2} and arterial pH and a decrease in P_{CO_2} prepares the fetus for initiating respirations immediately after its birth.

39. T   F   Because systolic blood pressure increases during a contraction, assessment of maternal blood pressure *between* contractions provides more accurate data.

40. T   F   The white blood cell count (WBC) increases in response to the stress, tissue trauma, and increased activity level associated with childbirth.

41. T   F   During labor, a woman should be encouraged to point her toes to reduce the incidence of leg cramps.

42. T   F   Endogenous endorphins secreted during labor raise a woman's pain threshold and produce sedation.

43. T   F   Fetal fibronectin is found in maternal plasma and cervicovaginal secretions of pregnant women before the onset of labor.

44. T   F   Effacement is more rapid during the active phase of the first stage of labor for the multiparous woman.

45. T   F   The average duration of the second stage of labor is approximately 20 to 50 minutes.

46. T   F   Women are expected to experience an urge to bear down as soon as the second stage of labor begins.

MULTIPLE CHOICE QUESTIONS: Circle the one correct option and state the rationale for the option chosen.

47. A vaginal examination during labor reveals the following information about the fetus: RMT, −2. An accurate interpretation of this data would be
   a. attitude: flexed.
   b. station: above the ischial spines.
   c. presenting part: vertex.
   d. lie: transverse.

48. Changes occur as a woman progresses through labor. Which of the following maternal adaptations would be expected during labor?
   a. Increase in both systolic and diastolic blood pressure during uterine contractions in the first stage of labor
   b. Decrease in white blood cell count
   c. Slight increase in heart rate during the first and second stage of labor
   d. Increase in gastric motility leading to vomiting during the latent phase of the first stage of labor

49. Duration of labor varies from woman to woman and is often influenced by a woman's obstetric history including parity. An expected duration for a nulliparous woman's stages of labor would be which of the following?
   a. First stage of labor: up to 12 hours for full dilation to be achieved
   b. Second stage of labor: average of 20 minutes or less
   c. Third stage of labor: 3 to 5 minutes, up to 1 hour
   d. Fourth stage of labor: 6 to 8 hours

50. When instructing a group of primigravid women about the onset of labor the nurse would tell them to be alert for
   a. urinary retention.
   b. weight gain of 2 kg.
   c. quickening.
   d. energy surge.

II. THINKING CRITICALLY

1. As part of their care of the laboring woman, nurses perform vaginal examinations and interpret the results. State the meaning of each of the following vaginal examination findings.

Exam I	Exam II	Exam III	Exam IV
ROP	RMA	LST	OA
−1	0	+1	+3
50%	25%	75%	100%
3 cm	2 cm	6 cm	10 cm

2. Brooke is a primigravida at 36 weeks of gestation. During a prenatal visit at 34 weeks of gestation, she asks you the following questions regarding her approaching labor. Describe how you would respond.

   a. "What gets labor to start?"

   b. "Are there things I should watch for that would tell me my labor is getting closer to starting?"

   c. "How long can I expect my labor to last once it gets started?"

   d. "My friend just had a baby and she told me the nurses kept helping her change her position and even encouraged her to walk! Isn't that dangerous for the baby and painful for the mom?"

16 Management of Discomfort

I. REVIEWING KEY CONCEPTS AND CONTENT

FILL IN THE BLANKS: Insert the term that corresponds to each of the following descriptions related to childbirth pain.

1. _____ pain originates in the body organs during labor and birth. This type of pain results from _____ changes, _____ of the lower uterine segment, and uterine _____ that predominates during the _____ stage of labor. It is located over the _____ of the abdomen.

2. _____ pain originates in the muscles and bones. During labor and birth, this type of pain occurs during the _____ stage of labor. It results from stretching and distention of _____ and the _____ to allow passage of the fetus, from distention and traction on the _____ and _____ supports during contractions, and from _____ of soft tissues.

3. _____ pain is felt in areas of the body other than the area of pain origin. During labor and birth, pain originating in the _____ radiates to the _____ wall, _____ area of the back, _____, _____ area, and down the _____.

4. According to the _____ theory of pain, pain sensations travel along sensory nerve pathways to the brain, but only a limited number of sensations or messages can travel through these nerve pathways at one time. Pain relief techniques based on this theory include _____ or _____, _____, _____, and _____. _____ work involving concentration on _____ and _____ techniques is also based on this theory.

5. _____ are endogenous opioids secreted by the pituitary gland that act on the central and peripheral nervous systems to reduce pain. It is thought that these opioid substances increase during pregnancy and birth in humans and may increase the ability of the woman in labor to tolerate acute pain.

FILL IN THE BLANKS: Insert the term that corresponds to each of the following descriptions of nonpharmacologic techniques for management of discomfort during childbirth.

6. Three methods or approaches are incorporated into most childbirth education classes today. These methods or approaches are _____, _____, and _____.

7. The basis of the _____ method, also known as the natural childbirth method, is that the pain of childbirth is caused by a _____ syndrome. Three techniques are emphasized with this method namely _____, _____, and _____ techniques.

8. The _____ method, also known as the psychoprophylactic method, is based on the belief that pain is a _____ response. This method prepares women to respond to uterine contractions with _____ techniques and _____ patterns.

9. The _____ method is also known as husband-coached childbirth. This method emphasizes working in _____ with the body using _____ control, _____, and promoting general body _____. The method stresses environmental factors such as _____, _____, and _____ to make childbirth a more natural experience.

10. Breathing techniques should be initiated when the laboring woman can no longer _____ or _____ through a contraction. _____ breathing is breathing at approximately _____ the woman's normal breathing rate. It is usually the first technique that is used in early labor.

11. As labor advances, _____ breathing is used with techniques becoming more _____ in depth and increasing to about _____ the normal breathing rate.

12. A routine _____ should begin each breathing pattern and end each contraction, exhaling to blow the contraction away.

13. A _____ breathing technique using a pattern of breaths and puffs in a ratio of 3:1, 4:1, 6:1, 8:1, or coach-called is used to enhance concentration during the _____ phase of the first stage of labor. An undesirable effect of this type of breathing may be _____ or rapid deep respirations that can result in respiratory _____ as exhibited by the symptoms of _____, _____, and _____ of fingers, or circumoral _____. It can be overcome by having the woman _____. This enables the woman to rebreathe _____. Maintaining the breathing rate at no more than _____ the normal rate will decrease the occurrence of this breathing-related problem.

14. _____ or light massage (stroking) of the abdomen or other body part in rhythm with breathing during contractions and _____ or steady pressure against the sacrum using the _____ or _____ of the hand, especially during back labor, are two examples of nonpharmacologic methods to relieve discomfort that are based on the _____ theory of pain.

15. _____ (i.e., bathing, showering, whirlpool baths) uses the buoyancy of the warm water to provide support for tense muscles, relief from discomfort, and general body relaxation. It should not be initiated until the laboring woman is in the _____ phase of the first stage of labor once uterine contractions are well established.

16. _____ uses two pairs of electrodes place on either side of the woman's _____ and _____ spine to provide continuous mild electrical currents that can be increased during a contraction. It may be effective because of a _____ effect that can stimulate the release of _____ in the woman's body, thereby alleviating discomfort.

17. Describe the factors that could influence the following nursing diagnosis identified for a woman in labor: Acute pain related to the processes involved in labor and birth.

18. Explain the theoretic basis for using such techniques as massage, stroking, music, and imagery to reduce the sensation of pain during childbirth.

MATCHING: Match the description in Column I with the appropriate pharmacologic method for discomfort management during childbirth in Column II.

COLUMN I

19. _____ Abolition of pain perception by interrupting nerve impulses going to the brain. Loss of sensation (partial or complete) and sometimes loss of consciousness occurs.

20. _____ Method used to repair a tear or hole in the dura mater around the spinal cord as a result of spinal anesthesia; the goal is to prevent or treat postdural puncture headaches (PDPH).

21. _____ Single-injection, subarachnoid anesthesia useful for pain control during birth but not for labor.

22. _____ Systemic analgesic that provides analgesia without causing maternal or neonatal respiratory depression.

23. _____ Provides rapid perineal anesthesia for performing and repairing an episiotomy.

24. _____ Anesthesia method used to relieve pain from uterine contractions and cervical dilation. It is associated with fetal bradycardia.

25. _____ Medication such as a barbiturate that can be used to relieve anxiety and induce sleep in prodromal or early latent labor.

26. _____ Analgesic potentiator such as a tranquilizer.

27. _____ Drug that reverses the effects of opioids, including neonatal narcosis (CNS depression of the newborn).

28. _____ Medication such as an opioid analgesic that is administered IM or IV for pain relief during labor.

29. _____ Alleviation of pain sensation or raising of the pain threshold without loss of consciousness.

30. _____ Relief from pain of uterine contractions and birth by injecting a local anesthetic and/or opioid into the peridural space.

31. _____ Anesthetic that relieves pain in the lower vagina, vulva, and perineum, making it useful for episiotomy, birth, and use of low forceps.

COLUMN II

a. Mixed opioid agonist-antagonist compound

b. Anesthesia

c. Analgesia

d. Ataractic

e. Epidural analgesia/anesthesia (block)

f. Autologous epidural blood patch

g. Local infiltration anesthesia

h. Spinal anesthesia (block)

i. Opioid antagonist

j. Paracervical (uterosacral) block

k. Pudendal nerve block

l. Systemic analgesic

m. Sedative

32. Complete the following table by listing the effects, criteria/timing for use, and nursing management for each of the following commonly used nerve block anesthetics.

Anesthetic	Effects	Criteria/Timing	Management
Local Infiltration			
Pudendal Nerve Block			
Spinal Block			
Epidural Anesthesia/ Analgesia (Block)			

33. Systemic analgesics cross the placenta and affect the fetus.

    a. List three factors that influence the effect systemic analgesics have on the fetus.

    b. Identify the fetal effects of systemic analgesics.

34. Complete the following table by giving one example for each of the following medication classifications and stating how each medication is administered and why it is used during the childbirth process.

Medication	Method of Administration	Purpose of Administration
Opioid Agonist Analgesic:		
Mixed Opioid Agonist-Antagonist:		
Ataractic:		
Opioid Antagonist:		

35. Explain why the intravenous route is preferred to the intramuscular route for the administration of systemic analgesics during labor.

TRUE OR FALSE: Circle T if true or F if false for each of the following statements. Correct the false statements.

36. T F With visceral pain, a woman usually experiences discomfort only during a uterine contraction.

37. T F A woman's perception of her birth experience as "good" or "bad" is influenced by the degree to which she believes she met her personal goals related to coping effectively with pain.

38. T F Water therapy cannot be used if the laboring woman's membranes are ruptured.

39. T F There is no limit on the time a laboring woman can spend in a whirlpool bath.

40. T F Acupressure is best applied over the skin without using lubricants.

41. T F Hyperventilation in labor can result in respiratory acidosis as the amount of carbon dioxide increases in the bloodstream.

42. T F Sedatives given without an analgesic when a laboring woman is experiencing pain can increase apprehension and lead to hyperactivity and confusion.

43. T F Intramuscular administration of opioid agonist analgesics during labor offers predictable and rapid onset of pain relief.

44. T F Naloxone (Narcan) should be used cautiously if a woman has a substance dependency because maternal opioid withdrawal can occur.

45. T F Before initiating epidural anesthesia/analgesia a woman should be adequately hydrated using an IV of 5% glucose in water.

46. T F Epidural anesthesia is useful as a pain relief measure for both labor and birth.

47. T F Keeping the woman in a flat position for at least 8 hours after birth is the most effective way to prevent headaches following a spinal block.

48. T F   The woman can be assisted into a sitting position for the induction of both spinal anesthesia and lumbar epidural blocks.

49. T F   Maternal hypotension is a major adverse reaction to both spinal and epidural blocks.

50. T F   When using nitrous oxide for pain relief during labor, a woman's oral intake is limited to ice chips to reduce the risk for aspiration.

MULTIPLE CHOICE QUESTIONS: Circle the one correct option and state the rationale for the option chosen.

51. In her birth plan, a woman requests that she be allowed to use the new whirlpool bath during labor. When implementing this woman's request the nurse would
    a. assist the woman to maintain a reclining position when in the tub.
    b. tell the woman she will need to leave the tub as soon as her membranes rupture.
    c. limit her to no longer than 1 hour in the tub.
    d. cool the water or have the woman step out of the tub if the fetal heart rate (FHR) or maternal temperature increases.

52. The use of ataractics can potentiate the action of analgesics. When preparing to administer an ataractic to a laboring woman, the nurse could expect to give
    a. naloxone (Narcan).
    b. hydroxyzine (Vistaril).
    c. butorphanol tartrate (Stadol).
    d. fentanyl (Sublimaze).

53. The doctor has ordered meperidine (Demerol) 25 mg IV q2-3hr prn for pain associated with labor. In fulfilling this order, the nurse should know which of the following:
    a. The onset of this analgesic's effect after IV administration would be approximately 10 minutes.
    b. The dosage of the analgesic is too high for IV administration, necessitating a new order.
    c. Respiratory depression of the woman or fetus is not a concern with this analgesic.
    d. The newborn should be observed for respiratory depression if birth occurs within 4 hours of the dose.

54. Following administration of fentanyl (Sublimaze) IV for labor pain, a woman's labor progresses more rapidly than expected. The physician orders that a stat dose of naloxone (Narcan) 1 mg be administered intravenously to the woman to reverse respiratory depression in the newborn after its birth. In fulfilling this order the nurse would
    a. question the route because this medication should be administered orally.
    b. recognize that the dose is too low.
    c. assess the woman's level of pain because it will return abruptly.
    d. observe maternal vital signs for bradycardia and hypertension because these are common side effects of this medication.

55. An anesthesiologist is preparing to begin a continuous epidural block using a combination local anesthetic and opioid analgesic as a pain relief measure for a laboring woman. Nursing measures related to this type of nerve block would be
    a. assist the woman into a modified Sims position or upright position with back curved.
    b. keep the woman in a semirecumbent position after administration to ensure equal distribution of the pharmacologic agents.
    c. assess the woman for headaches, especially after birth.
    d. assist the woman to the bathroom to urinate at least every 2 hours during labor to prevent bladder distention.

II. THINKING CRITICALLY

1. A nurse working with a group of expectant fathers is asked if there really is "a physical reason for all the pain women say they feel when they are in labor." Describe the response that this nurse should give.

2. On admission to the labor unit in the latent phase of labor, Mr. and Mrs. T. (2-0-0-1-0) tell you that they are so glad they took Lamaze classes and did so much reading about childbirth. "We will not need any medication now that we know what to do. But most importantly our baby will be safe." Describe how you would respond if you were their primary nurse for childbirth.

3. Imagine you are the nurse manager of a labor and birth unit. Major renovations are being planned for your unit and your input is required. You and your staff nurses believe that water therapy, including the use of showers and whirlpool baths, is a beneficial nonpharmacologic method to relieve pain and discomfort and to enhance the progress of labor. Discuss the rationale you would use to convince planners that installation of a shower and a whirlpool bath into each birthing room is cost effective.

4. Tara has been in labor for 4 hours. Her blood pressure had been stable, averaging 130/80 when assessed between contractions and the FHR pattern consistently exhibited criteria of a reassuring pattern. A lumbar epidural block was initiated. Shortly afterward during assessment of maternal vital signs and FHR, Tara's blood pressure decreased to 102/60 and the FHR pattern began to exhibit a decrease in rate and variability.

   a. State what Tara is experiencing. Support your answer and explain the physiologic basis for what is happening to Tara.

   b. Write a nursing diagnosis that reflects this occurrence.

   c. List the immediate nursing actions.

5. Moira, a primigravida, has elected a continuous epidural block as her pharmacologic method of choice during childbirth.

    a. Identify the assessment procedures that should be used to determine Moira's readiness for the initiation of the epidural block.

    b. Describe the preparation methods that should be implemented.

    c. Describe two positions you could help Moira assume for the induction of the epidural block.

    d. Outline the nursing care management interventions recommended while Moira is receiving the anesthesia to ensure her well-being and that of her fetus.

17 Fetal Assessment during Labor

I. REVIEWING KEY CONCEPTS AND CONTENT

FILL IN THE BLANKS: Insert the term that corresponds to each of the following descriptions related to fetal assessment.

1. The goals of intrapartum fetal heart rate (FHR) monitoring are to identify and differentiate the _____ patterns from the _____ patterns, which are indicative of fetal _____. _____ is characterized by a deficiency of oxygen in the arterial blood, whereas _____ is an inadequate supply of oxygen at the cellular level.

2. One method to assess fetal status is intermittent _____ using a _____ or _____ to listen to the FHR.

3. _____ is the method used to continuously assess the FHR pattern. Two modes can be used to accomplish this method of assessment. External monitoring uses an _____ to assess the FHR pattern and a _____ to monitor the frequency and duration of contractions. Internal monitoring uses a _____ attached to the fetal presenting part to assess the FHR pattern and an _____ to monitor the frequency, duration, and intensity of contractions.

4. _____ is an abnormally small amount of amniotic fluid or the absence of amniotic fluid. It can lead to compression of the umbilical cord, resulting in a _____ FHR pattern. _____ can be used to instill _____ or _____ solution into the uterine cavity via the intrauterine catheter for the purpose of adding fluid around the umbilical cord and thus preventing its compression during uterine contractions.

5. _____ therapy can be used when fetal compromise is associated with increased uterine activity. _____ improves _____ through the _____ by inhibiting _____.

6. It is critical that a nurse working on a labor unit be knowledgeable concerning factors associated with a reduction in fetal oxygen supply, characteristics of a reassuring FHR pattern, and characteristics of normal uterine activity. List the required information for each of the following:

   a. Factors associated with a reduction in fetal oxygen supply

   b. Characteristics of a reassuring FHR pattern

   c. Characteristics of normal uterine activity

7. Identify the characteristics of nonreassuring FHR patterns.

MATCHING: Match the definition in Column I with the appropriate term related to FHR pattern from Column II.

COLUMN I

8. _____ Average FHR during a 10-minute segment that excludes periodic or episodic changes, periods of marked variability, and segments of the baseline that differ more than 25 beats/min. It is assessed during the absence of uterine activity or between contractions.

9. _____ Absence of the expected irregular fluctuations in the baseline FHR.

10. _____ Persistent (10 minutes or longer) baseline FHR below 110 beats/min.

11. _____ Visually apparent decrease in the FHR of 15 beats/min or more below the baseline, which lasts more than 2 minutes but less than 10 minutes.

12. _____ Changes from baseline patterns in FHR that occur with uterine contractions.

13. _____ Persistent (10 minutes or longer) baseline FHR above 160 beats/min.

14. _____ Expected irregular fluctuations in the baseline FHR of two or more cycles per minute as a result of the interaction of the sympathetic and parasympathetic nervous systems.

15. _____ Visually apparent decrease in and return to baseline FHR in response to fetal head compression.

16. _____ Visually apparent gradual decrease in and return to baseline FHR in response to uteroplacental insufficiency; lowest point occurs after the peak of the contraction.

17. _____ Visually abrupt decrease in FHR below baseline, which can occur at any time during a contraction as a result of cord compression.

18. _____ Visually apparent abrupt increase in the FHR of 15 beats/min or more above the baseline, which lasts 15 seconds or more with return to baseline less than 2 minutes from the onset.

19. _____ Changes from baseline patterns in FHR that are not associated with uterine contraction.

COLUMN II

a. Acceleration

b. Early deceleration

c. Variability

d. Late deceleration

e. Variable deceleration

f. Tachycardia

g. Prolonged deceleration

h. Bradycardia

i. Baseline FHR

j. Undetected variability

k. Periodic changes

l. Episodic changes

FILL IN THE BLANKS: In general, the recommended frequency of FHR assessment depends on the risk status of the mother and the stage of labor. Insert the appropriate time for each of the following assessment recommendations:

20. Obtain a _____ minute strip by electronic fetal monitoring (EFM) on all women admitted to the labor unit.

21. Low risk patient (risk factors are absent during labor): auscultate FHR/assess tracing every _____ in the active phase of the first stage of labor and every _____ in the second stage of labor.

22. High risk patient (risk factors are present during labor): auscultate FHR/assess tracing every _____ in the active phase of the first stage of labor and every _____ in the second stage of labor.

23. Nurses caring for laboring women may need to use intermittent auscultation to assess fetal health and well-being during labor.

    a. State the advantages and disadvantages of intermittent auscultation as a method of fetal assessment during childbirth.

    b. Outline the guidelines that should be followed when monitoring the fetus using the intermittent auscultation method.

24. State the legal responsibilities related to fetal monitoring for nurses who care for women during childbirth.

TRUE OR FALSE: Circle T if true or F if false for each of the following statements. Correct the false statements.

25. T F A nonreassuring FHR pattern indicates that the fetus is compromised and is experiencing some degree of hypoxemia, hypoxia, or both.

26. T F Auscultation should be performed during a uterine contraction and for 10 seconds after the end of the contraction to detect periodic changes in pattern.

27. T F FHR variability can temporarily decrease when the fetus is in a sleep state.

28. T F When external monitoring is used, the tocotransducer should be repositioned every 4 hours and reddened skin areas gently massaged.

29. T F Maternal supine hypotensive syndrome reduces blood flow to the placenta, resulting in fetal hypoxia as reflected in fetal bradycardia, decreased variability, and late decelerations.

30. T F Acceleration of the FHR associated with fetal movement is a reassuring sign.

31. T F Decelerations of the FHR may be benign or nonreassuring in terms of fetal well-being.

32. T F Late deceleration patterns are characterized by a U or V shape with acceleration shoulders before and after the deceleration.

33. T F Early decelerations are nonreassuring patterns that typically occur when blood flow through the placenta is diminished.

34. T F The average intrauterine (intraamniotic) pressure range during a uterine contraction is 50 to 85 mm Hg.

35. T F The tocotransducer should be placed on the abdomen over the fundus.

36. T F The intrauterine pressure catheter (IUPC) is able to assess uterine contraction frequency, duration, and intensity.

37. T F Ritgen's maneuver is used to determine the correct placement of the ultrasound transducer.

38. T F Late deceleration patterns of any magnitude are considered to be nonreassuring FHR patterns.

39. A nurse caring for a woman in active labor notes a nonreassuring FHR pattern when evaluating the monitor tracing. Describe the action the nurse should take based on this finding.

40. Outline the nursing interventions that should be implemented when caring for a woman who is being monitored using an external monitor.

MULTIPLE CHOICE QUESTIONS: Circle the one correct option and state the rationale for the option chosen.

41. A laboring woman's uterine contractions are being internally monitored. When evaluating the monitor tracing, which of the following findings would be a source of concern and require further assessment?
    a. Frequency every 2 ½ to 3 minutes
    b. Duration of 80 to 85 seconds
    c. Intensity during a uterine contraction of 55 to 80 mm Hg
    d. Average resting pressure of 25 to 30 mm Hg

42. External electronic fetal monitoring will be used for a woman just admitted to the labor unit in active labor. A guideline the nurse should follow when implementing this form of monitoring would be to
    a. use Leopold's maneuvers to determine correct placement of the tocotransducer.
    b. apply contact gel to the ultrasound transducer before application over the point of maximum intensity.
    c. reposition the ultrasound transducer every hour and massage the site.
    d. apply a spiral electrode if nonreassuring FHR signs are noted.

43. The nurse caring for women in labor should be aware of signs characterizing reassuring FHR patterns. Which of the following would be a reassuring sign?
    a. Moderate baseline variability
    b. Average baseline FHR of 90 to 110 beats/min
    c. Transient episodic deceleration with movement
    d. Late deceleration patterns approximately every 3 or 4 contractions

44. A laboring woman's temperature is elevated as a result of an upper respiratory infection. The FHR pattern that reflects maternal fever would be
    a. diminished variability.
    b. variable decelerations.
    c. tachycardia.
    d. early decelerations.

45. A nulliparous woman is in the active phase of labor and her cervix has progressed to 6 cm dilation. The nurse caring for this woman evaluates the external monitor tracing and notes the following: decrease in FHR shortly after onset of several uterine contractions returning to baseline rate by the end of the contraction; shape is uniform. Based on these findings the nurse should
    a. change the woman's position to her left side.
    b. document the finding on the woman's chart.
    c. notify the physician.
    d. perform a vaginal examination to check for cord prolapse.

II. THINKING CRITICALLY

1. Darlene, a primigravida in active labor, has just been admitted to the labor unit. She becomes very anxious when external electronic monitoring equipment is set up. She tells the nurse that her father had a heart attack 2 months ago. "He was so sick they had to put him on a monitor too. Does this mean that my baby has a heart problem just like my father?" Describe the nurse's expected response.

2. Terry is a primigravida at 43 weeks of gestation. Her labor is being stimulated with oxytocin administered IV. Her contractions have been increasing in intensity with a frequency of every 2 to 2 ½ minutes and a duration of 80 to 85 seconds. She is currently in a supine position with a 30-degree elevation of her head. On observation of the monitor tracing, you note that during the last 2 contractions the FHR decreased after the contraction peaked and did not return to baseline until about 10 seconds into the rest period. A slight decrease in variability and baseline rate was observed.

    a. Identify the pattern described and the possible factors responsible for it.

    b. Describe the actions you would take. State the rationale for each action.

3. Analyze each of the following monitor tracings and document your findings. Describe each FHR pattern depicted and the criteria used to determine if the pattern is reassuring or nonreassuring. Indicate the possible causes, significance, and nursing actions required for each nonreassuring FHR pattern identified.

a.

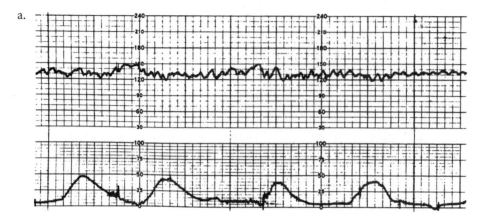

b.

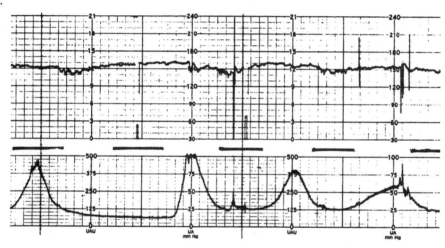

c.

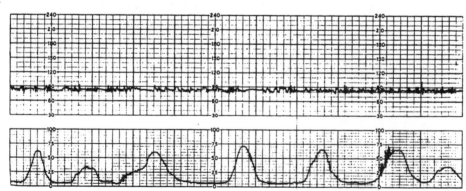

d.

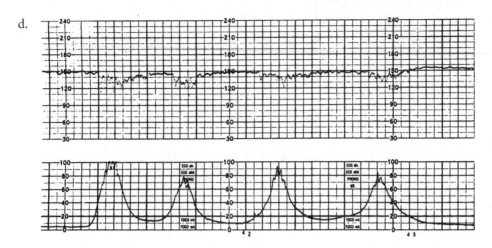

e.

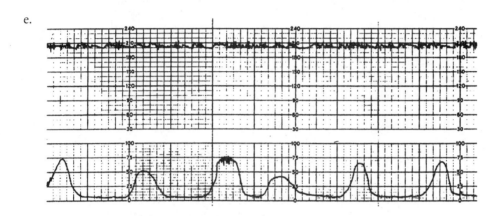

f.

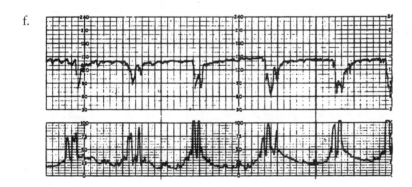

18 Nursing Care during Labor and Birth

I. REVIEWING KEY CONCEPTS AND CONTENT

Evaluate each of the following assessment findings that are used to distinguish true labor from false labor. Designate whether the assessment finding is associated with true labor (TL) or with false labor (FL).

1. _____ Contractions regular and progressive.

2. _____ Cervix soft and posterior.

3. _____ Contractions cease with ambulation.

4. _____ Cervix soft, 25%, 2 cm, midposition.

5. _____ Lightening occurs in multiparous woman.

6. _____ Discomfort present in abdomen above umbilicus.

7. _____ Contraction intensity increases with activity and ambulation.

8. _____ Presenting part is above ischial spines.

9. _____ Bloody show.

10. _____ Discomfort radiates from lower back to lower abdomen.

11. _____ Contractions continue even after a shower or back rub.

FILL IN THE BLANKS: Insert the term that corresponds to each of the following descriptions associated with stages of labor.

12. The first stage of labor begins with the onset of _____ and ends with complete _____, and full _____ of the cervix. A blood-tinged mucous discharge (bloody show) from the vagina usually indicates the passage of the _____.

13. During the latent phase of the first stage of labor the cervix dilates from _____ to _____ cm in approximately _____ to _____ hours. Cervical dilation progresses from _____ to _____ cm in about _____ to _____ hours during the active phase of the first stage of labor. The duration of the transition phase is approximately _____ to _____ minutes and the cervix dilates from _____ to _____ cm.

14. The second stage of labor is the stage in which the _____. It begins with full _____ and complete _____. It ends with the _____. Additional signs that the second stage of labor is beginning include _____, _____, _____, _____, _____, and _____. This stage is composed of three phases, namely _____, _____, and _____. A second stage that is longer than _____ may be considered prolonged in a woman without regional anesthesia and should be reported to the primary health care provider.

15. The third stage of labor lasts from the _____ until the _____. Detachment of the placenta from the wall of the uterus or _____ is indicated by a _____, change from a _____ shape to a _____ shape, a sudden _____ from the introitus, apparent _____, and the finding of _____ or of _____ at the introitus.

MATCHING: Match the description in Column I with the appropriate term from Column II.

COLUMN I	COLUMN II

COLUMN I

16. _____ Prolonged breath holding while bearing down (closed glottis pushing).

17 _____ Burning sensation of acute pain as vagina stretches and crowning occurs.

18. _____ Artificial rupture of membranes (AROM, ARM).

19. _____ Occurs when widest part of the head (biparietal diameter) distends the vulva just before birth.

20. _____ Incision into perineum to enlarge the vaginal outlet.

21. _____ Test to determine if membranes have ruptured by assessing pH of the fluid.

22. _____ Technique used to control birth of fetal head and protect perineal musculature.

23. _____ Expulsion of placenta with fetal side emerging first.

24. _____ Cord encircles the fetal neck.

25. _____ Method used to palpate fetus through abdomen.

26. _____ Occurs when pressure of presenting part against pelvic floor stretch receptors results in a woman's perception of an urge to bear down.

27. _____ Classification of medication that stimulates the uterus to contract.

28. _____ Expulsion of placenta with maternal surface emerging first.

29. _____ Protrusion of umbilical cord in advance of the presenting part.

COLUMN II

a. Ritgen maneuver

b. Episiotomy

c. Oxytocic

d. Ferguson reflex

e. Shultz mechanism

f. Valsalva maneuver

g. Ring of fire

h. Crowning

i. Duncan mechanism

j. Amniotomy

k. Nuchal cord

l. Prolapse of umbilical cord

m. Nitrazine test

n. Leopold's maneuvers

FILL IN THE BLANKS: Insert the term that corresponds to each of the following descriptions related to the characteristics of the powers of labor.

30. _____ The primary powers of labor that act involuntarily to expel the fetus and the placenta from the uterus.

31. _____ "Building up" of a contraction from its onset.

32. _____ The peak of a contraction.

33. _____ "Letting down" of a contraction.

34. _____ How often uterine contractions occur; the time that elapses from the beginning of one contraction to the beginning of the next or from the peak of one contraction to the peak of the next (if using electronic monitoring).

35. _____ The strength of a contraction at its peak.

36. _____ The time that elapses between the onset and the end of a contraction.

37. _____ The tension of the uterine muscle between contractions.

38. _____ Period of rest between contractions.

39. _____ An involuntary urge to push in response to the Ferguson reflex.

40. Assessment of the characteristics and patterns of uterine contractions is an important nursing responsibility.

   a. Label the following illustration that depicts the characteristics of uterine contractions.

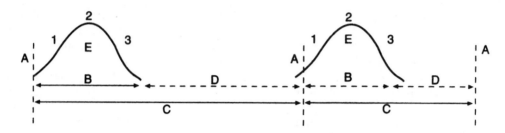

   b. Describe how you would assess each of these characteristics using the palpation method.

41. Laura (3-1-1-0-1) has just been admitted in the latent phase of the first stage of labor. As part of the admission procedure, you review her prenatal record and interview her regarding what she has observed regarding her labor and discuss her current health status.

   a. List the essential data you would need to obtain from her prenatal record to plan appropriate care for Laura.

   b. Identify the information required regarding the status of Laura's labor.

   c. State the information required regarding Laura's current health status.

TRUE OR FALSE: Circle T if true or F if false for each of the following statements. Correct the false statements.

42. T F   Amniotic fluid will turn Nitrazine test paper greenish yellow.

43. T F   A partogram is used to diagram the progress of uterine contractions.

44. T F   A laboring woman should be encouraged to void at least every 2 hours during labor.

45. T F   Ambulation should be encouraged only during the latent phase of the first stage of labor.

46. T F   A hands-and-knees position is recommended during contractions to facilitate the internal rotation of an occiput posterior position to a more anterior position.

47. T F   The nurse should perform a vaginal examination immediately, using strict sterile technique, if bright red, fresh vaginal bleeding is noted during active labor.

48. T F   Amniotic fluid is alkaline as compared to urine, which is usually acidic.

49. T F   Leopold's maneuvers can assist in the location of the point of maximum intensity (PMI) of the fetal heartbeat.

50. T F   Maternal body temperature should be monitored every 1 to 2 hours after the amniotic membranes rupture.

51. T F   Increased sensitivity to touch or hyperesthesia, which develops as labor progress, can result in a woman's rejection of her partner's or the nurse's touch with comfort measures.

52. T F   A woman should begin pushing as soon as the second stage of labor begins.

53. T F   In order for childbirth to progress safely and in a timely fashion, a woman's bearing-down efforts must be carefully regulated by the nurse and coach.

54. T F   For pushing to be effective, the woman should maintain a push and hold her breath for at least 10 seconds.

55. T F   The only certain objective sign of the onset of the second stage of labor is the woman's perception of an urge to bear down.

56. T F   During the descent phase of the second stage of labor, pressure of the presenting part on the pelvic floor stimulates release of oxytocin from the pituitary gland thus intensifying uterine contractions.

57. T F   During birth of the head, the woman must continue to fully bear down with uterine contractions to ensure prompt expulsion.

58. T F   If stirrups are used during birth, it is important to place the legs into the stirrups one leg at a time.

59. T F   The time of birth is recorded as the precise time when the newborn takes its first breath.

60. T F   The priority goal for a newborn in the immediate postbirth period is that the newborn's airway remains patent.

61. Complete the following table by identifying the stressors that a woman and her partner/coach experience during childbirth and the nursing measures that can be supportive and reduce stress.

Woman and Partner/Coach	Stressors	Support Measures
Laboring Woman		
Partner/Coach		

62. A nurse caring for a laboring woman needs to be alert for signs of potential complications. List these signs.

63. Complete the following table by identifying two advantages for each of the following labor positions.

Labor Position	Advantages
Semirecumbent	
Upright	
Lateral	
Hands and Knees	

64. Outline the critical factors to be included in the physical assessment of the maternal-fetal unit during labor.

65. Indicate the laboratory and diagnostic tests that are recommended during labor. State the purpose for each.

66. Complete the following table by identifying two support measures you would use during each phase of the second stage of labor. Validate your response with events and behaviors typical of that phase.

Phase	Events/Behaviors	Support Measures
Latent		
Descent		
Transition		

67. Identify the factors that can influence the duration of the second stage of labor.

68. Describe the maternal positions recommended to enhance the effectiveness of a woman's bearing-down efforts during the second stage of labor. State the basis for each position's effectiveness in facilitating the descent and birth of the fetus.

MULTIPLE CHOICE QUESTIONS: Circle the one correct option and state the rationale for the option chosen.

69. A primigravida calls the hospital and tells a nurse on the labor unit that she knows that she is in labor. The nurse's initial response would be
   a. "Tell me why you know that you are in labor."
   b. "How far do you live from the hospital?"
   c. "How far along are you in your pregnancy?"
   d. "Have your membranes ruptured?"

70. A woman's amniotic membranes have apparently ruptured. The nurse assesses the fluid to determine its characteristics and confirm membrane rupture. Which of the following would be an expected assessment finding?
   a. pH 5.5
   b. Absence of ferning
   c. Pale straw-colored fluid with white flecks
   d. Strong odor

71. A vaginal examination is performed on a multiparous woman who is in labor. The results of the examination were documented as 4 cm, 75%, +2, LOT. Which of the following would be an accurate interpretation of this data?
   a. Woman is in the latent phase of the first stage of labor
   b. Station is 2 cm above the ischial spines
   c. Presentation is vertex
   d. Lie is transverse

72. A nulliparous woman is in active labor. She is considered to be at low risk for complications. Which of the following is a standard recommendation for assessment during this phase of labor?
   a. Maternal blood pressure, pulse, respirations—every hour
   b. FHR—every 15 to 30 minutes
   c. Temperature—twice per shift once membranes rupture
   d. Vaginal examination to determine progress of dilation and effacement—every hour

73. A physical care measure for a laboring woman that has been identified as unlikely to be beneficial and may even be harmful would be
   a. allowing the laboring woman to drink fluids and eat light solids as tolerated.
   b. administering a Fleet enema at admission.
   c. ambulating periodically throughout labor as tolerated.
   d. using a whirlpool bath once active labor is established.

II. THINKING CRITICALLY

1. Alice, a primigravida, calls the labor unit. She tells the nurse that she thinks she is in labor. "I have had some pains for about 2 hours. Should my husband bring me to the hospital now?"

   a. Describe how the nurse should approach this situation.

   b. Write several questions the nurse could use to elicit the appropriate information required to determine the course of action required.

c. Based on the data collected during the telephone interview, the nurse determines that Alice is in very early labor. Since she lives fairly close to the hospital, she is instructed to stay home until her labor progresses. Outline the instructions and recommendations for care Alice and her husband should be given.

2. Analyze the assessment findings documented for each of the following women.

Denise	Teresa	Danielle
5 cm	9 cm	2 cm
moderate	very strong	mild
q4min	q2-3min	q6-8min
40-55 sec	65-75 sec	30-35 sec
0	+2	−1

a. Identify the phase of labor being experienced by each woman.

b. Describe the behavior and appearance you would expect to be exhibited by each woman.

c. Specify the physical care and emotional support measures you would implement if you were caring for each of these women.

3. Describe the procedure that should be followed before auscultating the FHR or applying an ultrasound transducer to the abdomen of a laboring woman. Explain the rationale for utilizing this procedure.

4. Tonya, a woman in active labor, begins to cry during a vaginal examination to assess her status. "Why not watch the monitor to see how I am progressing instead of doing these vaginal exams? They really hurt and they are embarrassing!"

a. Describe the response the nurse should make to Tonya's concern.

b. Discuss the measures the nurse could use to meet Tonya's safety and comfort needs during a vaginal examination.

5. Tasha is dilated 6 cm. Her coach comes to tell you that her "water just broke with a gush!" Identify each action you would take in this situation, in order of priority. State the rationale for the actions you have identified.

6. Sara, a 17-year-old primigravida, is admitted in the latent phase of labor. Her boyfriend, Dan, is with her as her only support. They appear committed to each other. During the admission interview, Sara tells you that they did not go to any classes because she was embarrassed about not being married. Both Sara and Dan appear very nervous and assessment indicates they know little about what is happening, what to expect, and how to work together with the process of labor. Identify the nursing diagnosis reflected in this data. State one expected outcome and list nursing measures appropriate for the diagnosis you identified.

Nursing Diagnosis	Expected Outcome	Nursing Measures

7. Identifying a laboring couple's cultural and religious beliefs and practices regarding childbirth is a critical factor in providing culturally sensitive care that enhances the couple's sense of control and eventual satisfaction with their childbirth experience.

   a. List the questions you would ask when assessing a couple's cultural and religious preferences for childbirth.

   b. Discuss the problems that can occur if the nurse does not consider the couple's cultural and religious preferences when planning and implementing care.

8. Cori (4-3-0-0-3) is in latent labor. She and her husband are being oriented to the birthing room. Their last birth occurred in a delivery room 10 years ago. Both she and her husband are amazed by the birthing room and the birthing bed that will allow her to give birth in an upright position. They are also informed that changes in bearing-down efforts now allow a woman to follow her own body feelings and even to vocalize with pushing. Both Cori and her husband state that with every other birth they put her legs in stirrups, she held her breath for as long as she could, and pushed quietly. "Everything turned out okay, so why should we change?" Describe the response the primary nurse caring for this couple should make to their concerns.

9. A nurse living in a rural area is called to her neighbor's home to assist his wife who is in labor. "Everything is happening so fast. She says she is ready to deliver!"

   a. Identify the measures the nurse can use to reassure and comfort the woman.

   b. Shortly after the nurse arrives, crowning begins. State what the nurse should do.

   c. Describe the action the nurse should take after the birth of the head.

   d. List the measures the nurse should use to prevent excessive neonatal heat loss after its birth.

   e. Identify the infection control measures that should be implemented during a home birth.

   f. Specify the measures the nurse should use to prevent excessive maternal blood loss or hemorrhage until the ambulance arrives.

   g. Outline the information the nurse should document regarding the childbirth.

10. Beth is in the descent phase of the second stage of labor. She is actively pushing/bearing down to facilitate birth. Indicate the criteria a nurse would use to evaluate the correctness of Beth's technique.

11. Molly is entering the second stage of labor. She states that she is experiencing some perineal pressure but refuses to start pushing because as she states, "I am just not ready to push yet."

   a. Discuss the factors that might be inhibiting Molly's desire to bear down and give birth to her baby.

   b. Describe what the nurse could do to help Molly reach the point of readiness to give birth.

12. Imagine that you are participating in a panel discussion on childbirth practices. Your topic is "Episiotomy—is it needed to ensure the safety and well-being of the laboring woman and her fetus?" Outline the information you would include in your presentation.

13. Imagine that you are a staff nurse on a childbirth unit. Your hospital is instituting a change in policy that would allow the participation of children in the labor and birth process of their mother. You are asked to be a part of the committee that will formulate the guidelines regarding sibling participation during childbirth. Discuss the suggestions you would make to help ensure a positive outcome for parents, children, and health care providers.

14. Annie is a primipara in the fourth stage of labor following a long and difficult labor and birth process. She seems disinterested in her baby. Annie looks him over quickly and then asks if you would take him back to the nursery.

    a. Identify the factors that could be accounting for Annie's behavior.

    b. Discuss the nursing measures you would use to encourage future maternal-newborn interactions and facilitate the attachment process.

19 Labor and Birth at Risk

I. REVIEWING KEY CONCEPTS AND CONTENT

FILL IN THE BLANKS: Insert the term that corresponds to each of the following descriptions.

1. _____ is any birth that occurs before the completion of 37 weeks of pregnancy.

2. _____ is defined as cervical changes and uterine contractions occurring between 20 weeks and 37 weeks of pregnancy.

3. Preterm birth describes _____, whereas low birth weight describes only _____.

4. Low birth weight can be caused by _____ or _____, a condition of fetal growth associated with pregnant women who are poorly _____ or who have various complications of pregnancy that interfere with _____ perfusion such as gestational _____.

5. _____ can be used to predict who might experience preterm labor. The two most commonly used are _____ and _____

6. _____ are glycoproteins found in plasma and produced during fetal life. Their reappearance in the _____ between _____ and _____ weeks of gestation could predict preterm labor. The negative predictive value is _____, whereas the positive predictive value is _____. The test is done during a _____ examination.

7. _____ is a form of estrogen produced by the fetus that is present in plasma at 9 weeks of gestation. Levels have been shown to _____ before preterm birth. The negative predictive value is _____, whereas the positive predictive value is _____.

8. A shortened _____ is another possible predictor of imminent preterm labor. Its measurement is determined by _____. A woman whose_____ measurement is _____ mm at _____ weeks is more likely to have a preterm birth than a woman whose measurement exceeds _____ mm.

9. _____ is the rupture of the amniotic sac and leakage of amniotic fluid beginning at least 1 hour before the onset of labor at any gestational age.

10. _____ is the rupture of the amniotic sac and leakage of fluid before 37 weeks of gestation. _____ often precedes this rupture but the etiology is unknown. _____ is an intraamniotic infection of the chorion and amnion that is potentially life-threatening for the fetus and the woman. Cord _____ and _____ leading to cord compression are serious complications of rupture of the amniotic sac.

11. _____ is defined as a long, difficult, or abnormal labor and is caused by various conditions associated with the _____.

12. _____ labor is described as abnormal uterine contractions that prevent the normal progress of cervical _____ and _____ (_____ powers), or _____ (_____ powers).

13. _____, or primary dysfunctional labor, often is experienced by an anxious first-time mother who is having _____ and _____ contractions that are ineffective in causing _____ or _____ to progress. These contractions usually occur in the _____ phase of the first stage of labor. _____ is usually prescribed for the management of this type of dysfunctional labor.

14. _____ or secondary uterine inertia usually occurs when a woman initially makes normal progress into the active phase of labor, then uterine contractions become _____ and _____ or _____.

15. _____ can occur whenever contractions of the pelvic diameters reduce the capacity of the bony pelvis, including the inlet, midpelvis, outlet, or any combination of these planes.

16. _____ results from obstruction of the birth passage by an anatomic abnormality other than that involving the bony pelvis. The obstruction may result from _____, _____, _____, and a full _____ or _____.

17. _____ may be caused by anomalies, excessive fetal size and malpresentation, malposition, or multifetal pregnancy. _____, also called _____, is related to excessive fetal size. The most common fetal malposition is persistent _____ position. _____ presentation is the most common form of malpresentation.

18. _____ is the gestation of twins, triplets, quadruplets, or more infants.

19. Six abnormal labor patterns have been identified and classified by Friedman (1989) according to the nature of cervical _____ and fetal _____. These patterns are _____, _____, _____, _____, _____, and _____. _____ is defined as a labor that lasts less than 3 hours from the onset of contractions to the time of birth. It may result from _____ that are _____ in intensity.

20. _____ is an attempt to turn the fetus from a breech or shoulder presentation to a vertex presentation for birth by exerting gentle, constant pressure on the abdomen.

21. A _____ is the observance of a woman and her fetus for a reasonable period of spontaneous active labor to assess the safety of a vaginal birth for the mother and infant.

22. _____ is the chemical or mechanical initiation of uterine contractions before their spontaneous onset for the purpose of bringing about the birth.

23. _____ is a rating system used to evaluate the inducibility of the cervix. The five characteristics assessed are _____, _____, _____, _____, and _____. If the score is low _____ can be applied to the cervix to soften and thin or _____ the cervix.

24. _____ is the artificial rupture of the membranes. It can be used to _____ labor when the cervix is ripe or to _____ labor if the progress begins to slow.

25. _____ is the stimulation of uterine contractions after labor has started spontaneously but progress is unsatisfactory. Common methods include _____ infusion, _____, and _____ stimulation.

26. A _____ birth is one in which an instrument with two curved blades is used to assist the birth of the fetal head.

27. _____ birth or _____ is a birth method involving the attachment of a vacuum cup to the fetal head, using negative pressure.

28. _____ is the birth of the fetus through a transabdominal incision of the uterus.

29. A _____ or _____ pregnancy is one that extends beyond the end of week 42 of gestation.

30. _____ is an uncommon obstetric emergency in which the head of the fetus is born but the anterior shoulder cannot pass under the pubic arch. Two major causes are _____ or maternal _____.

31. _____ occurs when the cord lies below the presenting part of the fetus. Contributing factors to its occurrence include a _____, _____, _____, or _____. When present, the woman is assisted into a position such as _____, _____, or _____. In these positions gravity keeps pressure of the _____ off of the cord.

32. An _____ occurs when amniotic fluid containing particles of debris enters the maternal circulation and obstructs pulmonary blood vessels, causing respiratory distress and circulatory collapse. Maternal death occurs most often when amniotic fluid contains thick _____ because it can clog the pulmonary veins more completely than other debris.

TRUE AND FALSE: Circle T if true or F if false for each of the following statements. Correct the false statements.

33. T   F   Preterm labor and birth are the most serious complications of pregnancy because they lead to approximately 90% of all neonatal deaths.

34. T   F   Preterm birth rates continue to rise.

35. T   F   Preterm birth is more dangerous than low birth weight because the shortened gestational time results in immature body systems.

36. T   F   The rate of preterm births among Caucasian women is nearly double the rate of African-American women in the United States.

37. T   F   Risk-scoring systems are excellent predictors of women who will go into labor prematurely.

38. T   T   Fetal fibronectin is more likely to predict women who will not go into preterm labor than women who will go into preterm labor.

39. T   F   Salivary estriol has a high positive predictive value for preterm labor.

40. T   F   Shortened endocervical length combined with a positive fetal fibronectin result increases the risk for spontaneous birth substantially.

41. T   F   Early recognition of preterm labor is essential if measures to suppress labor and enhance fetal lung maturation are to be successful.

42. T   F   Research evidence confirms that bed rest is highly effective in preventing preterm birth.

43. T   F   It is now thought that the best reason to use tocolytics is to gain the time needed to administer antenatal glucocorticoids.

44. T   F   Dysfunctional labor can occur as a result of maternal factors such as fatigue, fear, dehydration, and electrolyte imbalance.

45. T   F   The most common type of uterine dysfunction is hypotonic uterine dysfunction.

46. T   F   A breech presentation is most common in term pregnancies.

47. T   F   Women age 35 years and older are more likely to have a multifetal pregnancy with or without fertility enhancing drugs.

48. T   F   The incidence of prolonged labor patterns is slightly higher among women in their thirties.

49. T   F   A diagnosis of secondary arrest of active labor is made when there has been no change in cervical dilation for 2 hours or more for both nulliparous and multiparous women.

50. T   F   Ripening of the cervix with a prostaglandin preparation usually results in a higher success rate for induction of labor.

51. T   F   Prepidil gel is inserted into the posterior fornix of the vagina.

52. T   F   Oxytocin is discontinued immediately and the primary health care provider notified if uterine hyperstimulation or a nonreassuring fetal heart rate (FHR) occurs during labor stimulation.

53. T   F   Research has consistently proven that the one-on-one support provided by a doula reduces the risk for cesarean birth for laboring women who receive this support.

54. T   F   The incidence of postterm pregnancy in the United States is approximately 25%.

55. T   F   Assisting the laboring woman into a hands-and-knees position can help resolve shoulder dystocia.

56. T   F   The maternal mortality rate for amniotic fluid embolism (AFE) is as high as 50%.

57. Identify two factors for each of the following risk categories for preterm labor and birth.

Demographic factors

Biophysical risks

Behavioral and psychosocial risks

58. Explain why bed rest may be more harmful than helpful as a component of preterm birth care management.

MATCHING: Match the description of medications used as part of the management of preterm labor in Column I with the appropriate medication listed in Column II.

COLUMN I

COLUMN II

59. _____ Beta$_2$-adrenergic receptor agonist, often administered intravenously, is the only drug approved by the FDA for the purpose of suppressing uterine contractions.

60. _____ An antenatal glucocorticoid used to accelerate fetal lung maturity when there is risk for preterm birth.

61. _____ Beta$_2$-adrenergic receptor agonist often administered subcutaneously using a syringe or pump.

62. _____ A calcium channel blocker that relaxes smooth muscles including those of the contracting uterus; maternal hypotension is a major concern.

63. _____ Classification of drugs used to suppress uterine activity.

64. _____ A central nervous system (CNS) depressant used during preterm labor for its ability to relax smooth muscles; administered intravenously.

65. _____ A nonsteroidal antiinflammatory medication that relaxes smooth muscles as a result of prostaglandin inhibition; may be administered rectally or orally.

a. Tocolytic

b. Betamethasone

c. Ritodrine (Yutopar)

d. Terbutaline (Brethine)

e. Magnesium sulfate

f. Nifedipine (Procardia)

g. Indomethacin

MATCHING: Match the description of medications used during the management of labor complications in Column I with the medication listed in Column II.

COLUMN I

COLUMN II

66. _____ Tocolytic medication administered subcutaneously to suppress hyperstimulation of the uterus.

67. _____ Classification of hormones that can be used to ripen the cervix and/or stimulate uterine contractions.

68. _____ Cervical ripening agent in the form of a vaginal insert that is placed in the posterior fornix of the vagina.

69. _____ Cervical ripening agent in the form of a gel that is inserted into the cervical canal just below the internal os.

70. _____ Pituitary hormone used to stimulate uterine contractions in the augmentation or induction of labor.

71. _____ Natural cervical dilator made from seaweed.

72. _____ Cervical ripening agent, used in the form of a tablet, that is most commonly inserted intravaginally into the posterior fornix.

a. Oxytocin (Pitocin)

b. Misoprostol (Cytotec)

c. Dinoprostone (Cervidil)

d. Dinoprostone (Prepidil)

e. Terbutaline (Brethine)

f. Prostaglandin

g. Laminaria tent

73. Describe each of the five factors that cause labor to be long, difficult, or abnormal. Explain how they interrelate.

74. Explain the treatment approach of therapeutic rest.

75. Angela (1-0-0-0-0) is experiencing hypertonic uterine dysfunction, Bernice (3-1-0-1-1) is experiencing hypotonic uterine dysfunction, and Gloria (2-0-0-1-0) is having difficulty bearing down effectively. Complete the following table by contrasting each woman's labor in terms of causes/precipitating factors, maternal-fetal effects, change in pattern of progress, and care management.

	Angela (Hypertonic)	Bernice (Hypotonic)	Gloria (Inadequate Expulsion)
Causes/ Precipitating Factors			
Maternal-fetal Effects			
Changes in Progress of Labor			
Care Management			

76. List the signs of AFE.

77. Outline the recommended care management of a woman experiencing an AFE.

78. Identify four indications for oxytocin induction and four contraindications to the use of oxytocin to stimulate the onset of labor.

    Indications

    Contraindications

MULTIPLE CHOICE QUESTIONS: Circle the one correct option and state the rationale for the option chosen.

79. When assessing a woman during pregnancy, the nurse needs to be alert for signs that would indicate risk for preterm labor and birth. Which of the following factors exhibited by a pregnant woman is associated with preterm labor and birth?
    a. Age: 30
    b. Obstetric history: 3-2-0-0-2
    c. Children are 2 and 4 years of age
    d. Currently being treated for her second bladder infection in 4 months

80. A woman calls the prenatal clinic to report that she has been experiencing uterine contractions for the past hour at a frequency of every 8 to 10 minutes. Which one of the following actions would the nurse tell this woman to take?
    a. Lie down on her side
    b. Count contractions for 2 more hours
    c. Reduce fluid intake
    d. Report to the clinic for evaluation as soon as someone can bring her

81. Bed rest for prevention of preterm birth is least likely to result in
    a. Bone demineralization;
    b. Weight gain;
    c. Fatigue;
    d. Anxiety and depression.

82. A woman's labor is being suppressed using intravenous magnesium sulfate. Which of the following measures should be implemented during the infusion?
    a. Limit fluid intake to 1500 to 2500 ml per day.
    b. Assess FHR for tachycardia.
    c. Ensure that indomethacin is available should toxicity occur.
    d. Assist woman into a comfortable semirecumbent position.

83. The physician has ordered that dinoprostone (Cervidil) be administered to ripen a pregnant woman's cervix in preparation for an induction of her labor. In fulfilling this order, the nurse would
    a. insert the Cervidil into the cervical canal just below the internal os.
    b. tell the woman to remain in bed for at least 15 minutes.
    c. call the woman's physician if she reports a history of asthma.
    d. remove the Cervidil if the woman begins to experience uterine contractions.

84. A nulliparous woman experiencing a postterm pregnancy is admitted for labor induction. Assessment reveals a Bishop score of 9. The nurse would
    a. call the woman's primary health care provider to order a cervical ripening agent.
    b. mix 20 units of oxytocin (Pitocin) in 500 ml of 5% glucose in water.
    c. piggyback the Pitocin solution into the port nearest the drip chamber of the primary IV tubing.
    d. begin the infusion at a rate between 0.5 to 2 milliunits/min as determined by the induction protocol.

85. A woman's labor is being induced. The nurse assesses the woman's status and that of her fetus and the labor process just before an infusion increment of 2 milliunits/min. The nurse would discontinue the infusion and notify the woman's primary health care provider if which of the following had been noted during the assessment?
    a. Frequency of uterine contractions: every $1\frac{1}{2}$ minutes
    b. Variability of FHR: present
    c. Deceleration patterns: early decelerations noted with several contractions
    d. Intensity of uterine contractions at their peaks: 80 to 85 mm Hg

86. A multiparous woman is in the first stage of labor. In reviewing her partogram, the nurse midwife notes that the woman's cervix has dilated from 5 cm to 6 cm over 2 hours. The nurse midwife would recognize this woman's labor pattern as
    a. prolonged latent phase.
    b. protracted active phase.
    c. secondary arrest.
    d. precipitous labor.

87. A laboring woman's vaginal examination reveals the following: 3 cm, 50%, LSA, 0. The nurse caring for this woman would
    a. place the ultrasound transducer in the left lower quadrant of the woman's abdomen.
    b. recognize that passage of meconium would be a definitive sign of fetal distress.
    c. expect the progress of fetal descent to be slower than usual.
    d. assist the woman into a knee-chest position for each contraction.

II. THINKING CRITICALLY

1. Imagine that you are a nurse-midwife working at an inner-city women's health clinic. You are concerned about the rate of preterm labor and birth among the pregnant women who come to your clinic for care. Outline a preterm labor and birth prevention program that you would implement at your clinic to reduce the rate of preterm labors and birth.

2. Sara, a primiparous woman (2-0-1-0-1) at 22 weeks of gestation, comes to the clinic for her scheduled prenatal visit. She is anxious because her last labor began at 26 weeks and she is worried that this will happen again. "I had no warning the last time. Is there anything I can do this time to have my baby later or at least know that labor is starting so I can let you know?"
   a. Identify the signs of preterm labor that the nurse-midwife should teach Sara.

   b. Explain how the nurse-midwife could help Sara implement a plan to reduce her risk for preterm labor.

   c. Three weeks later, Sara calls the clinic and tells her nurse-midwife that she has been having uterine contractions about every 9 minutes or so for the last hour. Describe what the nurse-midwife should tell Sara to do.

   d. Conservative measures do not work and Sara's uterine contractions progress. She is admitted for possible tocolytic therapy. Specify the criteria that Sara must meet before tocolysis can be safely instituted.

   e. Sara is started on a tocolysis regimen that involves the intravenous administration of ritodrine. Outline the nursing care measures that must be implemented during the infusion to ensure the safety of Sara and her fetus.

   f. The nurse is preparing to give Sara a dose of betamethasone as ordered by the physician.

      1. State the purpose of this medication.

2. Explain the protocol that the nurse should follow in fulfilling this order.

3. Debra has been experiencing signs of preterm labor. After a period of hospitalization, her labor was successfully suppressed and she was discharged to be cared for at home. Debra is receiving terbutaline via a subcutaneous pump. She will palpate her uterine activity twice a day. Debra must also remain on bed rest with only bathroom privileges.

   a. Identify two nursing diagnoses that would be appropriate related to Debra's home care regimen for preterm labor suppression.

   b. Outline what the nurse should teach Debra regarding the care and maintenance of the terbutaline subcutaneous pump that is being used.

   c. Identify the side effects of terbutaline that the nurse should teach Debra before discharge.

   d. Describe the instructions that Debra should be given regarding palpating her uterus for contractions.

   e. Debra has 2 children who are 5 years old and 8 years old. Specify the suggestions you would give to help Debra and her children cope with the bed rest requirement ordered by Debra's primary health care provider.

4. Denise, a primigravida has reached the second stage of her labor with her fetus at zero station and positioned LOP. She is experiencing intense low back pain. Denise did not attend any childbirth classes and is having difficulty pushing effectively. No anesthesia has been used.

   a. Identify the factors that can have a negative effect on the secondary powers of labor (bearing-down efforts).

   b. Describe how you would help Denise use her expulsive forces to facilitate the descent and birth of her baby.

   c. Specify the positions that would be recommended based on the position of the presenting part of Denise's fetus.

5. Anne, a primigravida attended Lamaze classes with her husband, Mark. They were looking forward to working together during the labor and birth of their baby. Because of fetal distress, an emergency low-segment cesarean section with a transverse incision was performed after 18 hours of labor. Even though Anne and her son are in stable condition and she is glad that "everything turned out okay" for her son, she expresses a sense of failure stating, "I could not manage to give birth to my son in the normal way and now I never will!"

   a. List the preoperative nursing measures that should have been implemented to prepare Anne physically and emotionally for the unexpected cesarean birth.

   b. Specify the assessment measures that are critical when Anne is in the recovery room following her birth.

   c. State the postoperative nursing care measures that Anne requires.

   d. Identify the nursing diagnosis reflected in Anne's statement, "I could not manage to give birth to my baby in the normal way and now I never will." Specify the support measures the nurse could use to put her cesarean birth into perspective.

6. A vaginal examination reveals that Marie's fetus is RSA. Specify the considerations that the nurse should keep in mind when providing care for Marie.

7. Angela (2-0-0-1-0) is at 42 weeks of gestation and has been admitted for induction of her labor.

   a. Assessment of Angela at admission included determination of her Bishop score. State the purpose of the Bishop score and identify the factors that are evaluated.

   b. Angela's score was 5. Interpret this result in terms of the planned induction of her labor.

   c. Angela's primary health care provider ordered that dinoprostone (Cervidil) be inserted. State the purpose of the Cervidil, method of application, and potential side effects that can occur.

   d. Before induction of her labor, Angela's primary health provider performs an amniotomy. Specify the nursing responsibilities before, during, and after this procedure.

e. Indicate which of the following actions reflect appropriate care (A) for Angela during the induction of her labor with intravenous oxytocin. If the action is not appropriate (NA), state what the correct action would be.

1. _____ Assist Angela into a lateral or upright position.

2. _____ Apply an external electronic fetal monitor and obtain a 15- to 20-minute baseline strip of FHR and pattern.

3. _____ Explain to Angela what to expect and techniques used.

4. _____ Prepare a primary line with an isotonic electrolyte solution.

5. _____ Attach the secondary line of dilute oxytocin (10 units in 1000 ml) to the distal port (farthest from the venipuncture site) of the primary IV.

6. _____ Begin infusion at 4 milliunits/min.

7. _____ Increase oxytocin by 1 to 2 milliunits/min at 5- to 10-minute intervals after the initial dose until the desired pattern of contractions is achieved.

8. _____ Stop increasing the dosage and maintain level of oxytocin when contractions occur every 2 to 3 minutes, last 40 to 90 seconds, and reach an intrauterine pressure between 40 to 90 mm Hg if internal monitoring is being used.

9. _____ Monitor maternal blood pressure and pulse every 15 minutes and after every increment.

10. _____ Monitor FHR pattern and uterine activity every 15 minutes and before and after every increment.

11. _____ Limit IV intake to 1500 ml/8 hours.

f. State the major side effects of oxytocin (Pitocin) for which the nurse must be alert when managing Angela's labor.

g. The nurse notes a hyperstimulation pattern when evaluating Angela's monitor tracing. List the actions the nurse should take in order of priority.

8. Lora is a 37-year-old nulliparous woman beginning her forty-second week of pregnancy. She and her primary health care provider have decided on a conservative "watchful waiting" approach because both she and her fetus are not experiencing distress.

a. In helping Lora make this decision, the risks she and her fetus face as a result of a postterm pregnancy were explained. Identify the risks that Lora should have considered in making her decision.

b. State the clinical manifestations that Lora is likely to experience as her pregnancy continues.

c. State one nursing diagnosis appropriate for Lora's current situation.

d. Outline the typical care management measures that should be implemented to ensure the safety of Lora and her fetus.

e. Specify the instructions that the nurse should give to Lora regarding her self-care as she awaits the onset of labor.

Maternal Physiologic Changes

20

I. REVIEWING KEY CONCEPTS AND CONTENT

TRUE OR FALSE: Circle T if true or F if false for each of the following statements. Correct the false statements.

1. T   F   Within 12 hours of birth the fundus of the uterus may be 1 cm above the umbilicus.

2. T   F   The uterus is slightly smaller in size after every pregnancy.

3. T   F   Regeneration of the endometrium, including the placental site, is completed approximately 4 weeks after birth.

4. T   F   The external os of the cervix has a jagged, slit-like appearance in multiparous women.

5. T   F   Until estrogen levels rise, the postpartum woman is likely to experience discomfort during intercourse (dyspareunia) associated with inadequate secretion of lubricating mucus.

6. T   F   Breast milk is bluish white and has a skim milk–like appearance.

7. T   F   For most nonlactating women, ovulation resumes by 2½ months after birth.

8. T   F   During the first 24 hours after birth, an elevated temperature of 38° C is indicative of the onset of infection.

9. T   F   During the first 72 hours after birth, a decrease in the hematocrit is expected.

10. T   F   During the first 10 to 12 days of the postpartum period, a leukocytosis of 20,000/mm³ strongly suggests uterine or bladder infection.

11. T   F   Involution and the process of autolysis often produce a mild proteinuria of +1 for 1 to 2 days after birth.

12. T   F   An elevated follicle-stimulating hormone level in the postpartum period is responsible for the suppression of ovulation in lactating women.

13. T   F   Lochia normally has a fleshy odor similar to menstrual flow.

14. T   F   Most postpartum women will experience several anovulatory menstrual cycles before ovulation resumes.

15. When caring for a woman following vaginal birth, it is of critical importance for the nurse to assess the woman's bladder for distention.

   a. Explain why bladder distention is more likely to occur during the immediate postpartum period.

   b. Identify the problems that can occur if the bladder is allowed to become distended.

16. Cite the factors that can interfere with bowel elimination in the postpartum period.

17. Explain why hypovolemic shock is less likely to occur in the postpartum woman experiencing a normal or average blood loss.

18. Indicate the factors that place a postpartum woman at increased risk for the development of thrombophlebitis.

19. Compare and contrast the characteristics of lochial bleeding and nonlochial bleeding.

FILL IN THE BLANKS: Insert the term that corresponds to each of the following descriptions.

20. _____ Profuse sweating that occurs after birth, especially at night, to rid the body of fluid retained during pregnancy.

21. _____ Uncomfortable uterine cramping that occurs during the early postpartum period as a result of periodic relaxation and vigorous contractions.

22. _____ The lactogenic hormone secreted by the pituitary gland of lactating women. _____ is another pituitary hormone that is responsible for uterine contraction and the let-down reflex.

23. _____ Surgical incision of the perineum to facilitate birth.

24. _____ Failure of the uterine muscle to contract firmly. It is the most frequent cause of excessive postpartum bleeding.

25. _____ An anal varicosity.

26. _____ Term used to describe the return of the uterus to a nonpregnant state.

27. _____ Term used interchangeably with *postpartum* to refer to the period of recovery after childbirth.

28. _____ Separation of the abdominal wall muscles related to the effect of the enlargement of the uterus on the abdominal musculature.

29. _____ The pink to brownish uterine flow that begins about 3 to 4 days after birth.

30. _____ The bloody uterine flow that occurs for the first few days following birth.

31. _____ The yellowish white flow that begins about 10 days after birth and continues for 2 to 6 weeks.

32. _____ Term used to describe distended, firm, tender, and warm breasts during the postpartum period.

33. _____ Yellowish fluid produced in the breasts before lactation.

34. _____ Increased production of urine that occurs in the postpartum period to rid the body of fluid retained during pregnancy.

MULTIPLE CHOICE QUESTIONS: Circle the one correct option and state the rationale for the option chosen.

35. A nurse has assessed a woman who gave birth vaginally 12 hours ago. Which of the following findings would require further assessment?
    a. Bright to dark red uterine discharge
    b. Midline episiotomy—approximated, moderate edema, slight erythema, absence of ecchymosis
    c. Protrusion of abdomen with sight separation of abdominal wall muscles
    d. Fundus firm at 1 cm above the umbilicus and to the right of midline

36. A woman, 24 hours after giving birth, complains to the nurse that her sleep was interrupted the night before because of sweating and the need to have her gown and bed linen changed. The nurse's first action would be to
    a. assess this woman for additional clinical manifestations of infection.
    b. explain to the woman that the sweating represents her body's attempt to eliminate the fluid that was accumulated during pregnancy.
    c. notify her physician of the finding.
    d. document the finding as postpartum diaphoresis.

37. Which of the following women at 24 hours following birth is least likely to experience afterpains?
    a. Primipara who is breastfeeding her twins that were born at 38 weeks of gestation
    b. Multipara who is breastfeeding her 10-pound full-term baby girl
    c. Multipara who is bottle-feeding her 8-pound baby boy
    d. Primipara who is bottle-feeding her 7-pound baby girl

II. THINKING CRITICALLY

1. Describe how you would respond to each of the following typical questions/concerns of postpartum women.
   a. Mary is a primipara who is breastfeeding. "Why am I experiencing so many painful cramps in my uterus? I thought this happens only in women who have had babies before."

   b. Susan is being discharged after giving birth 20 hours ago. "For how many days should I be able to palpate my uterus to make sure it is firm?"

   c. June is a primipara. "My friend, who had a baby last year, said she had a flow for 6 weeks. Isn't that a long time to bleed after having a baby?"

   d. Jean is at 24 hours postpartum. "I cannot believe it—I look as if I am still pregnant! How can this be?"

   e. Marion is 1 day postpartum. "I perspired so much last night and I have such large amounts of urine when I go to the bathroom. I hope everything is okay and I can still go home!"

   f. Joan is a primipara who is breastfeeding her baby. "My friend told me that I cannot get pregnant as long as I continue to breastfeed. This is great because I do not like to use birth control."

   g. Alice, a multiparous woman, is concerned. She states, "My doctor is not going to give me a drug to dry up my breasts like I had with my first baby. How will my breasts ever get back to normal now?"

   h. Andrea, a primipara, is 1 day postpartum. While breastfeeding her baby she confides to the nurse that she does not know how long she will continue to breastfeed. "My husband and I have always had a satisfying sex life, but my friend told me that as long as I breastfeed, intercourse is painful."

21 Nursing Care during the Fourth Trimester

I. REVIEWING KEY CONCEPTS AND CONTENT

FILL IN THE BLANKS: Insert the term that corresponds to each of the following descriptions regarding the postpartum period.

1. _____ The first 1 to 2 hours after birth.

2. _____ Nursing care management approach in which one nurse cares for both the mother and her infant. It is also called _____.

3. _____ Term used for the decreasing hospital stays of mothers and their babies after low risk births. Other terms used are _____ and _____.

4. _____ Classification of medications that stimulate contraction of the uterine smooth muscle.

5. _____ Failure of the uterine muscle to contract firmly. It is the most frequent cause of _____ following childbirth.

6. _____ Perineal treatment that involves sitting in warm water for approximately 20 minutes to soothe and cleanse the site and to increase blood flow, thereby enhancing healing.

7. _____ Menstrual-like cramps experienced by many women as the uterus contracts after childbirth.

8. _____ Dilation of the blood vessels supplying the intestines as a result of the rapid decease in intraabdominal pressure after birth. It causes blood to pool in the viscera and thereby contributes to the development of _____ when the woman who has recently given birth sits or stands, first ambulates, or takes a warm shower.

9. _____ Complaint of pain in calf muscles when dorsiflexion of the foot is forced. The presence of pain is associated with the presence of a thrombus or thrombophlebitis. Additional signs include _____, _____, or _____ in the suspected leg.

10. _____ Exercises that can assist women to regain muscle tone that is often lost when pelvic tissues are stretched and torn during pregnancy and birth.

11. _____ Swelling of breast tissue caused by increased blood and lymph supply to the breasts before lactation.

12. _____ Vaccine that can be given to postpartum women whose antibody titer is less than 1:8 or whose EIA level is less than 0.8. It is used to prevent nonimmune women from contracting this TORCH infection during a subsequent pregnancy.

13. _____ Blood product that is administered to Rh-negative, antibody (Coombs')-negative women who have Rh-positive newborns. It is administered _____ within _____ hours after birth.

14. Explain to a woman who has just given birth why breastfeeding her newborn during the fourth stage of labor is beneficial to her and to her baby.

15. A postpartum woman at 6 hours after a vaginal birth is having difficulty voiding. List the measures that you would try to help this woman void spontaneously.

16. Identify the measures the nurse should teach a postpartum woman in an effort to prevent the development of thrombophlebitis.

17. State the criteria the nurse should use to determine the progress of a woman's recovery from each of the following types of anesthesia:

    a. General anesthesia

    b. Epidural or spinal anesthesia

18. Identify the measures you would teach a bottle-feeding mother to suppress lactation naturally and to relieve discomfort during breast engorgement.

19. State the two most important interventions that can be used to prevent excessive postpartum bleeding in the early postpartum period. Indicate the rationale for the effectiveness of each intervention you identified.

TRUE OR FALSE: Circle T if true or F if false for each of the following statements. Correct the false statements.

20. T F The effectiveness of the rubella vaccine may be reduced, if a postpartum woman receives both Rh immunoglobulin and a rubella vaccine.

21. T F Before sitting down in a sitz bath, the woman should relax her gluteal muscles to reduce discomfort when entering the bath, then tighten them after she is sitting in the bath.

22. T F Tucks are used to soothe sore hemorrhoids.

23. T F Medications such as estrogen and bromocriptine (Parlodel) are no longer used to suppress lactation for the bottle-feeding woman.

24. T F The most dangerous potential complication of the fourth stage of labor is infection.

25. T F Ice packs are most effective in minimizing perineal edema formation during the first 24 hours following birth.

26. T F A good time to administer pain medication to a breastfeeding woman would be immediately after a feeding session.

27. T F Rubella vaccine should not be given to a postpartum woman who is breastfeeding.

28. T F A woman should be expected to void at least 250 ml of urine spontaneously within 2 hours following vaginal birth.

29. T F RhoGAM should be administered intramuscularly into the deltoid or gluteal muscle.

30. T F A Chinese woman is likely to use hormonal preparations as her primary method of contraception.

31. T F Women who follow the cultural practice of balancing heat and cold will avoid bathing for a specified period of time after they have given birth.

32. T F A critical nursing action at the time of discharge is to carefully check the mother's and baby's identification bands.

33. T F A postpartum woman who is depressed and is experiencing thoughts of suicide or harming her child should call the warm line she learned about at discharge.

34. Tamara delivered vaginally 2 hours ago. She has a midline episiotomy.

    a. Describe the position that Tamara should assume in order to facilitate palpation of her fundus.

    b. Identify the characteristics of Tamara's fundus that should be assessed.

    c. Describe the position Tamara should assume in order to facilitate the examination of her episiotomy.

d. Identify the characteristics that should be assessed to determine progress of healing and adequacy of Tamara's perineal self-care measures.

e. State the characteristics of Tamara's uterine flow that should be assessed.

35. Imagine that you are the nurse who cared for a woman during her labor and birth and her recovery during the fourth stage of labor. Outline the information that you would report to the mother-baby nurse when you transfer the new mother and her baby to her room on the postpartum unit.

36. Infection control measures should guide the practice of nurses working on a postpartum unit.

   a. Discuss the measures designed to prevent transmission of infection from person to person.

   b. Discuss measures a postpartum woman should be taught to reduce her risk of infection.

37. Identify the signs of potential complications that may occur during the postpartum period.

MULITPLE CHOICE QUESTIONS: Circle the one correct option and state the rationale for the option chosen.

38. During the fourth stage of labor a woman experiences intense tremors that resemble shivers. Based on this finding the nurse would
   a. request an order for a sedative.
   b. assess the woman for signs of infection.

c. check the woman's rectal temperature to determine if she is becoming hypothermic.
   d. wrap the woman in warm blankets and reassure her.

39. The nurse is prepared to assess a postpartum woman's fundus. The nurse would tell the woman to
   a. elevate the head of the bed.
   b. place her hands under her head.
   c. flex her knees.
   d. lie flat with legs extended and toes pointed.

40. The expected outcome for care when methylergonovine (Methergine), an oxytocic, is administered to a postpartum woman during the fourth stage of labor would be: The woman will
   a. demonstrate expected lochial characteristics.
   b. achieve relief of pain associated with uterine cramping.
   c. remain free from infection.
   d. void spontaneously within 4 hours of birth.

41. A nurse is preparing to administer RhoGAM to a postpartum woman. Before implementing this care measure the nurse should
   a. ensure that medication is given at least 24 hours after the birth.
   b. verify that the Coombs' test results are negative.
   c. make sure that the newborn is Rh negative.
   d. cancel the administration of the RhoGAM if it was given to the woman during her pregnancy at 28 weeks of gestation.

42. When teaching a postpartum woman with an episiotomy about using a sitz bath, the nurse should emphasize
   a. using sterile equipment.
   b. filling the sitz bath basin with hot water (at least 42° C).
   c. taking a sitz bath once a day for 10 minutes.
   d. squeezing her buttocks together before sitting down, then relaxing them.

II. THINKING CRITICALLY

1. Tara is a breastfeeding woman at 12 hours postpartum. She requests medication for pain. Describe the approach that you would take when fulfilling Tara's request.

2. When caring for a woman who gave birth 4 hours earlier, the nurse notes an excessive rubra flow and early signs of hypovolemic shock.

   a. State the criteria that the nurse should have used to determine that the flow is rubra and excessive and that the early signs of hypovolemic shock are being exhibited.

   b. Identify the nurse's priority action in response to these assessment findings.

   c. Identify additional interventions that a nurse may need to implement to ensure this woman's safety and to prevent the development of further complications.

3. Carrie is a postpartum woman awaiting discharge. Because her rubella titer indicates that she is not immune, a rubella vaccination has been ordered before discharge. State what you would tell Carrie with regard to this vaccination.

4. The physician has written the following order for a postpartum woman: "Administer RhoGAM [Rh immunoglobulin] if indicated." Describe the actions the nurse should take in fulfilling this order.

5. Susan, a postpartum breastfeeding woman, confides to the nurse, "My partner and I have always had a very satisfying sex life even when I was pregnant. My sister told me that this will definitely change now that I have had a baby." Describe what the nurse should tell Susan regarding sexual changes and activity after birth.

6. Identify the priority nursing diagnosis as well as one expected outcome and appropriate nursing management for each of the following situations.

   a. Tina is 2 days postpartum. During a home visit the nurse notes that Tina's episiotomy is edematous, slightly reddened, with approximated wound edges, and no drainage. A distinct odor is noted and there is a buildup of secretions and the Hurricaine gel Tina uses for discomfort. During the interview Tina reveals that she is afraid to wash the area, "I rinse with a little water in my peri bottle in the morning and again at night. I also apply plenty of my gel."

      Nursing Diagnosis   **Expected Outcome**   **Nursing Management**

   b. Erin, who gave birth 3 days ago, has not had a bowel movement since a day or two before labor. She tells the visiting nurse during the interview that she has been avoiding "fiber" foods for fear that the baby will get diarrhea. Her activity level is low. "My family is taking good care of me. I do not have to lift a finger! Besides I would prefer to wait until my episiotomy is less sore before trying to have a bowel movement."

      Nursing Diagnosis   **Expected Outcome**   **Nursing Management**

   c. Mary gave birth 24 hours ago. She complains of perineal discomfort. "My hemorrhoids and stitches are killing me, but I do not want to take any medication because it will get into my breast milk and hurt my baby."

      Nursing Diagnosis   **Expected Outcome**   **Nursing Management**

7. Dawn gave birth 8 hours ago. Upon palpation, her fundus was found to be two fingerbreaths above the umbilicus and deviated to the right of midline. It was also assessed to be less firm than previously noted.

   a. State the most likely basis for these findings.

   b. Describe the action that the nurse should take based on these assessment findings.

8. Jill gave birth 3 hours ago. During labor, epidural anesthesia was used for pain relief. Jill's primary health care provider has written the following order, "Out of bed and ambulating when able." Discuss the approach the nurse should take in safely fulfilling this order.

9. Andrea gave birth 12 hours ago. She tells the nurse that she is ravenous. You check the chart, noting that Andrea's primary health care provider has ordered "diet as tolerated." State the criteria that should be met before fulfilling this order.

10. Dawn, a primiparous woman at 20 hours postpartum, is preparing for discharge within the next 4 hours. She is breastfeeding her new daughter.

   a. Describe the nurse's legal responsibility in terms of early discharge.

   b. List the criteria for discharge that Dawn and her newborn must meet before discharge from the hospital to home.

   Maternal criteria

   Newborn criteria

   General criteria

   c. Outline the essential content that must be taught before discharge. A home visit by a nurse is planned for Dawn's third postpartum day.

11. Cultural beliefs and practices must be considered when planning and implementing care in the postpartum period.

   a. Discuss the importance of using a culturally sensitive approach when providing care to postpartum women and their families.

   b. Kim, a Korean-American woman, has just given birth. Assessment reveals that she and her family are guided by beliefs and practices based on a balance of heat and cold. Describe how the nurse would adjust typical postpartum care in order to respect and accommodate Kim's cultural beliefs and practices.

   c. A Muslim woman has been admitted to the postpartum unit following the birth of her second son. Describe the approach you would use in managing this woman's care in a culturally sensitive manner.

Transition to Parenthood

(22)

I. REVIEWING KEY CONCEPTS AND CONTENT

1. Complete the following table by identifying the focus, characteristics (typical behaviors and concerns), and care requirements for postpartum women in each of the following phases of maternal adjustment.

Phase	Focus	Characteristics	Care Requirements
Dependent (Taking-In)			
Dependent-Independent (Taking-Hold)			
Interdependent (Letting-Go)			
Postpartum			

2. Describe the process of paternal adjustment to fatherhood and discuss the measures that nurses can use to facilitate this adjustment process.

3. Attachment of the newborn to parents and family is critical for optimum growth and development.

   a. Define the process of attachment and bonding.

   b. List conditions that must be present for the parent-newborn attachment process to begin favorably.

   c. Describe the acquaintance process.

   d. Discuss how you would assess the progress of attachment between parents and their new baby.

4. Identify several parental tasks and responsibilities that are part of parental adjustment to a new baby.

5. Discuss how each of the following forms of parent-infant contact can facilitate attachment and promote the family as a focus of care.

   a. Early contact

   b. Extended contact

FILL IN THE BLANKS: Insert the appropriate term for each of the following descriptions regarding parent-infant interaction and parenting.

6. _____ is the term used to refer to the process by which a parent comes to love and accept a child and a child comes to love and accept a parent. The term _____ is often used to refer to this process.

7. An important part of attachment is _____. Parents use _____, _____, _____, and _____ to get to know their baby during the immediate postpartum period.

8. _____, or _____, is a position in which the parent's face and the infant's face are approximately 8 inches apart and are on the same plane. Nursing actions to encourage this interaction would be _____, _____, and _____.

9. The _____ process is the identification of the new baby. The child is first identified in terms of _____ to other family members, then in terms of _____, and finally in terms of _____.

10. _____ is exhibited when newborns move in time with the structure of adult speech by _____ their arms, _____ their heads, and _____ their legs, seemingly _____ to a parent's voice.

11. One of the newborn's tasks is to establish a personal biorhythm or _____. Parents can help in this process by giving consistent _____ and using their infant's _____ state to develop _____ behavior and thereby

increase _____ and opportunities for _____.

12. _____ is a type of body movement or behavior that provides the observer with cues. The observer or receiver interprets those cues and responds to them. _____ refers to the "fit" between the infant's cues and the parents' response.

13. _____ is a father's absorption, preoccupation, and interest in his infant. Characteristics of this absorption include _____, _____, and awareness of _____.

14. Describe how each of the following factors influences the manner in which parents respond to the birth of their child. State two nursing implications/actions related to each factor.

   Adolescent parents

   Parental age over 35

   Social support

   Culture

   Socioeconomic conditions

   Personal aspirations

   Sensory impairment

MULTIPLE CHOICE QUESTIONS: Circle the one correct option and state the rationale for the option chosen.

15. During the final phase of the claiming process of a newborn, which of the following might a mother say?
    a. "She has her grandfather's nose."
    b. "His ears lay nice and flat against his head, not like mine and his sister's, which stick out."
    c. "She gave me nothing but trouble during pregnancy, and now she is so stubborn she won't wake up to breastfeed."
    d. "He has such a sweet disposition and pleasant expression. I have never seen a baby quite like him before."

16. Which of the following nursing actions would be least effective in facilitating parent attachment to their new infant?
    a. Referring the couple to a lactation consultant to ensure continuing success with breastfeeding
    b. Keeping the baby in the nursery as much as possible for the first 24 hours after birth so the mother can rest
    c. Extending visiting hours for the woman's partner or significant other as they desire
    d. Providing guidance and support as the parents care for their baby's nutrition and hygiene needs

17. Which of the following behaviors illustrates engrossment?
    a. A father is sitting in a rocking chair, holding his new baby boy, touching his toes, and making eye contact.
    b. A mother tells her friends that her baby's eyes and nose are just like hers.

    c. A mother picks up and cuddles her baby girl when she begins to cry.
    d. A grandmother gazes into her new grandson's face, which she holds about 8 inches away from her own; she and the baby make eye-to-eye contact.

18. A woman expresses a need to review her labor and birth experience with the nurse who cared for her while in labor. This behavior is most characteristic of which of the following phases of maternal postpartum adjustment?
    a. Taking-hold (dependent-independent phase)
    b. Taking-in (dependent phase)
    c. Letting-go (interdependent)
    d. Postpartum blues (baby blues)

19. Before discharge, a postpartum woman and her partner ask the nurse about the baby blues. "Our friend said she felt so let down after she had her baby, and we have heard that some women actually become very depressed. Is there anything we can do to prevent this from happening to us or at least to cope with the blues if they occur?" The nurse could tell this couple
    a. "Postpartum blues usually happen in pregnancies that are high risk or unplanned, so there is no need for you to worry."
    b. "Try to become skillful in breastfeeding and caring for your baby as quickly as you can."
    c. "Get as much rest as you can and sleep when the baby sleeps, because fatigue can precipitate the blues or make them worse."
    d. "I will call your doctor before you leave to get you a prescription for an antidepressant to prevent the blues from happening."

II. THINKING CRITICALLY

1. Jane and Andrew are parents of a newborn girl. Describe what you would teach them regarding the communication process as it relates to their newborn.

    a. Techniques they can use to communicate effectively with their newborn.

    b. The manner in which the baby is able to communicate with them.

2. Allison had a difficult labor that resulted in an emergency cesarean birth under general anesthesia. She did not see her baby until 12 hours after her birth. Allison tells the nurse who brings the baby to her room, "I am so disappointed. I had planned to breastfeed my baby and hold her close, skin to skin, right after her birth just like all the books say. I know that this is so important for our relationship." Describe how the nurse should respond to Allison's concern.

3. Angela is the mother of a 1-day-old boy and a 3-year-old girl. As you prepare Angela for discharge, she states, "My little girl just saw her brother. She says she loves him and cannot wait for him to come home. I am so glad that I do not have to worry about any of that sibling rivalry business!" Indicate how you would respond to Angela's comments?

4. Sara and Ben have just experienced the birth of their first baby. They are very happy with their baby boy but appear very unsure of themselves and are obviously anxious about how to tell what their baby needs. Sara is trying very hard to breastfeed and is having some success but not as much as she had hoped. Both parents express self-doubt about their ability to succeed at the "most important role in our lives."

   a. State the nursing diagnosis that is most appropriate for this couple.

   b. Describe what the nurse caring for this family can do to facilitate the attachment process.

5. Mary and Jim are the parents of three sons. They very much wanted to have a girl this time, but after a long and difficult birth they had another son who weighed 10 pounds. His appearance reflects the difficult birth process: occipital molding, caput succedaneum, and forceps marks on each cheek. Mary and Jim express their disappointment not only in the appearance of their son but also in the fact that they had another boy. "This was supposed to be our last child—now we just do not know what we will do." Discuss how you would facilitate Mary and Jim's attachment to their son and reconcile their fantasy ("dream") child with the reality of their actual child.

6. Dawn and Matthew have just given birth to their first baby. This is the first grandchild for both sets of grandparents. The grandmothers approach the nurse to ask how they can help the new family, stating, "We want to help Dawn and Matthew but at the same time not interfere with what they want to do." Discuss the role of the nurse in helping these grandparents to recognize their importance to the new family and to develop a mutually satisfying relationship with Dawn, Matthew, and the new baby.

7. Jane is 2 days postpartum. When the nurse makes a home visit, Jane is found crying. Jane states, "I have such a let-down feeling. I cannot understand why I feel this way when I should be so happy about the healthy outcome for myself and my baby." Jane's husband confirms her behavior and expresses confusion as well, stating, "I wish I knew what to do to help her." Identify the priority nursing diagnosis and one expected outcome for this situation. Describe the recommended nursing management for the nursing diagnosis you have identified.

   Nursing Diagnosis   **Expected Outcome**   **Nursing Management**

8. Imagine that you are a nurse teaching a group of expectant parents about caring for their newborns. How would you respond to each of the following questions posed by the parents?

   a. Dan and Cheryl ask: "We have heard that new babies cry all the time, especially at night. How on earth will we able to cope with this?"

   b. Sue and Tim ask: "A couple that we know took their baby to an infant massage class. What possible benefit could infant massage have?"

   c. Marie and Joseph ask: "Our friends tell us that they are always teaching their babies something new. How is this possible? Babies can't learn, can they?"

(23) Postpartum Complications

I. REVIEWING KEY CONCEPTS AND CONTENT

FILL IN THE BLANKS: Insert the term that corresponds to each of the following descriptions of postpartum complications.

1. _____ is the loss of 500 ml or more of blood following vaginal birth or 1000 ml or more of blood after cesarean birth. The leading cause is _____. _____ occurs within 24 hours after birth. _____ occurs more than 24 hours after birth but less than 6 weeks postpartum.

2. Marked hypotonia of the uterus is called _____.

3. A pelvic _____ is the accumulation of blood in the connective tissue as a result of blood vessel damage. _____ are the most common type. _____ are usually associated with a forceps-assisted birth, an episiotomy, or primigravidity.

4. _____ of the uterus refers to the turning of the uterus inside out after birth. The primary presenting signs are _____, _____, and _____. Contributing factors include _____ implantation of the placenta, _____ pressure, _____ applied to the umbilical cord, _____, _____, and abnormally adherent _____.

5. _____ is the delayed return of the enlarged uterus to normal size and function.

6. _____ is an emergency situation in which profuse blood loss (hemorrhage) can result in severely compromised perfusion of body organs. Death may occur.

7. A _____ is suspected when bleeding is continuous and there is no identifiable cause. _____ is a pathologic form of clotting that is diffuse and consumes large amounts of clotting factors.

8. A _____ is the formation of a blood clot or clots inside a blood vessel and is caused by _____ or partial _____ of the vessel. _____ involves the superficial saphenous venous system. For _____, involvement varies but can extend from the foot to the iliofemoral region. _____ occurs when part of a blood clot dislodges and is carried to the pulmonary artery, where it occludes the vessel and obstructs blood flow to the lungs.

9. _____ or _____ refers to any clinical infection of the genital canal that occurs within 28 days after miscarriage, induced abortion, or childbirth. The first symptom is usually a _____ of 38° C or more on _____. Common infection sites are _____, _____, _____, _____, and _____.

10. _____, or _____, is the most common cause of postpartum infection. It usually begins as a localized infection at the _____ site.

11. _____ is an infection of the breast affecting approximately 1% of women, soon after childbirth, most of whom are _____. This infection is almost always _____ and develops well after the _____ has been established.

12. _____ is a downward displacement of the uterus, with degrees of displacement from mild to complete.

13. _____ is the protrusion of the bladder downward into the vagina that develops when supporting structures in the vesicovaginal septum are injured.

14. _____ is the herniation of the anterior rectal wall through the relaxed or ruptured vaginal fascia and rectovaginal septum.

15. _____ is uncontrollable leakage of urine.

162

16. A _____ is an abnormal communication between one hollow viscus and another or from one hollow viscus to the outside. A _____ is an abnormal communication between the bladder and the genital tract. A _____ is an abnormal communication between the urethra and the vagina, whereas an abnormal communication between the rectum or sigmoid colon and the vagina is called a

    _____.

17. In the postpartum period, an intense and pervasive sadness with severe and labile mood swings is diagnosed as _____. It is more serious and persistent than postpartum blues. The incidence is from _____ to _____ of new mothers. These symptoms rarely disappear without outside help. A distinguishing feature of postpartum depression is _____, which often flares up with little provocation. Many of these outbursts are directed against_____ or the _____. A prominent feature of postpartum depression is _____ of the infant often caused by abnormal

    _____.

18. In the postpartum period, a syndrome most often characterized by depression, delusions, and thoughts by the mother of harming either herself or her infant is diagnosed as _____. Symptoms of this syndrome often begin within _____after birth, although the mean time to onset is _____ weeks and almost always within _____ weeks of the birth. Characteristically, the woman begins to complain of _____ and _____ and may have episodes of _____ and _____. Delusions, when present, often are related to the _____, and in severe cases auditory hallucinations may command the mother to _____.

TRUE OR FALSE: Circle T if true or F if false for each of the following statements. Correct the false statements

19. T F   Early postpartum hemorrhage is often the result of cervical lacerations.

20. T F   One of the major causes of late postpartum hemorrhage is retained placental fragments.

21. T F   When a woman hemorrhages, changes in her baseline vital sign values may not be reliable indicators of shock in the immediate postpartum

period because of the physiologic adaptations that occurred during pregnancy and in the postpartum period.

22. T F   Cervical lacerations are the most common of all injuries of the lower portion of the genital tract.

23. T F   Oxytocin (Pitocin) can be given orally for several days after birth to enhance uterine contraction in women who experienced early postpartum hemorrhage.

24. T F   Prostaglandin $F_{2\alpha}$ (Hemabate) should be avoided if the postpartum woman has asthma.

25. T F   Subinvolution of the uterus is the second major cause of early postpartum hemorrhage.

26. T F   Uterine inversion occurs most frequently in primiparous women with abruptio-placentae.

27. T F   The woman with a third-or fourth-degree laceration should not be given rectal suppositories or enemas.

28. T F   Aspirin or aspirin-containing analgesics can be safely used if a woman is receiving heparin because aspirin enhances its effect.

29. T F   Puerperal infection is the major cause of maternal morbidity and mortality in the United States.

30. T F   Mastitis usually develops in the second to fourth week postpartum.

31. T F   Lactation must be suppressed once mastitis is diagnosed.

32. T F   Once a woman has had a postpartum episode with psychotic features, there is little risk it will occur again with a subsequent pregnancy.

33. T F   Women with postpartum depression may experience suicidal ideation and obsessional thoughts regarding violence to their newborns.

34. T F   Women with postpartum depression almost always require pharmacologic intervention.

35. T F   Blue cohosh has been found to be effective in relieving postpartum depression

36. State the twofold focus of medical management of hemorrhagic shock.

37. Identify the priority nursing interventions for postpartum hemorrhage.

38. State the standard of care for bleeding emergencies.

39. Identify measures found to be effective in preventing genital tract infections during the postpartum period.

40. Mary, a pregnant woman at 24 weeks of gestation, has been admitted to the labor unit following a prenatal visit at her health care provider's office. Fetal death is suspected and eventually confirmed. Identify the phase of grief response represented by each of the comments made by Mary as she reacts to her loss. Describe each phase in terms of expected duration, behaviors typically exhibited, and emotions experienced.

    a. "The doctor says he cannot find my baby's heartbeat or feel my baby move. He thinks my baby has died. I know you will hear my baby's heartbeat since you have a monitor here. My baby is okay—I just know it!"

    b. "I know this never would have happened if I had quit my job as a legal secretary. My mom told me that pregnant women should take it easy. If I had listened I would have my baby in my arms right now!"

    c. "Since my baby died I just cannot seem to concentrate on even the simplest things at home and at work. I always seem to feel tired and out of sorts. Why did this happen to my baby? Why did it happen to me?"

    d. "It is going to be hard. I will always remember my little baby boy and the day he was supposed to be born. But I know that my husband and I have to go on with our lives."

41. Describe how you, as a nurse, would help parents and other family members actualize the loss of their newborn.

MULTIPLE CHOICE QUESTIONS: Circle the one correct option and state the rationale for the option chosen.

42. Methylergonovine (Methergine) 0.2 mg is ordered to be administered intramuscularly to a woman who gave birth vaginally 1 hour ago for a profuse lochial flow with clots. Her fundus is boggy and does not respond well to massage. She is still being treated for preeclampsia with intravenous magnesium sulfate at 1 g/hr. Her blood pressure, measured 5 minutes ago, was 155/98. In fulfilling this order the nurse would
    a. measure the woman's blood pressure again 5 minutes after administering the medication.
    b. question the order based on the woman's hypertensive status.
    c. recognize that Methergine will counteract the uterine relaxation effects of the magnesium sulfate infusion the woman is receiving.
    d. tell the woman that the medication will lead to uterine cramping.

43. A postpartum woman in the fourth stage of labor received prostaglandin $F_{2\alpha}$ (Hemabate) 0.25 mg intramuscularly. The expected outcome of care for the administration of this medication would be
    a. relief from the pain of uterine cramping.
    b. prevention of intrauterine infection.
    c. reduction in the blood's ability to clot.
    d. limitation of excessive blood loss that is occurring after birth.

44. The nurse responsible for the care of postpartum women should recognize that the first sign of puerperal infection would most likely be
    a. fever with body temperature at 38° C or higher after the first 24 hours following birth.
    b. increased white blood cell count.
    c. foul-smelling profuse lochia.
    d. bradycardia.

45. A breastfeeding woman's cesarean birth occurred 2 days ago. Investigation of the pain, tenderness, and swelling in her left leg led to a medical diagnosis of deep vein thrombosis (DVT). Care management for this woman during the acute stage of the DVT would involve
    a. explaining that she will need to stop breastfeeding until anticoagulation therapy is completed.
    b. administering heparin orally.
    c. placing the woman on bed rest with her left leg elevated.
    d. fitting the woman with an elastic stocking so that she can exercise her legs.

46. Which of the following would be a priority question to ask a woman experiencing postpartum depression?
    a. Have you thought about hurting yourself?
    b. Does it seem like your mind is filled with cobwebs?
    c. Have you been feeling insecure, fragile, or vulnerable?
    d. Does the responsibility of motherhood seem overwhelming?

47. A woman gave birth to twin girls, one of whom was stillborn. Which of the following nursing actions would be least helpful in supporting the woman as she copes with her loss?
    a. Remind her that she should be happy that one daughter survived and is healthy.
    b. Assist the woman in taking pictures of both babies.
    c. Encourage the woman to hold the deceased twin in her arms to say good-bye.
    d. Offer her the opportunity for counseling to help her with her grief and that of her surviving twin as she gets older.

48. During the acute distress phase of the grief response parents are most likely to experience
    a. fear and anxiety about future pregnancies.
    b. difficulty with cognitive processing.
    c. search for meaning.
    d. sadness and depression.

49. A 17-year-old woman experiences a miscarriage at 12 weeks of gestation. When she is informed about the miscarriage she begins to cry, stating that she was upset about her pregnancy at first and now she is being punished for not wanting her baby. Which of the following would be the nurse's best response?
    a. "You are still so young, you probably were not ready for a baby right now."
    b. "This must be so hard for you. I am here if you want to talk."
    c. "At least this happened early in your pregnancy before you felt your baby move."
    d. "God must have a good reason for letting this happen."

II. THINKING CRITICALLY

1. Andrea is a multiparous woman (6-5-1-0-7) who gave birth to full-term twins vaginally 1 hour ago. Pitocin was used to augment her labor when hypotonic uterine contractions protracted the active stage of her labor. Special forceps were used to assist the birth of the second twin. Currently her vital signs are stable, her fundus is at the umbilicus, midline and firm, and her lochial flow is moderate to heavy without clots.

   a. Early postpartum hemorrhage is a major concern at this time. State the factors that have increased Andrea's risk for hemorrhage at this time.

b. Identify the priority nursing diagnosis at this time.

c. During the second hour after birth the nurse notes that Andrea's perineal pad became saturated in 15 minutes and a large amount of blood had accumulated on the bed under her buttocks. Describe the nurse's initial response to this finding. State the rationale for the action you described.

d. The nurse prepares to administer 10 units of Pitocin intravenously as ordered by Andrea's physician. Explain the guidelines the nurse should follow in fulfilling this order.

e. During the assessment of Andrea, the nurse must be alert for signs of developing hypovolemic shock. Cite the signs the nurse would be watching for.

f. Describe the measures that the nurse should use to support Andrea and her family in an effort to reduce their anxiety.

2. Nurses working on a postpartum unit must be constantly alert for signs and symptoms of puerperal infection in their patients.

a. List the factors that can increase a postpartum woman's risk for puerperal infection.

b. State the typical clinical manifestations of endometritis for which the nurse should be alert when assessing postpartum women.

c. Identify two nursing diagnoses that would be appropriate for a woman diagnosed with endometritis.

d. Describe the critical nursing measures that are essential in care management related to puerperal infection.

3. Sara, a primiparous breastfeeding mother at 2 weeks postpartum, calls her nurse-midwife to tell her that her right breast is painful and she's not "feeling well."

   a. Explain the assessment findings the nurse-midwife would be alert for to indicate if Sara is experiencing mastitis.

   b. A medical diagnosis of mastitis of Sara's right breast is made. State two nursing diagnoses appropriate for this situation.

   c. Describe the treatment measures and health teaching that Sara needs regarding her infection and breastfeeding, since she wishes to continue to breastfeed.

   d. Identify several behaviors that Sara should learn to prevent recurrence of mastitis.

4. Susan is a 36-year-old obese multiparous woman (5-4-0-1-4) who experienced a cesarean birth 2 days ago. During this pregnancy, she was able to reduce her smoking to 2 packs of cigarettes every other day. Although she has never experienced a DVT or thrombophlebitis, she did develop varicose veins in both legs with her third pregnancy. A major complication of the postpartum period is the development of thromboembolic disease.

   a. State the risk factors for this complication that Susan presents.

   b. When assessing Susan on the afternoon of her second postpartum day, the nurse notes signs indicative of deep vein thrombosis (DVT). List the signs the nurse most likely observed.

c. A medical diagnosis of DVT is confirmed. State one nursing diagnosis appropriate for this situation.

d. Outline the expected care management for Susan during the acute phase of the DVT.

e. Upon discharge Susan will be taking warfarin for at least 3 months. Specify the discharge instructions that Susan and her family should receive.

5. Denise (6-5-0-1-5), a 60-year-old postmenopausal woman, has been diagnosed with cystocele and rectocele.

a. Describe the signs and symptoms Denise most likely exhibited to lead to this diagnosis.

b. Identify two priority nursing diagnoses related to the signs and symptoms Denise is most likely experiencing. Write one expected outcome for each of the nursing diagnoses identified.

c. Outline the care management approach recommended for Denise's health problem.

d. Denise will use a pessary during the day until a surgical repair can be accomplished. Identify one nursing diagnosis associated with pessary use and specify the instructions the nurse would give to Denise regarding the use and care of a pessary.

6. Mary, a 35-year-old primiparous woman beginning her second week postpartum, is bottle-feeding her baby. She and her husband, Tom, moved from Buffalo, where they lived all their lives, to Los Angeles 2 months ago to take advantage of a career opportunity for Tom. They live in a community with many other young couples who are also starting families. Last month they joined the Catholic church near their home. Tom tries to help Mary with the baby but he has to spend long hours at work to establish his position. Mary's prenatal record reveals that she often exhibited anxiety about her well-being and that of her baby. During a home visit by a nurse, as part of an early discharge program, Mary tells the nurse that she always wants to sleep and just cannot seem to get enough rest. Mary is very concerned that she is not being a good mother and states, "Sometimes I just do

not know what to do to care of my baby the right way, and I am not even breastfeeding my baby. It seems that Tom enjoys spending what little time he has at home with the baby and not with me. I even find myself yelling at him for the silliest things." The nurse recognizes that Mary is exhibiting behaviors strongly suggestive of postpartum depression.

a. Indicate the signs and symptoms that Mary exhibited to lead the nurse to suspect postpartum depression.

b. Specify the predisposing factors for postpartum depression that are present in Mary's situation.

c. Write several questions that the nurse could ask Mary to determine the depth of the postpartum depression that she is experiencing.

d. Write one nursing diagnosis that is reflective of Mary and Tom's current situation.

e. Describe the measures the nurse could use to help Mary and Tom cope with postpartum depression.

7. Jane (2-1-0-0-1) is a 21-year-old woman admitted with vaginal bleeding at 13 weeks of gestation. She experiences a miscarriage. Jane is accompanied by her husband, Tom. Her 5 year-old daughter is at home with Jane's mother.

a. Describe the approach you would take to develop a plan of individualized support measures for Jane as she and her family cope with their loss.

b. Cite questions and observations you would use to gather the information required to create an individualized plan of care.

c. Formulate three nursing diagnoses appropriate for Jane and her family.

d. Identify the therapeutic communication techniques you should use to help Jane and Tom acknowledge and express their feelings and emotions about their loss.

e. At discharge, Jane is crying. She tells you, "I know it must have been something I did wrong this time because my first pregnancy was okay. We wanted to give our daughter a baby brother or sister." Indicate whether the following responses would be therapeutic (T) or nontherapeutic (N). Specify how you would change the responses determined to be nontherapeutic.

_____ "You are still young. As soon as your body heals, you will be able to try to have another baby."

_____ "What can I do that would help you and Tom cope with what happened?"

_____ "Do not worry. I am sure you did everything you could to have a healthy pregnancy."

_____ "It was probably for the best. Fetal loss at this time is usually the result of defective development."

_____ "You sound like you are blaming yourself for what happened. Let's talk about it."

_____ "This must be difficult for you and your family."

_____ "If it had to happen it is best that it happened this early in the pregnancy before you and your family became attached to the fetus."

_____ "You really should concentrate on your little daughter rather than thinking so much about the baby you lost."

_____ "I feel sad about the loss that you and Tom are experiencing."

_____ "Would you and Tom like to speak to our hospital's chaplain before you are discharged?"

8. Angela gave birth vaginally to a stillborn fetus at 38 weeks of gestation. In addition to emotional support, her physical needs must be recognized and met. Identify these physical needs and how you would meet them.

9. Anita gave birth to a baby boy who died shortly thereafter as a result of multiple congenital anomalies, including anencephaly. She and her husband, Bill, are provided with the opportunity to see their baby.

   a. Discuss how the nurse can help Anita and Bill make a decision about seeing their baby that is right for them.

   b. Anita and Bill decide to see their baby. Specify the measures the nurse can use to make the time Anita and Bill spend with their baby as easy as possible and to provide them with an experience that will facilitate the grieving process.

24 Physiologic Adaptations of the Newborn

I. REVIEWING KEY CONCEPTS AND CONTENT

Neonatal nurses are responsible for the assessment of the physiologic integrity of newborns. As part of this responsibility the nurse must be aware of the significance of data collected. Label each of the following assessment findings, if present in a group of 3 full-term newborns who were born 12 hours ago, as N (reflective of normal adaptation or acceptable variation to extrauterine life) or P (reflective of potential problems with adaptation to extrauterine life).

Assessment Finding	Evaluation
1. Crackles upon auscultation of the lungs	_____
2. Respirations: 36, irregular, shallow	_____
3. Episodic apnea lasting 5 to 10 seconds	_____
4. Nasal flaring and sternal retractions	_____
5. Slight bluish discoloration of feet and hands	_____
6. Blood pressure 78/42	_____
7. Apical rate: 126 with murmurs	_____
8. Temperature 37.1° C axillary	_____
9. Head 34 cm and chest 36 cm	_____
10. Boggy, edematous swelling over occiput	_____
11. Overlapping of parietal bones	_____
12. White pimple-like spots on nose and chin	_____
13. Jaundice on face and chest	_____
14. Regurgitation of small amount of milk after feedings	_____
15. Liver palpated 1 cm below right costal margin	_____
16. Absence of bowel elimination since birth	_____
17. Spine straight with dimple at base	_____
18. Adhesion of prepuce—unable to fully retract	_____
19. Edema of scrotum and labia	_____

Assessment Finding	Evaluation
20. Hyperextension of toes with dorsiflexion of big toe when sole is stroked upward	_____
21. Hematocrit 36% and hemoglobin 12 g/dl	_____
22. White blood cell (WBC) count 23,000/mm³	_____
23. Blood glucose 40 mg/dl	_____

24. The most critical adjustment that a newborn must make at birth is the establishment of respirations. List the factors that are responsible for the initiation of breathing after birth.

FILL IN THE BLANKS: Insert the term that corresponds to each of the following descriptions related to temperature regulation in the newborn.

25. _____ is the maintenance of balance between heat loss and heat production. _____ from excessive heat loss is a common and dangerous problem in neonates. Heat production is referred to as _____. Nonshivering thermogenesis is accomplished primarily by _____, which is unique to the newborn and secondarily by increased _____ in the brain, heart, and liver.

26. Major factors that increase a newborn's risk for thermogenic problems when compared with a child or an adult include less of an ability to _____, _____ closer to body surface, and larger _____. The _____ position of the newborn helps guard against heat loss by decreasing the amount of _____ exposed to the environment.

27. _____ is the flow of heat from the body surface to cooler ambient air. Two measures to reduce heat loss by this method would be to keep the ambient air at _____ and _____ the infant.

28. _____ is the loss of heat from the body surface to a cooler, solid surface not in direct contact but in relative proximity. To prevent this type of heat loss, _____ and _____ are placed away from outside _____ and care is taken to avoid a direct _____.

29. _____ is the loss of heat that occurs when a liquid is converted to vapor. This heat loss can be intensified by failure to _____ the newborn directly after birth or by _____ the newborn too slowly after a bath.

30. _____ is the loss of heat from the body surface to cooler surfaces in direct contact. When admitted to the nursery, the newborn is placed in a _____ to minimize heat loss.

31. Specify the guidelines a nurse should follow to ensure accuracy of the findings and safety of the newborn when measuring the newborn. Indicate the expected range for the full-term newborn.

    a. Weight

    b. Head circumference

    c. Chest circumference

    d. Abdominal circumference

    e. Length

MATCHING: Match the description in Column I with the appropriate newborn reflex from Column II.

<table>
<tr><td align="center">COLUMN I</td><td align="center">COLUMN II</td></tr>
</table>

32. _____ Apply pressure to feet with fingers when the lower limbs are semi-flexed—legs extend.

    a. Rooting

33. _____ Place infant on flat surface and strike surface—symmetric abduction and extension of arms, fingers fan out, thumb and forefinger form a **C**, slight tremor may occur.

    b. Grasp

    c. Extrusion

34. _____ Place finger in palm of hand or at base of toes— infant's fingers curl around examiner's finger, toes curl downward.

    d. Glabellar (Myerson)

35. _____ Place infant prone on flat surface, run finger down side of back 4 to 5 cm lateral to spine—body flexes and pelvis swings toward stimulated side.

    e. Tonic neck

    f. Moro

36. _____ Tap over forehead, bridge of nose, or maxilla when eyes are open—blinks for first four to five taps.

    g. Stepping (walking)

37. _____ Use finger to stroke sole of foot beginning at heel, upward along lateral aspect of sole, then across ball of foot—all toes hyperextend, with dorsiflexion of big toe.

    h. Wink reflex

    i. Babinski

38. _____ Anal sphincter responds to touch by opening and closing.

    j. Truncal incurvation (Galant)

39. _____ Testes retract when infant is chilled.

    k. Magnet

40. _____ Touch infant's lip, cheek, or corner of mouth with nipple— turns head toward stimulus, opens mouth, takes hold, and sucks.

    l. Cremasteric

41. _____ Place infant in a supine position, turn head to side—arm and leg extend on side to which head is turned while opposite arm and leg flex.

42. _____ Hold infant vertically, allowing one foot to touch table surface—infant alternates flexion and extension of its feet.

43. _____ Touch or depress tip of tongue—tongue is forced outward.

FILL IN THE BLANKS: Insert the term that corresponds to each of the following descriptions of newborn behavioral characteristics.

44. Variations in the state of consciousness of newborn infants are called the _____ states.

45. The sleep states are _____ sleep and _____ sleep.

46. The wake states are _____, _____, _____, and _____. The optimum state of arousal is the _____ state in which the infant can be observed smiling, responding to voices, watching faces, vocalizing, and moving in synchrony.

47. The newborn sleeps about _____ hours a day, with periods of wakefulness gradually _____.

48. _____ is a protective mechanism that allows the infant to become accustomed to environmental stimuli. It is a psychologic and physiologic phenomenon in which the response to a constant or repetitive stimulus is decreased.

49. _____ refers to the quality of alert states and ability to attend to visual and auditory stimuli while alert.

50. _____ or
_____, refers to individual
variations in a newborn's primary reaction
pattern. The three major types are the
_____ child, _____
child, and _____ child.

51. Describe how each of the following factors can
influence a newborn's behavior.

a. Gestational age

c. Stimuli

b. Time

d. Medication

52. During the first 6 to 8 hours after birth, newborns experience a transitional period characterized by three
phases of instability. Complete the following table by identifying the timing/duration and typical behaviors
for each phase of this transitional period.

Phase	Timing/Duration	Typical Behaviors
First Period of Reactivity		
Period of Diminished Response		
Second Period of Reactivity		

**TRUE OR FALSE: Circle T if true or F if false for
each of the following statements. Correct the false
statements.**

53. T   F   Crackles, audible grunting, nasal flaring,
and retractions of the chest are often noted
during the second period of reactivity.

54. T   F   The white blood cell count increases
significantly when the newborn develops an
infection.

55. T   F   Vitamin K administered intramuscularly
(IM) to a newborn immediately after birth
enhances clotting, thereby preventing excessive
bleeding.

56. T   F   Blood-tinged mucus on the diaper of the
female newborn should be documented by the
nurse as pseudomenstruation and recognized as
an expected assessment finding related to the
withdrawal of maternal estrogen.

57. T   F   A newborn usually loses approximately
20% of its birth weight during the first 3 to
5 days of life as a result of fluid loss, limited fluid
intake, and an increased metabolic rate.

58. T F   Jitteriness and tremors may indicate that the newborn is experiencing hypoglycemia.

59. T F   Physiologic jaundice in the full-term newborn disappears by the end of the first week of life.

60. T F   Abdominal movements are counted when determining the respiratory rate of newborns.

61. T F   The first meconium stool often has a strong odor as a result of bacteria present in the fetal intestine during intrauterine life.

62. T F   The wink reflex can be used to test the anal sphincter.

63. T F   Breast tissue in full-term male and female newborns may be swollen and secrete a thin milky-type discharge.

64. T F   The presence of a click and asymmetric movement during Ortolani's maneuver indicates hip dislocation or dysplasia.

65. T F   Rectal thermometers should be avoided when assessing a newborn's temperature.

66. T F   Jaundice first appears when the serum bilirubin level reaches 12 mg/dl.

FILL IN THE BLANKS: Insert the term that corresponds to each of the following descriptions of typical newborn physical characteristics.

67. _____ Pinkish, easily blanched areas on the upper eyelids, nose, upper lip, back of head, and nape of neck. They are also known as stork bites.

68. _____ Overlapping of cranial bones to facilitate passage of the fetal head through the maternal pelvis during the process of labor and birth.

69. _____ Generalized, easily identifiable edematous area of the scalp usually over the occiput area.

70. _____ Collection of blood between skull bone and its periosteum as a result of pressure during birth.

71. _____ Bluish-black pigmented areas usually found on back and buttocks.

72. _____ Bluish discoloration of the hands and feet, especially when chilled.

73. _____ White, cheesy substance that coats and protects the fetus's skin while in utero.

74. _____ White facial pimples caused by distended sebaceous glands.

75. _____ Yellowish skin discoloration caused by increased levels of serum bilirubin.

76. _____ Thick, tarry, dark green–black stool usually passed within 24 hours of birth.

77. _____ Sudden, transient newborn rash characterized by erythematous macules, papules, and small vesicles.

78. _____ Transient cross-eyed appearance lasting until the third or fourth month of life.

79. _____ Color variation related to vasoconstriction on one side of the body and vasodilation on the other side of the body.

80. _____ Accumulation of fluid in the scrotum, around the testes.

81. _____ Monilial infection of the oral cavity resulting in white plaques on buccal mucosa and tongue that bleed when touched.

82. _____ Membranous area formed where skull bones join.

83. _____ Soft, downy hair on face, shoulders, and back.

MULTIPLE CHOICE QUESTIONS: Circle the one correct option and state the rationale for the option chosen.

84. A newborn, at 5 hours old, wakes from a sound sleep and becomes very active. He exhibits the following signs when assessed. Which one would require further assessment?
   a. Increased mucus production
   b. Passage of meconium
   c. Heart rate of 160 beats per minute
   d. Two apneic episodes of 20 and 24 seconds' duration

85. When assessing a newborn boy at 12 hours of age, the nurse notes a rash on his abdomen and thighs. The rash appears as irregular reddish blotches with pale centers. The nurse would
   a. document the finding as erythema toxicum.
   b. isolate the newborn and his mother until infection is ruled out.

c. apply an antiseptic ointment to each lesion.

d. request nonallergenic linen from the laundry.

86. A newborn girl is 12 hours old and is being prepared for early discharge. Which of the following assessment findings, if present, could delay discharge?

a. Dark green-black stool, tarry in consistency

b. Yellowish tinge in sclera and on face

c. Blood glucose level of 55 mg/dl

d. Rust stain on diaper after urination

87. As part of a thorough assessment of a newborn the nurse should check for hip dislocation and dysplasia. Which of the following techniques would the nurse most likely use?

a. Check for syndactyly bilaterally

b. Stepping or walking reflex

c. Magnet reflex

d. Ortolani's maneuver

88. When assessing a newborn after birth, the nurse notes flat, irregular, pinkish marks on the bridge of the nose, nape of neck, and over the eyelids. The areas blanch when pressed with a finger. The nurse would document this finding as

a. milia.

b. nevus vasculosus.

c. telangiectatic nevi.

d. nevus flammeus.

II. THINKING CRITICALLY

1. Newborns are at risk for cold stress.

a. State the dangers that cold stress poses for the newborn.

b. Identify one nursing diagnosis and one expected outcome related to this danger.

c. Describe care measures the nurse should implement to prevent cold stress from occurring.

2. After a long and difficult labor, baby boy James was born with a caput succedaneum and significant molding over the occipital area. Low forceps were used for the birth, resulting in ecchymotic areas on both cheeks. Describe what you would tell the parents of James about these assessment findings.

3. Mary and Jim are concerned that their baby boy who weighed 8 lb 6 oz at birth now, at 2 days of age, "weighs only 7 lb 14 oz." Describe how you would respond to their concern.

4. Susan and Allen are first-time parents of a baby girl. They ask the nurse about their baby's ability to see and hear things around her and to interact with them.

   a. Specify what the nurse should tell these parents about the sensory capabilities of their healthy full-term newborn.

   b. Name four stimuli Susan and Allen could provide for their baby that would help foster her development.

5. Tonya and Sam, an African-American couple, express concern that their new baby girl has several bruises on her back and buttocks. They ask if their baby was injured during birth or in the nursery. Describe the appropriate response of the nurse to this couple's concern.

Nursing Care of the Newborn (25)

I. REVIEWING KEY CONCEPTS AND CONTENT

TRUE OR FALSE: Circle T if true or F if false for each of the following statements. Correct the false statements.

1. T   F   Placing a dressed newborn under a radiant warmer facilitates a faster stabilization of body temperature after birth.

2. T   F   The thermistor probe of a radiant heat panel should be taped to the upper quadrant of the abdomen just below the intercostal margin (ribs) on the right or left side.

3. T   F   The nurse should wear gloves, gown, and mask when handling a newborn until blood and amniotic fluid have been removed.

4. T   F   Wearing gloves when caring for the newborn is the single most important measure in the prevention of neonatal infection.

5. T   F   For the first 12 hours after birth, a newborn's temperature should be taken rectally.

6. T   F   The Apgar Score is used to evaluate the newborn's transition to extrauterine life.

7. T   F   Umbilical cord separation from the abdomen usually occurs by the end of the first week after birth

8. T   F   Hearing screening should be done when the newborn is 2 weeks of age or older.

9. T   F   A newborn whose mother received magnesium sulfate during labor may be lethargic after birth.

10. T   F   The recommended site for intramuscular injections in the newborn is the dorsogluteal muscle.

11. T   F   A major preventive measure for hyperbilirubinemia is early feeding of the newborn.

12. T   F   If bleeding is noted after a circumcision, the nurse should apply gentle pressure to the site of bleeding using a folded sterile gauze pad.

13. T   F   To facilitate obtaining a heel stick blood sample, the loose application of a warm wet wash cloth around the foot for 5 to 10 minutes is sufficient to dilate the blood vessels in the heel.

14. T   F   An alcohol swab should be used to apply pressure to the heel after a blood sample is obtained.

15. T   F   Pressure with a dry gauze should be applied over an arterial puncture for at least 3 to 5 minutes to prevent bleeding from the site.

16. T   F   Before the application of a U bag, the genitalia, perineum, and surrounding skin should be sprinkled with talcum powder to prevent irritation of the skin.

17. T   F   Nonnutritive sucking with a pacifier or finger should be discouraged in the infant because it leads to malformation of the jaw and to dependency.

18. T   F   The ointment used for eye prophylaxis should be flushed out of the eyes with normal saline 5 minutes after instillation.

19. T   F   When using the neonatal postoperative pain scale, a score of greater than 4 indicates that the infant is experiencing significant pain.

20. T   F   A blood glucose level of less than 50 mg/dl during the early newborn period is indicative of hypoglycemia.

21. T   F   Hepatitis B vaccine should only be administered to newborns exposed to the hepatitis B virus.

22. T   F   The supine position should be used for the first few months of life to reduce the risk for sudden infant death syndrome (SIDS).

23. T   F   When using a bulb syringe, the nose should be suctioned before the mouth.

24. T   F   Infants should be placed in a rear-facing car seat that is secured in the back seat of the car.

FILL IN THE BLANKS: Insert the term that corresponds to each of the following descriptions of newborns and their care.

25. _____ or _____ ointment is used to prevent ophthalmia neonatorum. It should be instilled into the newborn's _____, from the _____ to the _____.

26. _____ is administered intramuscularly to newborns to prevent hemorrhage. It is administered in a dose of _____ using a _____ gauge, _____ inch needle.

27. The umbilical cord site should be assessed for _____, _____, and _____ at each diaper change. The skin around the base of the cord can be cleansed with _____, _____, _____, or _____. The clamp is removed approximately _____ when the cord is _____.

28. The _____ test is performed to distinguish cutaneous jaundice from normal skin color. It is performed by applying pressure with a finger over a bony area usually the _____, _____, or _____ for several seconds to empty all capillaries in the spot. The area will appear _____ when the finger is removed if jaundice is present.

29. _____ is the yellow staining of brain cells that may result in bilirubin encephalopathy.

30. _____ or _____ is that level of serum bilirubin, which if left untreated, can result in sensorineural _____, mild _____ delays, and _____.

31. CRIES is the _____. C refers to _____, R refers to _____, I refers to _____, E refers to _____, and S refers to _____.

32. EMLA refers to a topical method of pain management that involves application of _____ to reduce pain resulting from circumcision, venous or arterial puncture, and percutaneous venous catheter placement.

33. Gestational age assessment should be performed within the first _____ hours of life to ensure accuracy. When assessing gestational age _____ maturity and _____ maturity are determined using the New Ballard scale.

34. Outline the specific measures nurses should use when caring for newborns to ensure a safe and protective environment.

35. Birth trauma includes physical injury sustained by the newborn during labor and birth. Identify the predisposing factors for injury in each of the following categories.

    a. Maternal factors

    b. Fetal factors

    c. Factors related to intrapartum events and childbirth techniques

36. Nurses caring for newborns as they recover following their birth must be alert for signs of hypoglycemia and hypocalcemia. Complete the following table related to the signs, risk factors, and care management of hypoglycemia and hypocalcemia.

Imbalance	Signs	Risk Factors	Care Management
Hypoglycemia			
Hypocalcemia			

37. Preparing parents for the discharge of their newborn requires informing them about the essential aspects of newborn care. Identify three points that you would emphasize when teaching parents about each of the following aspects of newborn characteristics and care:

   a. Vital signs: temperature and respirations

   b. Feeding

   c. Elimination: urinary and bowel

   d. Positioning and holding

   e. Safety

   f. Hygiene: bathing, cord care, and skin care

38. Maintaining a patent airway and supporting respirations to ensure an adequate oxygen supply in the newborn are essential focuses of nursing care management of the newborn, especially in the early postbirth period.

   a. State the four conditions that are essential for maintaining an adequate oxygen supply in the newborn.

   b. List four signs that the nurse who is assessing a newborn would recognize as indicative of abnormal breathing.

   c. Describe three methods of relieving airway obstruction in an infant.

MULTIPLE CHOICE QUESTIONS: Circle the one correct option and state the rationale for the option chosen.

39. A newborn male is estimated to be at 40 weeks of gestation following an assessment using the New Ballard scale. Which of the following would be a Ballard scale finding consistent with this newborn's full-term status?
   a. Apical pulse rate of 120 beats per minute, regular, and strong
   b. Popliteal angle of 160°
   c. Weight of 3200 g, placing him at the 50th percentile
   d. Thinning of lanugo with some bald areas

40. The nurse evaluates the laboratory test results of a newborn who is 4 hours old. Which of the following results would require notification of the pediatrician?
    a. Hemoglobin 20 g/dl
    b. Hematocrit 54%
    c. Glucose 34 mg/dl
    d. Total serum bilirubin 0.6 mg/dl

41. A newborn male has been designated as large for gestational age. His mother was diagnosed with gestational diabetes late in her pregnancy. The nurse should be alert for signs of hypoglycemia. Which of the following assessment findings would be consistent with a diagnosis of hypoglycemia?
    a. Unstable body temperature
    b. Cyanosis
    c. Loose, watery stools
    d. Abdominal distention

42. A radiant warmer will be used to help a newborn girl to stabilize her temperature. The nurse implementing this care measure should
    a. undress and dry the infant before placing her under the warmer.
    b. set the control panel between 35° to 38° C.
    c. place the thermistor probe on her abdomen just above her umbilical cord.
    d. assess her rectal temperature every hour until her temperature stabilizes.

43. A newborn male has been scheduled for a circumcision. Essential nursing care measures as part of this surgical procedure would include which one of the following?
    a. Feed the infant just before the procedure to help him remain relaxed and quiet.
    b. Apply petroleum jelly or A&D ointment to the site with every diaper change until site is healed.
    c. Check the penis for bleeding every 15 minutes for the first 4 hours.
    d. Teach the parents to remove the yellowish exudate that forms over the glans using a diaper wipe.

II. THINKING CRITICALLY

1. Apgar scoring is a method of newborn assessment used in the immediate postbirth period, at 1 and 5 minutes. Indicate the Apgar score for each of the following newborns.

    a. Baby boy Smith at 1 minute after birth:
       Heart rate—160 beats/min
       Respiratory effort—good, crying vigorously
       Muscle tone—active movement, well flexed
       Reflex irritability—cries with stimulus to soles of feet
       Color—body pink, feet and hands cyanotic
          Score: _____
          Interpretation:

b. Baby girl Doe at 5 minutes after birth:
   Heart rate—102 beats/min
   Respiratory effort—slow, irregular with weak cry
   Muscle tone—some flexion of extremities
   Reflex irritability—grimace with stimulus to soles of feet
   Color—pale
      Score: _____
      Interpretation:

2. Baby girl June was just born.

   a. Outline the protocol that the nurse should follow when assessing June's physical status during the first 2 hours after her birth.

   b. State the nurse's legal responsibility regarding identification of June and her mother after birth.

   c. Cite two priority nursing diagnoses appropriate for June during the first 2 hours after birth.

   d. Identify the priority nursing care measures that the nurse must implement to ensure June's well-being and safety during the first 2 hours after birth.

3. Baby boy Tim is 24 hours old. The nurse is preparing to perform a physical examination of this newborn before his discharge.

   a. List the actions the nurse should take in order to ensure safety and accuracy. Include the rationale for the actions identified.

   b. Identify the major points that should be assessed as part of this physical examination.

   c. Support the premise that Tim's parents should be present during this examination.

4. Baby girl Susan has an accumulation of mucus in her nasal passages and mouth, making breathing difficult.

   a. State the nursing diagnosis represented by the assessment findings.

   b. List the steps that the nurse should follow when clearing Susan's airway using a bulb syringe.

   c. If mucus accumulation continues and breathing is compromised, use of a nasopharyngeal catheter with mechanical suction may be required. List the guidelines a nurse should follow when using this method to clear the newborn's airway.

5. Susan and James are taking their newly circumcised (6 hours postprocedure) baby home. This is their first baby and they express anxiety concerning care of both the circumcision and the umbilical cord.

   a. State one nursing diagnosis related to this situation.

   b. State one expected outcome related to the nursing diagnosis identified.

   c. Specify the instructions that the nurse should give to Susan and James regarding assessment of both sites and the care measures required to facilitate healing.

6. Andrew and Marion are parents of a newborn, 30 hours old, who has developed hyperbilirubinemia. They are very concerned about the color of their baby and the need to put the baby under special lights. "A relative was yellow just like our baby and later died of liver cancer!"

   a. Describe how the nurse should respond to Andrew and Marion's concern.

   b. Describe the blanch test as a method of assessment for jaundice.

   c. Identify the expected assessment findings and physiologic effects related to hyperbilirubinemia.

   d. List the precautions and care measures required by the newborn undergoing phototherapy in order to prevent injury to the newborn yet maintain the effectiveness of the treatment. State the rationale for each action identified.

7. Angela, the mother of a newborn, tells the nurse, "I know that I should get my baby immunized, but I have heard that each shot is so expensive and there are so many. Since I am breastfeeding, my baby is protected from infection anyway. Do you think it would be all right to wait until the baby's first birthday? Then he will need fewer shots." Describe how the nurse should reply to Angela.

8. A newborn is scheduled for a circumcision. The nurse caring for this newborn is aware that he will experience pain as a result of this procedure.

   a. Describe the most common behavioral responses to pain.

   b. State the factors that should be assessed if the nurse uses the Neonatal Postoperative Pain Scale to determine the level of pain this newborn is experiencing as part of the circumcision. Explain how the pain score is calculated.

c. State the nursing diagnosis reflective of this pain experience.

d. Outline the nonpharmacologic and pharmacologic measures the nurse could use or suggest be used to minimize the pain experience and its effects and maximize the newborn's ability to cope with the pain and recover.

Newborn Nutrition and Feeding 26

I. REVIEWING KEY CONCEPTS AND CONTENT

1. Calculate the daily energy (kcal) and fluid requirements for each of the following infants.

Infant	Calories (Kcal)	Fluid
a. Jim: 1 month 4 kg		
b. Sue: 4 months 6 kg		
c. Sam: 7 months 7.5 kg		

2. Development and function of lactation structures within the breast are critical to the success of lactogenesis.

   a. Label the following illustration as indicated.

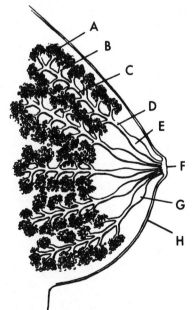

Lactation Structures of the Female Breast

b. FILL IN THE BLANKS: Insert the lactation structure that corresponds to the following descriptions:

(1). _____ Structures in the breast that are composed of alveoli, milk ductules, and myoepithelial cells.

(2). _____ Cluster of milk-producing cells.

(3). _____ Breast structure that connects several alveoli.

(4). _____ Breast structure that connects a duct to the lactiferous sinus.

(5). _____ Milk collection structures that narrow to form many openings or pores in the nipple. They are compressed with infant sucking and the milk is ejected. _____ is another name used for these structures.

(6). _____ Cells surrounding alveoli; these cells contract in response to oxytocin, resulting in the milk ejection reflex or let-down.

(7). _____ Rounded, pigmented section of tissue surrounding the nipple.

3. A nurse has been asked to participate in a women's health seminar for women of childbearing age in the community. Her topic is "Breastfeeding: The Goals for *Healthy People 2010* and Beyond." Outline the points that this nurse should emphasize to help women appreciate the benefits of breastfeeding and seriously consider breastfeeding when they have a baby.

4. It is important that a breastfeeding woman alter the position she uses for breastfeeding as one means of preserving nipple and areolar integrity. Describe four breastfeeding positions the nurse should demonstrate to a woman who is breastfeeding her newborn.

5. Infants exhibit feeding readiness cues as they recognize and express their hunger.

   a. Identify feeding readiness cues of the infant.

   b. State why the new mother should be guided by these cues when determining the timing of feeding sessions.

6. Indicate the differences between foremilk and hindmilk.

7. Label each of the following illustrations depicting the maternal breastfeeding reflexes.

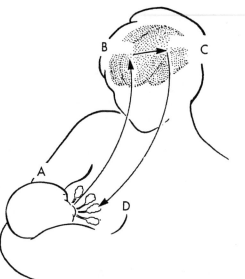

Milk Production Reflex

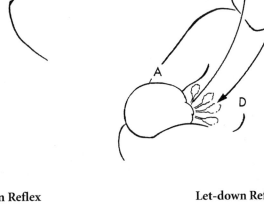

Let-down Reflex

8. There are three stages of lactogenesis. State expected time of occurrence for each stage and describe the events typical of each stage.

    a. Stage I

    b. Stage II

    c. Stage III

9. Proper latch-on is essential for effective breastfeeding and preservation of nipple and areolar tissue integrity.

    a. Indicate the steps the nurse should teach a breastfeeding woman to follow to ensure a proper latch-on.

b. When observing a woman breastfeeding, it is essential that the nurse determine the effectiveness of the latch-on. State the signs a nurse should look for that would indicate a proper latch-on.

c. Describe the way a woman should remove her baby from her breast after feeding is completed.

TRUE OR FALSE: Circle T if true or F if false for each of the following statements. Correct the false statements.

10. T   F   Approximately 75% of infants in the United States are breastfed at birth.

11. T   F   A newborn should lose no more than 15% of his or her birth weight.

12. T   F   The birth weight of a full-term newborn is usually regained within 10 to 14 days of life.

13. T   F   To prevent fat-related cardiovascular problems later in life, bottle-fed infants should be

given low-fat or skim milk after the first 6 months of life.

14. T F   Infants who are entirely breastfed should receive iron supplementation in the form of iron-containing foods such as cereals, after the first 6 months of life.

15. T F   Milk production depends primarily on the secretion of estrogen and progesterone.

16. T F   Women from some cultures avoid breastfeeding until their milk comes in because they believe that colostrum may harm the baby.

17. T T   Early and frequent feeding facilitates the elimination of bilirubin in feces, thereby reducing the incidence or severity of hyperbilirubinemia.

18. T F   Women with diabetes should avoid breastfeeding because insulin requirements are increased.

19. T F   Colostrum acts as a laxative to remove meconium from the newborn's intestine.

20. T F   Breastfed babies require vitamin C supplementation.

21. T F   Maternal smoking may impair milk production.

22. T F   When breastfeeding a newborn, mothers should avoid using a bottle for supplementary feedings until breastfeeding is well established, in about 3 to 4 weeks.

23. T F   Uterine cramping during breastfeeding indicates that oxytocin is being secreted.

24. T F   Fluoride supplementation should begin at 2 months for breastfed and bottle-fed babies not receiving fluoridated water.

25. T F   A woman with mastitis should stop breastfeeding as soon as a diagnosis of infection is made.

26. A breastfeeding woman has been having difficulty calming down her fussy baby daughter in order to feed her. Identify several techniques that the nurse could teach this woman to calm her baby in preparation for feeding.

27. Complete the following table by identifying the factors that should be assessed before and during breastfeeding and the factors for ongoing assessment as related to the infant and the breastfeeding mother.

Infant/Mother	Assessment Before and During Breastfeeding	Ongoing Assessment
Infant		
Mother		

FILL IN THE BLANKS: Insert the term that corresponds to each of the following descriptions regarding breastfeeding.

28. _____ is an infection of the breast, which may be manifested by a swollen, tender breast and sudden onset of flu-like symptoms.

29. _____ is manual application of gentle but deep pressure to the breasts in order to trigger the let-down reflex and facilitate expression of milk.

30. The process of milk production is termed _____.

31. Exposing the newborn to both breast and bottle nipples can lead to _____, a difficulty in knowing how to latch on to the breast after having taken a bottle.

32. A _____ is a health care professional who specializes in breastfeeding and may be available to assist a new mother with breastfeeding while in the hospital or after discharge.

33. _____ occurs around the third to fifth day, when the "milk comes in" and blood supply to the breasts increases. The breasts become tender, swollen, hot and hard, and even shiny and red.

34. _____ are newborn behaviors that indicate hunger and a desire to eat.

35. _____ is a process whereby the infant is gradually introduced to drinking from a cup and eating solid food while breastfeeding is reduced by gradually decreasing the number of feedings.

36. An _____ nipple becomes hard, erect, and protrudes upon stimulation, thereby facilitating latch-on. An _____ nipple remains flat and soft and does not protrude even when stimulated. A breast _____ is a plastic device that can be placed over the nipple and areola to keep clothing off the nipple and put pressure around the base of the nipple to promote protrusion of the nipple.

37. _____ is a very concentrated, high-protein, antibody-rich substance present in the breasts before the formation of milk.

38. Pituitary hormones play an essential role in lactation. _____ is the lactogenic hormone secreted by the anterior pituitary gland in response to the infant's suck and emptying of the breast. _____ is the posterior pituitary hormone that triggers the let-down reflex.

39. At times, infants cease to respond to stimulation when their feeding needs are not met and withdraw into sleep even after several attempts to awaken them for feeding. This behavior is termed _____.

40. _____ is an infection that is caused by a fungus or yeast. The newborn may exhibit signs of _____ in its mouth. Both of the mother's nipples and the baby's mouth must be treated simultaneously.

41. For the _____ position, the mother holds the baby's head and shoulders in her hand with the baby's back and body tucked under her arm. For the _____ position, the baby's head is positioned in the crook of the arm and the mother and baby are "tummy to tummy."

42. The _____ reflex, also known as the _____ reflex, is triggered by the contraction of myoepithelial cells. Colostrum, and later milk, is ejected toward the nipple.

43. The _____ reflex is stimulated when a hungry baby's lower lip is touched. The baby opens its mouth and begins to suck.

44. _____ occurs when the baby is positioned onto the breast with the mouth open wide and the tongue down. The nipple and some of the areola should be in the baby's mouth.

MULTIPLE CHOICE QUESTIONS: Circle the one correct option and state the rationale for the option chosen.

45. During a home visit, the mother of a 1-week old infant son tells the nurse that she is very concerned about whether her baby is getting enough breast milk. The nurse would tell this mother that at 1 week of age a well-nourished newborn should exhibit
    a. weight gain sufficient to reach his birth weight.
    b. a minimum of 3 bowel movements each day.
    c. approximately 10 to 12 wet diapers each day.
    d. breastfeeding at a frequency of every 4 hours or about 6 times each day.

46. A woman is trying to calm her fussy baby daughter in preparation for feeding. She exhibits a need for further instruction if she does which of the following?
    a. Removes all clothing from infant except the diaper
    b. Dims lights in the room and turns off the television
    c. Gently rocks the baby and talks to her in a low voice
    d. Allows the baby to suck on her finger

47. The nurse should teach breastfeeding mothers about breast care measures to preserve the integrity of the nipples and areola. Which of the following should the nurse include in these instructions?
    a. Cleanse nipples and areola twice a day with mild soap and water.
    b. Apply vitamin E cream to nipples and areola at least four times each day before a feeding.
    c. Insert plastic-lined pads into the bra to absorb leakage and protect clothing.
    d. Apply modified lanolin to both dry and sore nipples.

48. A breastfeeding woman asks the nurse about what birth control she should use during the postpartum period. Which is the best recommendation for a safe, yet effective method during the first 6 weeks after birth?
    a. Combination oral contraceptive that she used before she was pregnant
    b. Barrier method using a combination of a condom and spermicide foam
    c. Progestin-only contraceptive such as Depo-Provera
    d. Complete breastfeeding—baby only receives breast milk for nourishment

49. A woman has determined that bottle-feeding is the best feeding method for her. Instructions the woman should receive regarding this feeding method should include which of the following?
    a. Check nipple before feeding to ensure that it allows passage of formula in a slow stream.
    b. Sterilize water by boiling, then cool and mix with formula powder or concentrate.
    c. Expect a 1-week-old newborn to drink approximately 30 to 60 ml of formula at each feeding.
    d. Microwave refrigerated formula before feeding the newborn.

II. THINKING CRITICALLY

1. Evaluate each of the following actions of Janet, a breastfeeding mother. Determine if the action indicates competency (+) or a need for further instruction (−). Indicate what information you would give Janet to correct actions that require further instruction.

   a. _____ Washes her breasts and nipples thoroughly with soap and water twice a day.

   b. _____ Massages a small amount of breast milk into her nipple and areola before and after each feeding.

   c. _____ Lines her bra with a thick plastic-lined pad to absorb leakage.

   d. _____ Positions baby supporting back and shoulders securely and then brings her breast toward the baby putting the nipple in the baby's mouth.

   e. _____ Alternates breastfeeding positions among football, cradle, modified cradle, and lying-down holds.

   f. _____ Limits breastfeeding at the first breast to a maximum of 10 minutes then switches to the second breast.

   g. _____ Supports her breast with the thumb on top and four fingers underneath the breast at the back edge of the areola.

   h. _____ Inserts her finger into the corner of her baby's mouth between the gums before removing him from the breast.

   i. _____ Awakens the baby every 2 to 3 hours day and night to feed.

j. _____ Increases her fluid intake to 3 L/day by drinking water, coffee, herbal teas, juice, milk, cola, and wine.

k. _____ Increases her caloric intake by approximately 500 calories each day with a gradual weight loss noted.

l. _____ Plans to use the "pill" for birth control beginning at 3 weeks postpartum.

2. Tonya is bottle-feeding her baby. She expresses concern to the nurse at the well-baby clinic about heart disease and cholesterol levels as they relate to her 2-month-old baby. She tells the nurse that her family has a history of cardiac disease and hypertension and she has already changed her diet and wants to do the same for her baby. Tonya asks, "When should I start giving my baby skim milk instead of the prepared formula that I am using, which seems to contain quite a bit of fat?" Discuss how the nurse should respond to Tonya's question.

3. Elise and her husband, Mark, are experiencing their first pregnancy. During one of their prenatal visits, they tell the nurse that they are as yet unsure about the method they want to use for feeding their baby. "Everyone has an opinion—some say breastfeeding is best, yet others tell us that bottle feeding is more convenient, especially because the father can help. What should we do?"

a. Identify one nursing diagnosis and one expected outcome appropriate for this situation.

b. Discuss why it is important for the pregnant couple to make this decision together.

c. Indicate why is it preferable to make this decision during the prenatal period rather than waiting until the baby is born.

d. Describe how the nurse could use the decision-making process to assist Elise and Mark to choose the method that is best for them.

4. Mary, as a first-time breastfeeding mother, has many questions. Describe how you would respond to the following questions and comments.

a. "I am so afraid that I will not make enough milk for my baby. My breasts are not as large as some of my friends who breastfeed."

b. "Everyone keeps talking about this let-down that is supposed to happen. What is it and how will I know I have it?"

c. "How can I possibly know if breastfeeding is going well and my baby is getting enough if I cannot tell how many ounces he gets with each feeding?"

d. "It is only the first day that I am breastfeeding and my nipples already feel sore. What can I do to relieve this soreness and prevent it from getting worse?"

e. "My friends all told me to watch out for the fourth day and engorgement. What can I do to keep it from being too bad and to take care of myself when it occurs?"

f. "Every time I breastfeed, I get cramps and my flow seems to get heavier. Is there something wrong with me?"

g. "I am so glad I do not have to worry about getting pregnant again as long as I am breastfeeding. I hate using birth control and my friend told me I do not have to as long as I am breastfeeding."

h. "What should I do when I am ready to stop feeding my baby?"

5. Susan is 2 days old. She last fed 5 hours ago. Her mother tells the nurse that Susan is so sleepy that she just does not have the heart to wake her.

a. Identify one nursing diagnosis and one expected outcome appropriate for this newborn.

b. Discuss the approach the nurse should take with regard to this situation.

6. Alice has decided that for personal and professional reasons, bottle-feeding with a commercially prepared formula is the feeding method that is best for her. She tells the nurse that she hopes she made a good decision for her baby. "I hope she will be well nourished and feel that I love her even though I am bottle-feeding."

   a. Describe how the nurse should respond to Alice's concern.

   b. State three guidelines for bottle-feeding technique that the nurse should teach Alice to ensure the safety and health of her baby.

27 Infants with Gestational Age-Related Problems

I. REVIEWING KEY CONCEPTS AND CONTENT

FILL IN THE BLANKS: Insert the term that corresponds to each of the following descriptions related to gestational age and intrauterine growth.

1. An infant whose birth weight is less than 2500 g, regardless of gestational age is described as being _____. An infant whose birth weight is less than 1500 g is described as being _____, whereas an infant whose birth weight is less than 1000 g is described as being _____.

2. An infant born before completion of 37 weeks of gestation, regardless of birth weight is described as being _____ or _____.

3. An infant born between the beginning of 38 weeks and the completion of 42 weeks of gestation, regardless of birth weight is described as being _____.

4. An infant born after 42 weeks of gestational age, regardless of birth weight is described as being _____ or _____.

5. An infant whose birth weight falls above the 90th percentile on intrauterine growth curves is described as being _____.

6. An infant whose birth weight falls between the 10th and the 90th percentiles on intrauterine growth curves is described as being _____.

7. An infant whose rate of intrauterine growth was restricted and whose birth weight falls below the 10th percentile on intrauterine growth curves is described as being _____ or _____.

8. _____is found in infants whose intrauterine growth is restricted. Growth restriction in which the weight, length, and head circumference are all affected is termed _____. Growth restriction in which the head circumference remains within normal parameters and the birth weight falls below the 10th percentile is termed _____.

9. _____ is a birth in which the neonate manifests any heartbeat, breathes, or displays voluntary movement, regardless of gestational age.

10. _____ is a death of a fetus after 20 weeks of gestation and before delivery, with absence of any signs of life after birth.

11. _____ is a death that occurs in the first 27 days of life; _____ occurs in the first week of life, and _____ occurs at 7 to 27 days.

12. _____ refers to the total number of fetal and early neonatal deaths per 1000 live births.

TRUE OR FALSE: Circle T if true or F if false for each of the following statements. Correct the false statements.

13. T F   An extremely-low-birth-weight (ELBW) infant is one whose weight at birth is 2000 g or less.

14. T F   Eight months after birth, an infant born at 28 weeks of gestation would be considered to be the corrected age of 5 months.

15. T F   The incidence of physical and emotional abuse is higher in infants who, because of preterm birth or illness, were separated from their parents for a time after birth.

16. T F   Preterm infants are at risk for polycythemia.

17. T F   Neonatal respiratory distress with hypoxemia can result in opening up of the ductus arteriosus.

18. T   F   For preterm infants a PaO_2 of less than 60 mm Hg or an oxygen saturation of less than 92% indicates the need for oxygen therapy.

19. T   F   Surfactant is administered intravenously to a preterm infant.

20. T   F   Infants born before 36 weeks of gestation require exogenous surfactant administration to survive extrauterine life.

21. T   F   Infants who need oxygen should have their respiratory status assessed accurately every 1 to 2 hours.

22. T   F   Acrocyanosis is an assessment finding indicative of an underlying respiratory disorder.

23. T   F   A preterm newborn's temperature should be monitored rectally to enhance accuracy.

24. T   F   High risk infants usually have lower caloric, nutrient, and fluid requirements than those of the full-term, normal newborn.

25. T   F   The flow rate for a gavage tube feeding should approximate that of an oral feeding (1 ml/minute).

26. T   F   Nonnutritive sucking during gavage feedings can facilitate the preterm newborn's transition to nipple feeding.

27. T   F   The weight of most postmature infants is appropriate for gestational age (AGA).

28. T   F   When meconium is present in the amniotic fluid at birth, the infant should be suctioned below the vocal cords before the infant takes its first breath.

29. T   F   Preterm infants should have blood glucose values equal to 36 mg/dl within the first few hours of life.

30. T   F   Excessive hair growth on the external ear (hypertrichosis) has been noted in infants of diabetic mothers who are affected by caudal regressive syndrome.

31. T   F   The fetal mortality rate from an episode of maternal ketoacidosis can be as high as 50% or more.

32. T   F   Glucose control early in pregnancy has little effect on the incidence of congenital anomalies in the infants of women with pregestational diabetes.

33. Explain the purpose of exogenous surfactant administration to the preterm newborn.

34. Describe kangaroo care.

35. The preterm infant is vulnerable to a number of complications related to immaturity of body systems. Complete the following table by identifying the potential problems and their physiologic basis for each of the physiologic functions listed.

Physiologic Function	Potential Problems	Physiologic Basis
Respiratory Function		
Cardiovascular Function		
Maintaining Body Temperature		
Central Nervous System Function		
Maintaining Adequate Nutrition		
Maintaining Renal Function		
Maintaining Hematologic Status		
Resisting Infection		

MATCHING: Match the description in Column I with the appropriate complication associated with prematurity in Column II.

COLUMN I

36. _____ Complex, multicausal disorder that affects the developing blood vessels in the eyes; it is often associated with oxygen tensions that are too high for the level of retinal maturity initially resulting in vasoconstriction and continuing problems after the oxygen is discontinued.

37. _____ Acute inflammatory disease of the gastrointestinal mucosa commonly complicated by perforation.

38. _____ Occurs when the fetal shunt between the pulmonary artery and the aorta fails to constrict after birth or reopens after constriction has occurred.

COLUMN II

a. Chronic lung disease (CLD)

b. Retinopathy of prematurity (ROP)

c. Patent ductus arteriosus (PDA)

d. Periventricular-intraventricular hemorrhage (PV-IVH)

e. Necrotizing enterocolitis (NEC)

39. _____ Chronic pulmonary iatrogenic condition caused by barotrauma from pressure ventilation and oxygen toxicity.

40. _____ One of the most common types of brain injury encountered in the neonatal period and among the most severe in both short-term and long-term outcomes.

41. Respiratory distress syndrome (RDS) is a lung disorder usually associated with preterm birth.

    a. Respiratory distress syndrome (RDS) is caused by a lack of pulmonary _____, which leads to progressive _____, loss of functional _____, and _____ imbalance, with an uneven distribution of _____.

    b. Clinical signs of RDS include _____, _____, _____, intercostal or subcostal _____, _____, respiratory or mixed _____, _____, and _____. These respiratory symptoms usually occur immediately after _____ or within _____ hours. Physical examination reveals _____, poor _____, _____, use of _____, and occasionally _____.

    c. RDS is usually self-limiting with respiratory symptoms abating after_____ hours. The disappearance of symptoms coincides with _____ production.

    d. Treatment for RDS is supportive. It involves establishment and maintenance of adequate_____ and _____, administration of exogenous _____, and maintenance of a _____ environment.

    FILL IN THE BLANKS: Insert the term that corresponds to the following descriptions of diabetes mellitus during pregnancy and the effect on the newborn.

42. Infants born to mothers with diabetes are at increased risk for some complications.

    a. The incidence of congenital anomalies for infants born to mothers with pregestational diabetes is _____ higher than for infants born to mothers without diabetes.

During early pregnancy, congenital anomalies are believed to be caused by fluctuations in _____ levels and episodes of _____. Later in pregnancy, maternal _____ forces high levels of _____ to cross the placenta, stimulating the fetal pancreas to secrete increased amounts of _____. This event results in excessive fetal _____ called _____. In addition, if the blood of a pregnant diabetic woman becomes more _____ than fetal blood, as occurs during _____, _____ or _____ exchange will be diminished. There are indications that some neonatal conditions, namely _____, _____, _____, _____, and perhaps fetal _____ may be eliminated or the incidence decreased if maternal _____ levels are maintained within the narrow limits of _____ to _____ mg/dl.

    b. Identify the most common congenital anomalies experienced by infants with diabetic mothers in terms of each of the following:

    Cardiac

    Central nervous system

    Musculoskeletal

43. Baby boy Robert, weighing 11 pounds 4 ounces, was born 1 hour ago. His mother had gestational diabetes mellitus.

    a. Describe the typical characteristics exhibited by a macrosomic infant such as Robert.

    b. Robert, as a macrosomic infant, is most at risk for the complications of

    _____,
    _____,
    _____, and
    _____.

    c. Describe the warning signs for each of the potential complications of which the nurse should be aware when assessing Robert during the first 24 hours after birth.

MULTIPLE CHOICE QUESTIONS: Circle the one correct option and state the rationale for the option chosen.

44. Preterm infants are at increased risk for developing respiratory distress. The nurse should assess for signs that would indicate that the newborn is having difficulty breathing. Which of the following is a sign of respiratory distress?
    a. Use of abdominal muscles to breathe
    b. Respiratory rate of 40 breaths/min or greater
    c. Periodic breathing pattern with a 5- to 10-second respiratory pause followed by 10 to 15 seconds of rapid breathing
    d. Suprasternal retraction

45. When caring for a preterm infant at 30 weeks of gestation, the nurse should recognize which of the following as the newborn's primary nursing diagnosis?
    a. Risk for infection related to decreased immune response
    b. Impaired gas exchange related to deficiency of surfactant
    c. Ineffective thermoregulation related to immature thermoregulation center
    d. Imbalanced nutrition: less than body requirements related to ineffective suck and swallow

46. A nurse is preparing to insert a gavage tube and feed a preterm newborn. As part of the protocol for this procedure the nurse would
    a. determine the length of tubing to be inserted by measuring from tip of nose to lobe of ear to midpoint between xiphoid process and umbilicus.
    b. coat the tube with water-soluble lubricant to ease passage.
    c. insert the tube through the nose as the preferred route for most infants.
    d. check placement of the tube by injecting 2 to 3 ml of sterile water into the tube and listening for gurgling with a stethoscope.

47. The nurse is caring for a newborn whose mother had gestational diabetes. His estimated gestational age is 41 weeks, and his weight indicates that he is macrosomic. When assessing this newborn, the nurse should be alert for which of the following?
    a. Fracture of the femur
    b. Hypercalcemia
    c. Blood glucose level less than 40 mg/dl
    d. Signs of a congenital heart defect

II. THINKING CRITICALLY

1. Oxygen therapy is a vital component in the care of the newborn experiencing respiratory distress.

    a. Identify the criteria that should be used to determine if there is a need for supplemental oxygen.

b. Create a set of general guidelines that reflects the recommended principles for safe and effective administration of oxygen to a compromised newborn.

c. Complete the following table by specifying the indications for each of the following methods of oxygen therapy and describing the care measures required to ensure their safe and effective administration.

Method	Indications	Nursing Measures
Oxygen Hood		
Nasal Cannula		
Continuous Distending Pressure		
Mechanical Ventilation		

2. Baby girl Jane has been receiving oxygen therapy. Her health care providers are preparing to begin the process of weaning her from the oxygen.

   a. Describe signs that would indicate that Jane is ready to be weaned from oxygen therapy.

   b. Outline the guidelines that should be followed when weaning Jane from oxygen therapy.

3. Anne, a 3 pound 12 ounce (1705 g) preterm newborn at 32 weeks of gestation, is admitted to the neonatal intensive care unit (NICU) after her birth for observation and supportive care. Anne's nutritional needs are a critical concern in her care. Oral formula feedings are attempted first.

   a. State the assessment data that the nurse should document after each of Anne's feedings to indicate feeding method effectiveness.

b. The nurse determines that Anne's suck is weak and she becomes too fatigued during oral feedings to obtain sufficient nutrients and fluid. The nurse confers with the neonatologist and a decision is made to provide intermittent gavage feedings with occasional oral feedings. Describe the guidelines the nurse should follow when inserting the gavage tube.

c. State the priority nursing diagnosis for Anne.

d. Discuss the principles the nurse should follow before, during, and after a gavage feeding to ensure safety and maximum effectiveness.

e. Outline the protocol that should be followed when advancing Anne back to full oral feeding.

4. The NICU is a stressful environment for preterm infants and their families.

a. Identify the common sources of stress facing infants and their families in an intensive care environment.

Infant stressors

Family stressors

b. Nurses working in the NICU must be aware of infant cues and adjust stimuli accordingly. List infant cues that indicate overstimulation and infant cues that indicate a relaxed state.

Overstimulation

Relaxed state

c. Identify specific measures that can be used to protect infants from overstimulation and yet provide appropriate stimulation to meet the developmental and emotional needs of infants.

d. Specify the guidelines that should be followed regarding infant positioning.

e. Describe the nursing measures that should be used to support the parents of an infant who is being cared for in a NICU.

5. Marion is beginning her 43rd week of pregnancy.

a. Support this statement: Perinatal mortality is significantly higher in the postmature fetus and neonate.

b. State the assessment findings that are typical of a postmature infant.

c. Discuss the two major complications that can be experienced by a postmature infant.

6. Janet, a pregnant woman at term, is in labor. On the basis of serial ultrasound findings, her fetus is estimated to be smaller than it should be as a consequence of Janet's heavy smoking during pregnancy and her high risk status related to preeclampsia.

a. Identify three major complications facing Janet's baby during labor, birth, and the postpartum period.

b. Describe the physiologic basis for each potential complication and the signs and symptoms indicative of its presence.

7. Marion is at 24 weeks of gestation and is in preterm labor. Her primary health care provider determines that preterm birth is inevitable and has elected to transport Marion to a tertiary center before she gives birth to maximize the survival potential of her unborn infant.

a. Explain the advantages of transport before birth.

b. Marion gives birth before she can be transported. Her baby will now be transported to the tertiary center once stable. Indicate the needs of this preterm baby that must be stabilized before transport.

c. Identify the measures that the nurse should use to support Marion and her family as her newborn is transported to the tertiary center.

The Newborn at Risk: Acquired and Congenital Problems (28)

I. REVIEWING KEY CONCEPTS AND CONTENT

TRUE OR FALSE: Circle T if true or F if false for each of the following statements. Correct the false statements.

1. T   F   Some birth injuries may not be readily apparent even at the initial examination of the newborn.

2. T   F   Most birth injuries can be prevented with careful assessment for risk factors and with birth planning.

3. T   F   Cephalhematoma is a birth injury that can occur during a forceps- or vacuum-assisted birth.

4. T   F   Plexus injury results from forces that alter the normal position and relationship of the leg, hip, and spine.

5. T   F   Linear fractures of the skull can result in increased intracranial pressure if an artery is damaged.

6. T   F   The bone most frequently fractured during the birth process is the femur.

7. T   F   Neonatal spinal cord injuries are almost always a result of a difficult birth from the breech presentation.

8. T   F   The woman infected with toxoplasmosis during pregnancy has a 90% chance of transmitting the infection to her fetus.

9. T   F   Newborns infected with toxoplasmosis in utero are at risk for developing severe psychomotor problems or mental retardation.

10. T   F   A major mode of transmission of gonorrhea to the fetus/newborn is via passage through an infected birth canal during birth.

11. T   F   Maternal infection with syphilis is most dangerous during the first trimester when organogenesis takes place.

12. T   F   Penicillin is the antibiotic choice for treating syphilis.

13. T   F   Even with adequate treatment, the neonate infected with syphilis may experience complications as late as 15 years of age.

14. T   F   Infants born to mothers who had chickenpox 5 days before birth should be given varicella-zoster immune globulin (VZIG) at birth.

15. T   F   Women positive for the hepatitis B virus should not breastfeed their newborn.

16. T   F   Prenatal, intrapartum, and neonatal treatment has reduced the incidence of neonatal HIV infection to 5% to 8%.

17. T   F   Congenital anomalies associated with rubella are most severe if the mother becomes infected during the first trimester.

18. T   F   The infant infected with the rubella virus may be a serious source of infection to susceptible individuals, particularly women in their childbearing years.

19. T   F   Newborns infected with cytomegalovirus must begin receiving penicillin therapy within 24 hours of birth.

20. T   F   Snuffles is a common assessment finding exhibited by infants infected with herpes simplex virus (HSV).

21. T   F   A primary maternal infection with HSV after 32 weeks of gestation presents a greater risk to the fetus/newborn than a recurrent HSV infection.

22. T   F   The most common cause of early onset neonatal sepsis and meningitis in the United States is group B streptococcus.

23. T   F   Hepatitis B during pregnancy is associated with an increased risk for preterm birth.

24. T   F   To prevent a chlamydial infection of the eyes, silver nitrate should be instilled over the cornea of the newborn's eyes immediately after birth.

25. T   F   Infants diagnosed with alcohol-related neurodevelopmental disorder could develop learning, speech, and behavioral problems.

26. T   F   Maternal heroin use, especially during the first trimester, results in a high rate of congenital anomalies.

27. T   F   Marijuana use during pregnancy may result in shortened gestation and a higher incidence of intrauterine growth restriction (IUGR).

28. T   F   Newborns exposed to cocaine in utero begin a process of withdrawal within 24 hours of birth.

29. T   F   If the mother is Rh negative and the father of the baby is Rh positive and homozygous for the Rh factor, all offspring will be Rh positive.

30. T   F   If the mother of an Rh-negative infant is Rh positive, she will require RhoGAM within 24 hours of giving birth.

31. T   F   First-born infants are unlikely to be affected by an ABO incompatibility disorder.

32. T   F   At the first prenatal visit of an Rh-negative woman, an indirect Coombs' test should be done to determine if her fetus will be Rh-negative or Rh positive.

33. T   F   ABO incompatibility is more common than Rh incompatibility but causes less severe problems in the affected infant.

34. T   F   At birth an indirect Coombs' test is performed on the newborn's cord blood to determine if the fetus has produced antibodies to its mother's blood.

35. T   F   Major congenital defects are the leading cause of death among infants in the United States.

36. T   F   The etiology for congenital heart defects is readily identified in the majority of diagnosed infants.

37. T   F   Closure of spina bifida cystica is usually delayed until the infant is approximately 6 months of age.

38. T   F   Infants born with a diaphragmatic hernia often experience respiratory distress.

39. T   F   Clubfoot is treated with serial casting beginning shortly after birth before discharge.

40. Birth injuries (trauma) are an important cause of neonatal morbidity.

    a. Identify the factors that increase fetal vulnerability to injury (trauma) at birth.

    b. Baby boy Timothy's right clavicle was fractured during birth as a result of shoulder dystocia. Describe the signs Timothy most likely exhibited to alert the nurse that his clavicle was fractured.

    c. Explain to Timothy's parents the most likely care approach related to his injury.

41. State the infections(s) represented by each letter in the acronym TORCH.

    T

    O

    R

    C

    H

42. Sepsis is one of the most significant causes of neonatal morbidity and mortality.

    a. When caring for newborns, nurses must be alert for factors that increase the newborn's risk for sepsis. Identify the major risk factors that, if present, should alert the nurse to the increased potential for infection in the neonate.

b. Early diagnosis is critical for successful treatment. List the signs a neonate might exhibit that would indicate sepsis is present.

c. Describe two effective nursing measures for each of the following categories.

Prevention

Care

43. Describe the physiologic basis for ABO incompatibility.

44. Indicate how each of the following types of postnatal tests can be used to diagnose an infant with a congenital anomaly.

a. Newborn screening

b. Cytogenetic studies

c. Dermatoglyphics

45. Congenital heart defects (CHD) are a major cause of death in the first year of life.

a. List several maternal factors associated with a higher incidence of CHDs.

b. Describe the signs that may be exhibited at birth by an infant with a severe congenital heart defect.

FILL IN THE BLANKS: Insert the congenital disorder represented by each of the following descriptions.

46. _____ A group of disorders caused by a defect that results from the absence of, or a change in, a protein, usually an enzyme and mediated by the action of a single gene. Examples include phenylketonuria and galactosemia.

47. _____ A head circumference that measures more than three standard deviations below the mean for age and gender; brain growth is usually restricted and mental retardation is common.

48. _____ Urethral meatus opens below the glans penis or anywhere along the ventral surface of the penis, scrotum, or peritoneum. _____ Urethral meatus opens on the dorsal surface of the penis. _____ Abnormal development of the bladder, abdominal wall, and symphysis pubis that causes the bladder, urethra, and ureteral orifices to be exposed.

49. _____ Enlargement of the ventricles of the brain usually as a result of an imbalance between production and absorption of cerebrospinal fluid (CSF). It is characterized by a bulging anterior fontanel, an abnormal increase in the circumference of the head, and an increasing CSF pressure.

50. _____ Ventricular septal defects and tetralogy of Fallot are two common forms of this type of congenital disorder.

51. _____ The most common form of clubfoot. The foot points downward and inward in varying degrees of severity.

52. _____ The most common congenital anomaly of the nose requiring emergency surgery after birth. It consists of a bony or membranous septum located between the nose and the pharynx.

53. _____ A form of spina bifida cystica (a neural tube defect) in which an external sac containing the meninges and spinal fluid protrudes through a defect in the vertebral column.

54. _____ A covered defect of the umbilical ring into which varying amounts of the abdominal organs may herniate. It is covered with a peritoneal sac. _____ Herniation of the bowel through a defect in the abdominal wall to the right of the umbilical cord. No membrane covers the contents.

55. _____ The passageway from the mouth to the stomach ends in a blind pouch or narrows into a thin cord; thus, a continuous passageway to the stomach is not

present._____ An abnormal connection between this passageway and the trachea.

56. _____ A type of neural tube defect characterized by the absence of both cerebral hemispheres and the overlying skull. It is incompatible with life.

57. _____ Disorder characterized by displacement of the abdominal organs into the thoracic cavity.

58. _____ A form of spina bifida cystica (a neural tube defect) in which an external sac containing the meninges, spinal fluid, and nerves protrudes through a defect in the vertebral column.

MULTIPLE CHOICE QUESTIONS: Circle the one correct option and state the rationale for the option chosen.

59. When assessing a newborn after birth, the nurse notes the following: limited movement of left arm with crepitus at the shoulder, absence of Moro reflex on left side. The nurse suspects
    a. brachial paralysis.
    b. fracture of the clavicle.
    c. phrenic nerve injury.
    d. intracranial hemorrhage on right side of the brain.

60. The care management of a newborn whose mother is HIV positive would most likely include which of the following?
    a. Isolating the newborn in a special nursery
    b. Telling her that she should not breastfeed
    c. Wearing gloves for routine care measures such as feeding
    d. Initiating zidovudine treatment once the newborn's HIV status is determined

61. An Rh-negative woman (2-2-0-0-2) just gave birth to an Rh-positive baby boy. The direct and indirect Coombs' test results are both negative. The nurse should
    a. prepare to administer $Rh_o(D)$ immune globulin (RhoGAM) to the newborn within 24 hours of his birth.
    b. observe the newborn closely for signs of pathologic jaundice.
    c. recognize that RhoGAM is not needed because both Coombs' test results are negative.
    d. administer $Rh_o(D)$ immune globulin intramuscularly to the woman within 72 hours of her baby's birth.

62. The nurse will be assisting the physician with an exchange transfusion to be performed for a newborn male with pathologic jaundice that has been unresponsive to phototherapy. As part of the protocol for this procedure the nurse would
    a. monitor the newborn for hypertension.
    b. expect that 95% to 100% of the newborn's blood will be exchanged with donor blood.
    c. implement measures to maintain the newborn's body temperature to prevent hypothermia.
    d. observe the newborn closely for signs of hypercalcemia.

63. A newborn female has been diagnosed with myelomeningocele. Which of the following would be an important nursing measure to protect the newborn from injury and further complications during the preoperative period?
    a. Maintain the newborn in a lateral or prone position.
    b. Tell the parents that they cannot hold their newborn.
    c. Cover the sac with Vaseline gauze to keep it moist and intact.
    d. Avoid touching the skin around the defect to prevent accidental rupture.

II. THINKING CRITICALLY

1. Baby girl Susan was born 2 hours ago. Her mother tested positive for HBsAg antibodies as a result of infection with hepatitis B virus (HBV).

   a. Describe the protocol that should be followed in providing care for Susan.

   b. Susan's mother asks the nurse if she can breastfeed her baby daughter. Discuss the nurse's response to this mother's question.

2. Baby boy Andrew is a full-term newborn who was just born by spontaneous vaginal birth. Genital herpes recurred in his mother, and her membranes ruptured before the onset of labor.

   a. Identify the four modes of transmission for HSV to the newborn. Indicate the mode most likely to have transmitted the infection to Andrew.

   b. List the clinical signs Andrew would exhibit as evidence of a disseminated and localized HSV infection.

   c. Describe the recommended nursing measures related to each of the following:

   • Management after birth, before discharge

   • Vidarabine or acyclovir therapy

3. Baby girl Mary is 1 day old. Her mother is HIV positive but received no treatment during pregnancy.

   a. Discuss Mary's potential for HIV infection.

   b. Identify the modes of transmission of HIV to Mary.

   c. Name the opportunistic/secondary infections that, if contracted by Mary, would strongly suggest that she is infected with HIV.

   d. Describe the care measures recommended for Mary.

   e. Mary's mother wishes to breastfeed Mary because she has read that it can prevent infection and help her bond with her infant. Discuss the nurse's response to this mother's question.

4. Baby boy Thomas, at 2 days of age, has developed thrush.

    a. Describe the signs most likely exhibited by Thomas that led to this diagnosis.

    b. Name the modes of transmission for this infection.

    c. Discuss the care management required by Thomas as a result of his infection.

5. Jane, a newborn, has been diagnosed with fetal alcohol syndrome (FAS) as a result of her mother's moderate to sometimes heavy binge drinking throughout the pregnancy.

    a. Describe the characteristics Jane most likely exhibited to establish the diagnosis of FAS.

    b. State three long-term effects Jane could experience as she gets older.

    c. Describe two nursing measures that could be effective in promoting Jane's growth and development.

6. Maternal substance abuse can be harmful to fetal and newborn health status, as well as growth and development.

    a. Describe the assessment findings associated with newborn withdrawal from each of the following substances.

    Heroin

    Methadone

b. Susan has just been born. Her mother used cocaine during pregnancy. Identify the effects Susan may exhibit as a result of exposure to cocaine while in utero.

7. Tony is a 2-hour-old newborn. It is suspected that his mother abused drugs during pregnancy.

a. List the signs associated with neonatal abstinence syndrome that the nurse should observe for when assessing Tony.

b. Tony begins to exhibit signs that confirm that his mother used heroin during pregnancy. Cite two nursing diagnoses that would be appropriate for Tony.

c. Outline the care management that Tony and his mother will require.

8. Angela, who is Rh negative, had a spontaneous abortion at 13 weeks of gestation, which resulted in what she said was just a heavier than usual menstrual period. Six months later she becomes pregnant again.

a. Describe the physiologic basis for Rh incompatibility and the occurrence of sensitization.

b. An indirect Coombs' test is positive. State the meaning of this finding.

c. Indicate whether Angela is a candidate for RhoGAM. Support your answer.

d. Describe RhoGAM (Rh immunoglobulin) and its use.

e. Angela's fetus is at risk for erythroblastosis fetalis and hydrops fetalis. Explain each of these conditions.

Erythroblastosis fetalis

Hydrops fetalis

f. Describe the treatment approaches that can be used to prevent intrauterine fetal death and early neonatal death for Angela's baby.

9. Baby girl Jennifer was born with spina bifida cystica, myelomeningocele. Describe the measures the nurse should use to manage Jennifer's care and help her parents cope with this congenital anomaly.

10. Baby girl Denise was born with a cleft lip and palate.

a. State three nursing diagnoses faced by Denise and her parents. Discuss the rationale for each nursing diagnosis stated.

b. Outline several nursing measures that will need to be implemented to ensure Denise's well-being until surgical repair can be accomplished.

Contemporary Pediatric Nursing (29)

I. LEARNING KEY TERMS

MATCHING: Match each term with its corresponding definition.

1. _____ The person affected by a disease.

2. _____ Figures describing rates of occurrence for events such as death in children.

3. _____ Lack of awareness of available health care services, for example.

4. _____ The time and place a disease occurs.

5. _____ Illness.

6. _____ A care delivery system that balances cost and quality; created to provide care in a more cost-effective manner in response to pressure from payers.

7. _____ Interaction with patients where boundaries are blurred and the nurse's personal needs may be served rather than the patient's.

8. _____ Figures describing the incidence or number of individuals who have died over a specific period of time.

9. _____ Death.

10. _____ Individuals who are trained to provide care activities as delegated by and under the supervision of the registered professional nurse.

11. _____ The object that is the direct cause of a disease.

12. _____ An advanced practice role for nurses that includes history taking, physical diagnosis, and pharmacologic management.

13. _____ The prevalence of a specific illness in the population at a particular time.

14. _____ An advanced practice role for nurses that includes role modeling, consultation, and research.

a. Mortality

b. Morbidity

c. Vital statistics

d. Mortality statistics

e. Host

f. Environment

g. Agent

h. Morbidity statistics

i. Financial barriers

j. System barriers

k. Knowledge barrier

l. Family-centered care

m. Empowerment

n. Atraumatic care

o. Therapeutic care

p. Primary nursing

q. Case management

r. Therapeutic relationship

s. Nontherapeutic relationships

t. Pediatric nurse practitioner (PNP)

u. Clinical nurse specialist (CNS)

v. Advanced nurse practitioners (ANP or ARNP)

w. Standard of practice

x. Unlicensed assistive personnel (UAP)

15. _____ A merged role of clinical nurse specialist and nurse practitioner.

16. _____ An example is inadequate health insurance.

17. _____ Therapeutic care that minimizes the psychologic and physical distress experienced by children and their families.

18. _____ An example is great travel distance to any health care facility.

19. _____ A care delivery system in which one nurse has 24-hour responsibility and accountability for the care of a small group of patients.

20. _____ Describes the interaction that maintains or helps families acquire a sense of control over their lives.

21. _____ The philosophy that recognizes the family as the constant in a child's life that service systems must support and enhance.

22. _____ Meaningful interaction with caring, well-defined boundaries separating the nurse from the client.

23. _____ Care that encompasses the prevention, diagnosis, treatment, or palliation of chronic or acute conditions.

24. _____ The level of performance that is expected of a professional.

MATCHING: Match each term with its corresponding definition.

25. _____ Symptoms severe enough to limit activity or require medical attention.

26. _____ The number of infant deaths per 1000 live births that occur before the twenty-eighth day of life.

27. _____ The leading cause of death in children over 1 year of age; responsible for more childhood deaths and disabilities than all causes of disease combined.

28. _____ The number of infant deaths per 1000 live births that occur between the twenty-eighth day of life and age 11 months.

29. _____ The number of deaths during the first year of life per 1000 live births.

30. _____ The third leading cause of death among adolescents and young adults 15 to 19 years old.

31. _____ Can be measured in days absent from school or days confined to bed.

a. Injuries

b. Prospective payment system

c. Accident

d. Justice

e. Standard of practice

f. Infant mortality rate

g. Beneficence

h. Neonatal mortality

i. Disability

j. Evidence-based practice

k. Postneonatal mortality

32. _____ A chaotic, random event related to "luck" or "chance."

33. _____ Increasing in number among young people ages 10 through 25 years, especially among African-American males.

34. _____ The level of performance that is expected of a professional.

35. _____ Based on diagnosis-related groups (DRGs). The DRG categories define pretreatment billing for hospitals reimbursed by Medicare.

36. _____ A key factor in its higher neonatal mortality rates when compared with other countries.

37. _____ The concept that involves analyzing and translating published clinical research into everyday nursing practice.

38. _____ The patient's right to be self-governing.

39. _____ The obligation to minimize or prevent harm.

40. _____ The obligation to promote the patient's well-being.

41. _____ The concept of fairness.

l. Suicide

m. Low birth weight (LBW)

n. Nonmaleficence

o. Acute illness

p. Violent deaths

q. Autonomy

II. REVIEWING KEY CONCEPTS AND CONTENT

42. Which of the following objectives would not be considered a priority area for *Healthy People 2010?*
    a. Improving nutritional and infant health
    b. Technologic advances to treat neonates
    c. Reducing violent and abusive behavior
    d. Expanding health promotion programs

43. Mortality rates are calculated from a
    a. survey of physicians.
    b. sample of hospital records.
    c. registry of all deaths.
    d. sample of death certificates.

44. Infant mortality for infants less than 1 year of age
    a. has been steadily increasing.
    b. is low when compared with death rates at other ages.
    c. is high when compared with death rates at other ages.
    d. is lower in the neonatal period than postneonatally.

45. Which of the following statements about injuries in childhood is false?
    a. Developmental stage determines the prevalence of injuries at a given age.
    b. Most fatal injuries occur in children younger than the age of nine.
    c. Developmental stage helps direct preventive measures.
    d. The older the child, the greater the risk of death from injury.

46. List three factors that contribute to increasing the morbidity of any disorder in children.

47. Another term for the new morbidity is
    a. pediatric social illness.
    b. pediatric noncompliance.
    c. learning disorder.
    d. dyslexia.

48. Two basic concepts in the philosophy of family-centered pediatric nursing care are:
    a. enabling and empowerment.
    b. empowerment and bias.
    c. enabling and curing.
    d. empowerment and self-control.

49. An example of atraumatic care would be to
    a. eliminate all traumatic procedures.
    b. restrict visiting hours to adults only.
    c. perform invasive procedures only in the treatment room.
    d. permit only traditional clinical practices.

50. A care delivery system that balances quality with cost and that has been shown to improve satisfaction, decrease fragmentation, and measure patient outcomes best describes
    a. case management.
    b. primary nursing.
    c. family-centered nursing.
    d. functional nursing.

MATCHING: Match each federal program with the corresponding impact it has on maternal and child health.

51. _____ Created in 1965; the largest maternal-child health program; includes the Child Health Assessment Program (CHAP), which provides services for pregnant women and children; variable eligibility from state to state.

52. _____ Created in 1935 as a cash grant to aid needy children without fathers.

53. _____ Provides services to reduce infant mortality, disease, and handicaps and to increase access to care.

54. _____ Established in 1981 to fund projects related to substance abuse and to treat mentally disturbed children.

55. _____ Provides funds for child protective services, family planning, and foster care.

56. _____ Started in 1974 to provide nutritious food and education to low-income childbearing women, infants, and children up to age 5 years.

57. _____ Passed in 1975 to provide free public education to handicapped children.

58. _____ The first-ever federal privacy standards to protect patients' medical records and other health information.

59. _____ Provides funding for multidisciplinary programs for handicapped infants and toddlers.

60. _____ Allows employees to take unpaid leave (1993).

a. Education of the Handicapped Act Amendments of 1886 (P.L. 99-457)

b. Social Services block grant

c. Alcohol, drug abuse, and mental health block grants

d. Education for All Handicapped Children Act (P.L. 94-1432)

e. Medicaid

f. Family and Medical Leave Act (FMLA)

g. Aid to Families with Dependent Children (AFDC)

h. MCH service block grant

i. Women, Infants and Children (WIC)

j. Health Insurance Portability and Accountability Act (HIPAA)

Match each role of the pediatric nurse with its corresponding description.

61. _____ A mutual exchange of ideas and opinions.

62. _____ Extending to include the community or society; influence the decision-making body of government.

63. _____ Health maintenance strategies; the role of the pediatric nurse practitioner was developed for this purpose.

64. _____ Using patient/family/societal values in care.

Determining actions for difficult situations by assigning different weight to the competing moral values

a. Family advocacy/caring

b. Disease prevention/health promotion

c. Health teaching

d. Support

65. _____ Using a unified interdisciplinary approach to provide holistic care; working together as a member of the health team.

66. _____ Attention to emotional needs (listening/physical presence).

67. _____ Transmitting information about health

68. _____ Validation of nursing contributions through systematic recording and analysis

69. _____ Acting in the child's best interest; the responsibility of the nurse that aims to preserve the rights of the child and ensure that children receive optimum care.

e. Counseling

f. Coordination/collaboration

g. Ethical decision-making

h. Research

i. Health care planning

70. List three expected future trends in pediatric nursing.

71. Define the term *unlicensed assistive personnel (UAP).*

III. THINKING CRITICALLY

1. Generate at least one idea that could be implemented by pediatric nurses to meet the three goals for public health as outlined by *Healthy People 2010.*

2. Using examples from a wide variety of practice areas, describe ways that the pediatric nurse currently fulfills the responsibilities of each of the following broad roles of the nurse.

   a. Family advocacy/caring

   b. Disease prevention/health promotion

   c. Health teaching

   d. Support/counseling

e. Coordination/collaboration

f. Ethical decision making

g. Research

h. Health care planning

3. It is the year 2020, and you have been a pediatric nurse since the year 2000. Your local news service has asked you to compare your profession with what it was like 20 years ago. Your thoughts will be used for a feature article for *Nurse's Week*. Write a description of what your response might be.

Community-Based Nursing Care of the Child and Family 30

I. LEARNING KEY TERMS

MATCHING: Match each term with its corresponding definition.

1. _____ Responsible for causing a disease; may be an infectious agent such as *Mycobacterium tuberculosis*.

2. _____ Involves a collaboration of individuals and groups, including health care providers, advocates, government, managed care organizations, businesses, children and families within a specific community.

3. _____ Groups of people who live in a community.

4. _____ Groups of people toward whom health care workers direct their activities to improve the health status of individuals in the group.

5. _____ Identifies the distribution and causes of disease, injury, or illness and determines the levels of prevention; science of population health applied to the detection of morbidity and mortality in a population.

6. _____ Measures the occurrence of new events in a population during a period of time.

7. _____ Measures existing events in a population during a period of time.

8. _____ Classified into environmental, behavioral, and biologic categories.

9. _____ Method of problem solving that shifts from the individual child and family to the target population and uses the stages of assessment, diagnosis, planning, implementation, and evaluation.

10. _____ Collection of information that includes what community members say and data collected by direct observation.

11. _____ The reflection of health status risks or needs, as determined by a causative agent.

12. _____ An increased probability of developing a disease, injury or illness

13. _____ Interventions aimed at health promotion and prevention of disease or injury.

14. _____ Focuses on screening and early diagnosis of disease.

a. Tertiary prevention

b. Secondary preventions

c. Target populations/subpopulations

d. Primary prevention

e. Prevalence

f. Incidence

g. Epidemiology

h. Populations

i. Community nursing process

j. Community needs assessment

k. Community health diagnosis

l. Community care

m. Causative agents

n. Public Health Core functions

o. Demography

p. Risk

q. Agent

15. _____ The study of population characteristics.

16. _____ Focuses on optimizing function for children with a disability or chronic disease.

17. _____ Population-wide services that include assessment of health status monitoring, disease surveillance, policy development, and assurance.

II. REVIEWING KEY CONCEPTS AND CONTENT

18. Community nursing is best defined as nursing that
    a. empowers children and families to advocate effectively for resources.
    b. provides care to individuals, families, groups, and communities.
    c. assists the patient to cope with health problems.
    d. coordinates care throughout the course of a patient's illness.

19. The children with asthma in a midsize rural town are an example of a(n)
    a. environmental agent.
    b. behavioral agent.
    c. target population.
    d. biologic population.

20. *Healthy People 2010* is an example of a health promotion and disease prevention program that was developed using the
    a. community assessment.
    b. epidemiologic process.
    c. nursing process.
    d. community nursing assessment.

21. The pediatric continuum of care system contains the subsystems of
    a. assessment, planning, implementation, and evaluation.
    b. health promotion and disease protection and prevention.
    c. rehabilitation and disease management programs.
    d. wellness, acute illness, chronic illness, and end-of-life care.

22. In the community nursing process, the focus shifts from the
    a. community to the individual child and family.
    b. individual child and family to the target population.
    c. target population to the individual in the community.
    d. individual child to the family in a community.

23. An example of a secondary prevention activity is a(n)
    a. cardiac rehabilitation program.
    b. immunization program.
    c. mammography screening program.
    d. nutrition education program.

24. Nurses participate more fully in decision making about community health programs when they become knowledgeable about
    a. diagnostic-related groups.
    b. health care economics.
    c. private health insurance programs.
    d. patient safety issues.

III. THINKING CRITICALLY

1. Describe at least one example (other than those in the textbook) of a way to collect subjective and objective information for a community needs assessment.

2. Using community nursing examples, describe ways that the pediatric nurse currently fulfills the responsibilities of each of the following broad roles of the nurse.

    a. Family advocacy/caring

    b. Disease prevention/health promotion

    c. Health teaching

    d. Support/counseling

    e. Coordination/collaboration

    f. Ethical decision making

    g. Research

    h. Health care planning

31 Family Influences on Child Health Promotion

I. LEARNING KEY TERMS

MATCHING: Match each term with its corresponding description.

1. _____ Establishment of the rules or guidelines for behavior.

2. _____ Laissez-faire approach; exerting little or no control over children's actions.

3. _____ A refinement of the practice of sending the child to his or her room; based on the premise of removing the reinforcer and using the strategy of unrelated consequences.

4. _____ A system of rules governing conduct.

5. _____ Democratic approach; combining childrearing practices and emphasizing the reason for rules.

6. _____ Resources for dealing with stress, such as community services, social support, and the adoption of a future orientation.

7. _____ Family situation in which each parent is awarded custody of one or more of the children, thereby separating siblings.

8. _____ Family situation in which the children reside with one parent, with both parents acting as legal guardians and both participating in childrearing.

9. _____ A group of people, living together or in close contact, who take care of one another and provide guidance for their dependent members.

10. _____ Dictatorial approach; trying to control behavior and attitudes through unquestioned mandates.

a. Family

b. Coping strategies

c. Authoritarian

d. Permissive

e. Authoritative

f. Discipline

g. Limit-setting

h. Time-out

i. Divided, or split, custody

j. Joint custody

11. _____ The descriptive term used that accommodates a variety of family styles, including communal families, single-parent families and homosexual families.

12. _____ The unit of care ("the patient") when working with children.

13. _____ Marital relationships.

14. _____ Family unit a person is born into.

15. _____ Blood relationships.

16. _____ The term used to describe the concept that parents rear their own children in much the same way as they themselves were reared.

a. Consanguineous

b. Affinal

c. Family of origin

d. Household

e. The family

f. Role discontinuity

g. Generational continuity

h. Internal family resources

17. _____ The term used to describe the support of the family from within, such as adaptability and integration.

18. _____ The term used when role behavior expected of children conflicts with the desirable adult behavior.

II. REVIEWING KEY CONCEPTS AND CONTENT

19. Which of the following descriptions would *not* be correct using the current definition of the term *family?*
    a. The family is what the patient considers it to be.
    b. The family may be related or unrelated.
    c. The family members are always related by legal ties or genetic relationships and live in the same household.
    d. The family members share a sense of belonging to their own family.

20. Parenting practices differ between small and large families. Which one of the following characteristics is *not* found in small families?
    a. Emphasis is placed on the individual development of the child, with constant pressure to measure up to family expectations.
    b. Adolescents identify more strongly with their parents and rely more on their parents for advice.
    c. More emphasis is placed on the group and less on the individual.
    d. Children's development and achievement are measured against children in the neighborhood and social class.

21. Because age differences between siblings affect the childhood environment, the nurse recognizes that there may be more affection and less rivalry and hostility between children that are spaced how many years apart?
    a. 4 or more years
    b. 4 or fewer years
    c. 3 or fewer years
    d. 2 or fewer years

22. One sibling has always been viewed by his parents as being less dependent than his brother or his sister. This sibling is described as affectionate, good-natured, and flexible in his thinking. He identifies with his peer group and is very popular with classmates. His parents tend to place fewer demands on him for household help. From this description, the nurse would expect this sibling to have what birth position within the family?
    a. Firstborn child
    b. Middle child
    c. Youngest child
    d. Any of the above (Birth position does not affect personality.)

23. Monozygotic twins are
    a. the result of fertilization of two ova.
    b. the result of fertilization of one ovum that became separated early in development.
    c. different physically and genetically.
    d. of dissimilar behaviors with greater sibling rivalry.

24. Which of the following is *not* a description of the discipline "time-out"?
    a. Allows the reinforcer to be maintained
    b. Involves no physical punishment
    c. Offers both parents and child "cooling-off" time
    d. Facilitates the parent's ability to consistently apply the punishment

25. Which of the following is a correct interpretation in the use of reasoning as a form of discipline?
    a. Used for older children when moral issues are involved
    b. Used for younger children to "see the other side" of an issue
    c. Used only in combination with scolding and criticism
    d. Used to allow children a greater degree of attention from parents

26. Areas of concern for parents of adoptive children include
    a. the initial attachment process.
    b. telling the children that they are adopted.
    c. identity formation of the children during adolescence.
    d. all of the above.

27. T   F   Research has shown that children of divorce suffer no lasting psychological and social difficulties.

28. T   F   One outcome found in children of divorce is a heightened anxiety about forming enduring relationships as young adults.

29. T   F   Children of divorce cope better with their feelings of abandonment when there is continuing conflict between parents.

30. T F Preschoolers assume themselves to be the cause of the divorce and interpret the separation as punishment.

31. T F School-age children's teachers and school counselors should be informed about divorce because these children will often display altered behaviors.

32. T F Adolescents have concerns and heightened anxiety about their own future as marital partners and the availability of money for future needs.

33. Which of the following is not an important consideration for parents when telling their children about the decision to divorce?
   a. Initial disclosure should include both parents and siblings.
   b. Time should be allowed for discussion with each child individually.
   c. The initial disclosure should be kept simple and reasons for divorce should not be included.
   d. Parents should physically hold or touch their child to provide feelings of warmth and reassurance.

MATCHING: Single-parenting, step parenting, and dual-earner family parenting add stress to the parental role. Match each family type with an expected stressor or concern.

34. _____ Managing shortages of money, time, and energy are major concerns.

35. _____ Overload is a common source of stress, and social activities are significantly curtailed with time demands and scheduling seen as major problems.

36. _____ Competition is a major area of concern among adults, with reduction of power conflicts a necessity.

a. Single-parenting

b. Stepparenting

c. Dual-earner families

III. THINKING CRITICALLY

1. Ester and Roberto Garcia are the proud new parents of twin boys, Timothy and Thomas. Ester and Roberto have been married less than 1 year. Ester is 17 years old and plans to return to finish school next year. Roberto finished high school and works with his father in a local auto repair shop. He is taking a week off from work to help Ester at home with Timothy and Thomas. Neither of the parents attended child-parenting classes. You are making a home visit to the couple 1 day after they have brought Timothy and Thomas home from the hospital. As you arrive at the house, you see that both Timothy and Thomas are crying. Ester is trying to give Timothy his bath while Roberto is busy trying to get Thomas to take his formula. Both new parents appear tired, and Roberto admits that they have been up all night with the infants and that either Timothy or Thomas seems to be crying, "all the time" and "something must be terribly wrong with them."

   a. Identify three possible basic goals of parenting for this family.

   b. Identify the family's immediate needs.

   c. Identify long-term goals for this family.

d. Discuss nursing interventions that would foster achievement of these long-term goals.

2. Compare and contrast the following types of consequences, and give an example of a discipline technique for each type.

   a. Natural consequences

   b. Logical consequences

   c. Unrelated consequences

3. Discuss the disadvantages of using corporal punishment as a form of discipline to decrease or stop certain behaviors.

32 Social, Cultural, and Religious Influences on Child Health Promotion

I. LEARNING KEY TERMS

MATCHING: Match each term with its corresponding definition.

1. _____ The emotional attitude that one's own ethnic group is superior to others; that one's values, beliefs, and perceptions are the correct ones; and that the group's ways of living and behaving are the best way.

2. _____ The affiliation of a set of people who share a unique cultural, social, and linguistic heritage.

3. _____ The concept that any behavior must be judged first in relation to the context of the culture in which it occurs.

4. _____ The process by which children acquire the beliefs, values, and behaviors of a given society in order to function within that group.

5. _____ Those gradual changes produced in a culture by the influence of another culture that cause one or both cultures to be more similar to the other.

6. _____ Those smaller groups within a culture that possess many characteristics of the larger culture while contributing their own particular values.

7. _____ A pattern of assumptions, beliefs, and practices that unconsciously frames or guides the outlook and decisions of a group of people.

8. _____ The condition in which a person lacks resources and community ties necessary to provide for their own adequate shelter.

9. _____ The relative lack of money, material resources, social or cultural opportunities.

10. _____ The orientation to nursing that includes an awareness of the nurse's own culture; the nurse learns about and becomes able to assess from and share the culture of others.

11. _____ A division of mankind possessing traits that are transmissible by descent and sufficient to characterize it as a distinct human type.

12. _____ The observable components of a culture, such as material objects (objects, art, utensils, and other artifacts) and actions.

a. Culture

b. Ethnicity

c. Socialization

d. Subculture

e. Ethnocentrism

f. Poverty

g. Homelessness

h. Acculturation

i. Culture relativity

j. Transcultural nursing

k. Race

l. Manifest culture

m. Nonmaterial covert culture

n. Primary group

o. Secondary group

p. Ethnic stereotyping

q. Cultural diversity

r. Assimilation

s. Cultural pluralism

t. Cultural shock

u. Cultural sensitivity

v. Cultural competency

13. _____   Refers to those aspects of culture that cannot be observed directly, such as the ideas, beliefs, customs and feelings of the culture.

14. _____   Characterized by intimate, continued, face-to-face contact; mutual support of members; and the ability to order or constrain a considerable proportion of individual member's behavior. Family and peer group are examples.

15. _____   Groups that have limited, intermittent contact and in which there is generally less concern for members' behavior; examples are professional associations and church organizations.

16. _____   Feelings of helplessness and discomfort and a state of disorientation experienced by an outsider attempting to comprehend or effectively adapt to a different cultural group because of differences in cultural practices, values, and beliefs.

17. _____   Labeling that stems from ethnocentric views of people; implies that the groups are inferior if different.

18. _____   Refers to the differences that exist among various groups of people, particularly the minority and majority populations.

19. _____   The process of developing a new cultural identity.

20. _____   Supports the rights of group differences and promotes a mutual respect for the existence of cultural differences.

21. _____   An awareness of cultural similarities and differences.

22. _____   An interactive care process that requires a change in the way the nurse understands and interacts within the work environment to address core cultural issues.

II. REVIEWING KEY CONCEPTS AND CONTENT

23. When considering the impact of culture on the pediatric patient, the nurse recognizes that culture
    a. is synonymous with race.
    b. affects the development of health beliefs.
    c. refers to a group of people with similar physical characteristics.
    d. refers to the universal manner and sequence of growth and development.

24. The use of guilt and shame by a culture provides
    a. feelings of comfort about wrongdoing.
    b. outlets following wrongdoing.
    c. rewards for culturally acceptable social behavior.
    d. internalization of the cultural norms.

25. Currently in North America there is less reliance on tradition, families are fragmented, and transmission of customs is limited because of
    a. a growing proportion of ethnic minorities.
    b. more emphasis on ethnic diversity.
    c. the frontier background of the American culture.
    d. increasing geographic and economic mobility.

26. Which country has more racial, ethnic, and religious minority groups than any other country?
    a. United States
    b. Mexico
    c. Canada
    d. India

27. Which of the following groups is the fastest growing minority group in the United States?
    a. African-American
    b. Hispanic
    c. Asian-American
    d. Latino

28. A child has become acculturated when
    a. a gradual process of ethnic blending occurs.
    b. the child identifies with traditional heritage.
    c. ethnic and racial pride emerges.
    d. counter-aggressive behavior is eliminated.

29. Which of the following strategies would be likely to produce the most conflict when considering the concept of cultural shock?
    a. Teaching the family some of the dominant culture's customs
    b. Using the child to translate for the parent
    c. Identifying some of the usual family customs
    d. Learning tolerance of others' values and beliefs

30. Cultural beliefs and practices are an important part of nursing assessment, because when analyzed and incorporated into the nursing process, beliefs
    a. may sometimes expedite the plan of care.
    b. can be manipulated more easily if known.
    c. must be in unison with standard health practices.
    d. are very similar from one culture to another.

31. An innate susceptibility is acquired through
    a. the child's general physical status.
    b. exposure to environmental factors.
    c. long-term proximity to disease.
    d. generations of evolutionary changes.

MATCHING: Match each disease with the ethnic group that corresponds most closely.

32. _____ Greek

33. _____ Arab

34. _____ Jewish

35. _____ Native American

36. _____ African-American

37. _____ English/Scottish

a. Tay-Sachs disease

b. Cystic fibrosis

c. Sickle cell disease

d. Lactase deficiency

e. G6PD deficiency

f. Tuberculosis

MATCHING: Match each custom or belief with the ethnic group that corresponds most closely.

38. _____ Eye contact often considered sign of hostility.

39. _____ Nonverbal communication as a practiced art.

40. _____ A desire to avoid disharmony.

41. _____ A focus on time and use of the expression "time flies."

42. _____ Belief that the male child will take care of his parents in their old age.

43. _____ Belief that infants can develop symptoms of the "evil eye."

a. Jewish

b. Caucasian (dominant culture)

c. Hispanic

d. Asian

e. Native

f. Asian-American

44. All of the following factors have been shown to affect food preferences and traditions *except*
    a. age.
    b. availability.
    c. religion.
    d. gender.

45. Adopting a multicultural perspective means that the nurse
    a. explains that biomedical measures are usually more effective.
    b. uses the patient's traditional health and cultural beliefs.
    c. realizes that most folk remedies have a scientific basis.
    d. uses aspects of the cultural beliefs to develop a plan.

46. Which of the following terms is not used to describe a kind of folk healer?
    a. Asafetida
    b. Curandera
    c. Curandero
    d. Kahunas

47. To provide culturally sensitive care to children and their families, the nurse should
    a. disregard his or her own cultural values.
    b. identify behavior that is abnormal.
    c. recognize characteristic behaviors of certain cultures.
    d. rely on his or her own feelings and experiences for guidance.

48. In planning and implementing transcultural patient care, nurses need to strive to
    a. adapt the family's ethnic practices to the health need.
    b. change the family's long-standing beliefs.
    c. use traditional ethnic practices in every patient's care.
    d. teach the family only how to treat the health problem.

49. Generalizations about cultural groups are important for nurses to know, because this information helps the nurse to
    a. learn the similarities among all cultures.
    b. learn the unique practices of various groups.
    c. stereotype groups' characteristics.
    d. categorize groups according to their similarities.

50. During assessment, a patient reveals that her family uses an acupuncturist occasionally. Based on this information, the nurse would realize that another health practice commonly found in the same cultural group would be
    a. voodoo.
    b. moxibustion.
    c. santeria.
    d. kampo.

III. THINKING CRITICALLY

1. As a staff nurse for an acute care pediatric unit, discharge instructions to the family of the child must be communicated in such a way that the family member is able to carry out the care of the child in the home. Describe how you would adapt your discharge instructions to reflect the usual cultural beliefs and practices of 3-year-old pediatric patients from each of the following ethnic groups who are discharged and need to follow a bland diet.

   a. Hispanic

   b. African-American

c. Asian-American

2. Liseth is a 3-month-old Mexican-American child. She comes to the immunization clinic with her 25-year-old mother, Noemi, her 18-month-old brother, and her 3-year-old sister. One of your goals is to promote continuation of the immunization schedule.

a. List the questions you should ask to determine whether there are cultural influences that affect Noemi's intent to have her children immunized.

b. Describe specific strategies you would use to communicate with Noemi.

c. Identify the Hispanic beliefs and practices regarding childrearing that may influence Noemi's approach to childrearing in general and immunization in particular.

3. You are a clinical nurse at a large community health clinic. You are assigned to the pediatric clinic where infants and children receive their first 2 years of health care. The clinic has a very well-developed education program in which the child's caregiver receives age-appropriate education at each clinic visit. The clinic serves a multicultural population.

a. Describe the approach you would use to facilitate culturally sensitive communication between you and your patients during the educational process.

b. Identify at least three different cultural beliefs or practices regarding childrearing and how they may influence the caregiver's reaction to the education program.

Developmental Influences on Child Health Promotion $\boxed{33}$

I. LEARNING KEY TERMS

MATCHING: Match each term with its corresponding definition.

1. _____ A set of skills and competencies peculiar to each developmental stage that children must accomplish or master in order to deal effectively with the environment.

2. _____ An increase in competence and adaptability; aging; usually used to describe a qualitative change.

3. _____ Specific ways in which children deal with stresses.

4. _____ The processes by which developing individuals become acquainted with the world and the objects it contains.

5. _____ Processes by which early cells and structures are systematically modified and altered to achieve specific and characteristic physical and chemical properties.

6. _____ A special class of individual reactions to stressors.

7. _____ The most widely accepted theory of personality development, advanced by Erikson and emphasizing a healthy personality; uses the biologic concepts of critical periods and epigenesis, describing key conflicts or more problems that the individual strives to master during critical periods in personality development.

8. _____ Term used by Freud to describe any sensual pleasure.

9. _____ Both children who are abused and those who are depressed exhibit these same behaviors.

10. _____ According to Chess and Thomas, a term defined as the manner of thinking, behaving, or reacting that is characteristic of an individual; the way in which a person deals with life.

11. _____ The rate of metabolism when the body is at rest.

12. _____ The universal medium in which children learn about their world and how to deal with their environment.

13. _____ The most accurate measure of general development; the radiologic determination of osseous maturation.

14. _____ A personal, subjective judgment of one's worthiness derived from and influenced by the social groups in the immediate environment and individuals' perceptions of how they are valued by others.

a. Maturation

b. Differentiation

c. Developmental task

d. Cephalocaudal

e. Proximodistal

f. Sensitive period

g. Skeletal age

h. Basal metabolic rate

i. Temperament

j. Psychosexual development

k. Psychosocial development

l. Cognition

m. Self-concept

n. Body image

o. Self-esteem

p. Play

q. Signs of stress

r. Coping

s. Coping strategies

t. Coping styles

15. _____   Limited times during a process of growth when the organism is more susceptible to positive or negative influences.

16. _____   A vital component of self-concept, referring to the subjective concepts and attitudes that individuals have toward their own bodies.

17. _____   The directional pattern of growth and development that proceeds from near to far.

18. _____   Relatively unchanging personality characteristics or outcomes of coping.

19. _____   The term that includes all the notions, beliefs, and convictions that constitute an individual's self-knowledge and influence that individual's relationships with others.

20. _____   The directional trend of growth and development that proceeds from head to tail.

II. REVIEWING KEY CONCEPTS AND CONTENT

21. Categorizing growth and behavior into approximate age stages
    a. helps to account for individual differences in children.
    b. can be applied to all children with some degree of precision.
    c. provides a convenient means to describe the majority of children.
    d. determines the speed of each child's growth.

22. Which of the following is an example of a cephalocaudal directional trend in development?
    a. Infants stand after they are able to hold the back erect.
    b. Fingers and toes develop after embryonic limb buds.
    c. Infants manipulate fingers after they are able to use the whole hand as a unit.
    d. Infants begin to have fine muscle control after gross random muscle movement is established.

23. The directional trend that predicts orderly and continuous development is known as
    a. cephalocaudal.
    b. proximodistal.
    c. sequential.
    d. differentiation.

24. Which of the following is considered fixed and precise in the development of children?
    a. The pace and rate of development
    b. The order of development
    c. Physical growth—in particular, height
    d. Growth during the vulnerable period

25. Sensitive periods in development are those times when the child is
    a. more likely to respond to beneficial stimulation.
    b. more likely to require specific stimulation for physical growth.
    c. less likely to acquire a specific skill if it is not learned during this time.
    d. less likely to be harmed by external conditions.

MATCHING: Match each developmental trend in external proportions with its corresponding age group.

26. _____   Rapid growth and growth of the trunk with a high center of gravity predominates in this age group.

27. _____   The lower limbs constitute one-half of the total body height and 30% of the total body weight.

28. _____   The head is the fastest growing part of the body; at one point during this stage the head constitutes 50% of the total body length.

29. _____   The legs are the most rapidly growing part of the body, and the slender, long-legged build is characteristic of both sexes during this stage.

a. Fetal

b. Newborn

c. Infancy

d. Childhood

e. Adolescence

f. Adulthood

30. _____ The lower limbs are one-third of the total body length but only 15% of the total body weight in this age group.

31. _____ A large portion of the increase in height during this stage is the result of trunk elongation. The feet and hands also grow rapidly and may appear large and ungainly in proportion to the rest of the body.

32. The lordosis that a 15-month-old child develops would be considered a secondary curvature that is
    a. located in the cervical region.
    b. fused and permanently fixed.
    c. a sign of a developmental delay.
    d. a compensatory lumbar curve exaggeration.

33. If the height of a 2-year-old is measured as 88 cm, his height at adulthood would be estimated as
    a. 132 cm.
    b. 176 cm.
    c. 172 cm.
    d. 190 cm.

34. If a newborn measures 19 inches at birth, the expected height at age 4 years would be approximately
    a. 28.5 inches.
    b. 38 inches.
    c. 43.5 inches.
    d. 48 inches.

35. At 17 years of age, a girl will be considered to be at her
    a. midgrowth height.
    b. terminal height.
    c. growth spurt.
    d. transitory height.

36. Dentition is often used as an indicator of
    a. physical development.
    b. maturity.
    c. linear growth.
    d. certain endocrine problems.

37. The best estimate of biologic age can be made using measurements obtained from
    a. nasal bone height.
    b. facial bone radiography.
    c. hand and wrist radiography.
    d. mandibular size.

38. One probable reason for large lymph node development in the child is that lymph tissue growth patterns reflect the
    a. parallel development of the nervous system.
    b. general growth patterns of the child.
    c. repeated exposure to new infectious agents.
    d. parallel development of the thymus gland.

39. The nurse determines that a 7-month-old infant who weighs 10 kg needs about
    a. 450 kcal per day.
    b. 700 kcal per day.
    c. 1000 kcal per day.
    d. 1200 kcal per day.

40. The basal metabolic rate (BMR) is highest in the
    a. adult male.
    b. infant over 6 months of age.
    c. school-age child.
    d. infant under 6 months of age.

41. The energy requirement to build tissue
    a. fluctuates randomly.
    b. fluctuates based on need.
    c. steadily decreases with age.
    d. steadily increases with age.

42. Body temperature in young children and infants responds to
    a. changes in the environment.
    b. exercise.
    c. emotional upset.
    d. all of the above.

43. A mother asks whether her 11-month-old child's sleep behavior is abnormal because he usually sleeps through the night and takes two naps a day. The nurse's response should indicate that the infant probably
    a. has normal sleep behavior.
    b. has periods of sleeplessness at night.
    c. is slow to return to sleep during the night.
    d. is overly fatigued.

MATCHING: Match each attribute of temperament with its corresponding description.

44. _____ Amount of stimulation required to evoke a response.

45. _____ Nature of initial responses to a new stimulus: positive or negative.

46. _____ Regularity in the timing of physiologic functions such as hunger, sleep, and elimination.

47. _____ Energy level of the child's reactions.

48. _____ Level of physical motion during activity.

49. _____ Ease or difficulty with which the child adapts or adjusts to new situations.

50. _____ Length of time a child pursues a given activity and continues it.

51. _____ Ease with which attention can be diverted.

52. _____ Amount of pleasant behavior compared with the unpleasant.

a. Activity

b. Rhythmicity

c. Approach-withdrawal

d. Adaptability

e. Threshold of responsiveness

f. Intensity of reaction

g. Mood

h. Distractibility

i. Attention span and persistence

53. Personality development as viewed by Freud focuses on
    a. the significance of sexual instincts.
    b. the suppression of psychosexual instincts.
    c. direct observations of adults.
    d. retrospective studies of children.

54. Erikson's theory provides a framework for
    a. clearly indicating the experience needed to resolve crises.
    b. emphasizing pathologic development.
    c. coping with extraordinary events.
    d. explaining children's behavior in mastering developmental tasks.

55. Erikson's stage of trust vs. mistrust corresponds to Freud's
    a. anal stage.
    b. oral stage.
    c. phallic stage.
    d. guilt stage.

56. For adolescents, their struggle to fit the roles they have played and those they hope to play is best outlined by
    a. Freud's latency period.
    b. Freud's phallic stage.
    c. Erikson's identity vs. role confusion stage.
    d. Erikson's intimacy vs. isolation stage.

57. The best-known theory regarding cognitive development was developed by
    a. Sullivan.
    b. Kohlberg.
    c. Erikson.
    d. Piaget.

58. An important prerequisite for all other mental activity is the child's awareness that an object exists even though it is no longer visible. According to Piaget, this awareness is called
    a. object permanence.
    b. logical thinking.
    c. egocentricity.
    d. reversibility.

59. The predominant characteristic of Piaget's preoperational period is egocentricity, which according to Piaget, means
    a. concrete and tangible reasoning.
    b. selfishness and self-centeredness.
    c. inability to see another's perspective.
    d. ability to make deductions and generalize.

60. The stages of moral development that allow for prediction of behavior but not for individual differences are outlined in the moral development theory according to
    a. Fowler.
    b. Holstein.
    c. Gilligan.
    d. Kohlberg.

61. The difference between religion and spirituality is that spirituality
    a. requires an organized set of practices.
    b. affects the whole person: mind, body, and spirit.
    c. ensures the individual's desire to differentiate right from wrong.
    d. extends beyond religion.

MATCHING: Match each type of play with the corresponding example of that type of play.

62. _____ Coloring a picture.

63. _____ Rocking a doll.

64. _____ Daydreaming.

65. _____ Playing peekaboo/patty-cake.

66. _____ Watching a children's puppet show on television.

67. _____ Preparing a puppet show.

68. _____ Learning to ride a bicycle.

69. _____ Swinging.

70. _____ Playing with dolls.

71. _____ Toddlers playing blocks in the same room.

a. Sense pleasure

b. Skill play

c. Unoccupied behavior

d. Dramatic play

e. Games

f. Onlooker play

g. Solitary play

h. Parallel play

i. Associative play

j. Cooperative play

72. Which of the following functions of play may be hindered by increasing the early academic achievements of a child?
    a. Intellectual development
    b. Creative development
    c. Sensorimotor development
    d. Moral development

73. Based on documented research, which of the following behaviors can be attributed more to girls than to boys during childhood?
    a. Higher analytic skills
    b. Lower self-esteem
    c. Physical aggressiveness
    d. Verbal aggressiveness

74. The medium that has the most impact on children in America today is
    a. television.
    b. movies.
    c. comic books.
    d. newspapers.

II. THINKING CRITICALLY

Use the following scenario to respond to questions 1 through 3.

An 8-year-old child arrives at the clinic for a checkup for school. He has historically been in the 50th percentile for both height and weight and is generally considered healthy. He watches television for about 4 to 5 hours each day. He has a family history of heart disease. His mother is concerned about an increase in her son's physical aggressiveness lately. Today the child's height is noted to be in the 50th percentile, but his weight is in the 95th percentile. His serum cholesterol is elevated.

1. Delineate the factors in this patient's history that need to be addressed.

2. Describe at least three strategies this child's parents can use to deal with the child's aggressiveness.

3. Describe what outcomes the nurse could encourage the child and his parents to aim for.

Communication and Health Assessment of the Child and Family $\boxed{34}$

I. LEARNING KEY TERMS

MATCHING: Match each term with its corresponding description.

1. _____ The pitch, pause, intonation, rate, volume, and stress apparent in speech.

2. _____ An essential parameter of nutritional status; the measurement of height, weight, head circumference, proportions, skinfold thickness, and arm circumference.

3. _____ The capacity to understand what another person is experiencing from within that person's frame of reference.

4. _____ Takes the form of play, artistic expression, symbols, photographs, and choice of clothing.

5. _____ Refers to the composition of the family.

6. _____ Involves having feelings or emotions in common with another person rather than merely understanding those feelings.

7. _____ Often called body language and includes gestures, movements, facial expressions, postures, and reactions.

8. _____ A drawing that indicates the significant people in an individual's life.

9. _____ Refers to all those individuals who are considered by the family member to be significant to the nuclear unit.

10. _____ Involves language and its expression; vocalizations.

11. _____ Concerned with how family members behave toward one another and with the quality of the relationships.

a. Verbal communication

b. Nonverbal communication

c. Abstract communication

d. Paralanguage

e. Empathy

f. Sympathy

g. Family

h. Family structure

i. Sociogram

j. Family function

k. Anthropometry

237

II. REVIEWING KEY CONCEPTS AND CONTENT

12. Which nursing action would negatively affect the communication process between the nurse and the patient?
    a. Verbal and nonverbal messages delivered to the patient are congruous.
    b. Communication includes the child as well as the parent.
    c. The nurse uses verbal and nonverbal communication to reflect approval of the patient's statement.
    d. The nurse uses a slow, even, steady voice to convey instruction.

13. Mrs. Green has brought her daughter Karen to the clinic as a new patient. Karen, age 12 years, requires a physical examination so that she can play volleyball. Which of the following techniques used by the nurse to establish effective communication during the interview process is *not* correct?
    a. The nurse introduces himself or herself and asks the name of all family members present.
    b. After the introduction, the nurse is careful to direct questions about Karen to Mrs. Green because she is the best source of information.
    c. After the introduction and explanation of her role, the nurse begins the interview by saying to Karen, "Tell me about your volleyball team."
    d. The nurse chooses to conduct the interview in a quiet area with few distractions.

14. While conducting an assessment of the child, the nurse communicates with the child's family. Which of the following does the nurse recognize as *not* productive in obtaining information?
    a. Obtaining input from the child, verbal and nonverbal
    b. Observing the relationship between parents and child

c. Using broad, open-ended questions
d. Avoiding the use of guiding statements to direct the focus of the interview

15. The nurse's role in problem solving is to
    a. give advice.
    b. act as a facilitator.
    c. guide the focus of the interview.
    d. offer reassurance.

16. Anticipatory guidance should
    a. view family weakness as a competence builder.
    b. focus on problem resolution.
    c. base interventions on needs identified by the nurse.
    d. empower the family to use information to build parenting ability.

17. T F   Nonverbal components of the communication process do not convey significant messages.

18. T F   Children are alert to their surroundings and attach meaning to gestures.

19. T F   Active attempts to make friends with children before they have had an opportunity to evaluate an unfamiliar person increases their anxiety.

20. T F   The nurse should assume a position that is at eye level with the child.

21. T F   Communication through transition objects such as dolls or stuffed animals delays the child's response to verbal communication offered by the nurse.

MATCHING: Match each development stage with its corresponding description of appropriate communication guidelines to be used.

22. _____ Children focus communication on themselves; experiences of others are of no interest to them.

23. _____ Children primarily use and respond to nonverbal communication.

24. _____ Children require explanations and reasons why procedures are being done to them.

25. _____ Children are often willing to discuss their concern with an adult outside the family and often welcome the opportunity to interact with a nurse.

a. Infancy

b. Early childhood

c. School-age years

d. Adolescence

26. Which of the following best describes the appropriate use of play as a communication technique in children?
    a. Small infants have little response to activities that focus on repetitive actions like patting and stroking.
    b. Few clues about intellectual or social developmental progress are obtained from the observation of children's play behaviors.
    c. Therapeutic play has little value in reduction of trauma from illness or hospitalization.
    d. Play sessions serve as assessment tools for determining children's awareness and perception of illness.

27. List eight components of a complete pediatric health history.

28. In eliciting the chief complaint, it would be inappropriate for the nurse to
    a. limit the chief complaint to a brief statement restricted to one or two symptoms.
    b. use labeling-type questions such as "How are you? Are you sick?" to facilitate information exchange.
    c. record the chief complaint in the child's or parent's own words.
    d. use open-ended neutral questions to elicit information.

29. Which component of the pediatric health history is illustrated by the following? "Nausea and vomiting for 3 days. Started with abdominal cramping after eating hamburger at home. No pain or cramping at present. Unable to keep any foods down but able to drink clear liquids without vomiting. No temperature elevation, no diarrhea."
    a. Chief complaint
    b. Past history
    c. Present illness
    d. Review of systems

30. Which of the following components is *not* a part of the past history in a pediatric health history?
    a. Symptom analysis
    b. Allergies
    c. Birth history
    d. Current medications

31. The nurse knows that the best description of the sexual history for a pediatric health history
    a. includes a discussion of plans for future children.
    b. allows the patient to introduce sexual activity history.
    c. includes a discussion of contraception methods only when the patient discloses current sexual activity.
    d. alerts the nurse to the need for sexually transmitted disease screening.

32. Assessment of family structure is best conducted
    a. after the first meeting with the patient.
    b. only when a problem is suspected within the family.
    c. toward the end of the interview when rapport has been established.
    d. by interviewing the patient about other family members' roles within the family.

33. Assessment of family interactions and roles, decision making and problem solving, and communication is known as assessment of
    a. family structure.
    b. family function.
    c. family composition.
    d. home and community environment.

34. The dietary history of a pediatric patient includes
    a. a 12-hour dietary intake recall.
    b. a more specific, detailed history for the older child.
    c. financial and cultural factors that influence food selection.
    d. criticism of parents' allowance of nonessential foods.

35. To effectively establish a setting for communication, the nurse, upon entering the room with a child and his mother, introduces herself and explains the purpose of the interview. The child is included in the interaction as the nurse asks his name and age and what he is expecting at his visit today. The nurse next tells them both, "The child is 25 pounds overweight, and his diet and exercise plan must be dreadful for him to be in such appalling shape." Which aspect of effective communication has the nurse disregarded that will most significantly impact the exchange of information during this interview?
    a. Assurance of privacy and confidentiality
    b. Preliminary acquaintance
    c. Directing the focus away from the complaint of fatigue to one of obesity
    d. Injecting her own attitudes and feelings into the interview

36. Mrs. Jones brings her 11-month-old daughter to the clinic because she is "sleeping poorly and tugging at her ear when she is awake." Based on the information provided, the nurse can correctly record which of the following?
    a. Chief complaint
    b. Present illness
    c. Past medical history
    d. Symptom analysis

37. The brief screening questionnaire designed to reflect a family member's satisfaction with the state of the family is called the
    a. HOME screening tool.
    b. family Apgar.
    c. home screening questionnaire.
    d. sociogram.

38. Which of the following ways to record dietary intake would the nurse suggest as most reliable?
    a. 12-hour recall
    b. 24-hour recall
    c. Food diary for 3-day period
    d. Food frequency questionnaire

39. Part of any nutritional status examination will include measurements of skinfold thickness and arm circumference. These measures reflect _____ nutritional status and are part of the clinical examination known as _____.

III. THINKING CRITICALLY

1. Compare and contrast between adults and children in the following nursing situations:

   a. The guidelines for communicating with and interviewing adults vs. the guidelines for communicating with and interviewing children

   b. Communicating with families vs. communicating with adults

   c. Taking a health history from an adult vs. taking a health history from a child

Physical and Developmental Assessment of the Child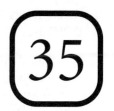

I. LEARNING KEY TERMS

MATCHING: Match each term with its corresponding definition.

1. _____ Small, distinct, pinpoint hemorrhages 2 mm or less in size; can denote a type of blood disorder such as leukemia.

2. _____ Hyperextension of the neck and spine that is accompanied by pain when the head is flexed.

3. _____ Lateral curvature of the spine.

4. _____ An individual's distinct and detailed hand prints and footprints.

5. _____ Redness that may be a result of increased blood flow from climatic conditions, local inflammation, infection, skin irritation, allergy, or other dermatoses or may be caused by increased numbers of red blood cells as a compensatory response to chronic hypoxia.

6. _____ Response of the testes to stimulation by cold, touch, emotional excitement, or exercise.

7. _____ Yellow staining of the skin usually caused by bile pigments.

8. _____ Bowel sounds.

9. _____ The amount of elasticity in the skin; determined by grasping the skin on the abdomen between the thumb and index finger, pulling it taut, and quickly releasing it.

10. _____ Large diffuse area usually black and blue; caused by hemorrhage of blood into skin; typically a result of injuries.

11. _____ Placing the hands against the skin to feel for abnormalities and tenderness.

12. _____ Paleness that may be a sign of anemia, chronic disease, edema, or shock.

13. _____ Using the stethoscope to evaluate breath sounds.

14. _____ A person's standing height.

15. _____ Occurs when one eye deviates from the point of fixation; sometimes called "cross eye."

16. _____ A patient's length measured while the patient is lying down.

17. _____ The ability to visually fixate on one visual field with both eyes simultaneously.

18. _____ A bluish tone through skin indicating reduced (deoxygenated) hemoglobin.

a. Recumbent length

b. Stature

c. Tissue turgor

d. Cyanosis

e. Pallor

f. Erythema

g. Ecchymosis

h. Petechiae

i. Jaundice

j. Dermatoglyphics

k. Opisthotonos

l. Binocularity

m. Strabismus

n. Auscultation

o. Palpation

p. Peristalsis

q. Cremasteric reflex

r. Scoliosis

II. REVIEWING KEY CONCEPTS AND CONTENT

19. In examining pediatric patients, the normal sequence of head-to-toe direction is often altered to accommodate the patient's developmental needs. With this approach, the nurse will
    a. increase the stress and anxiety associated with the assessment of body parts.
    b. record the findings according to the normal sequence.
    c. hinder the trusting nurse-child relationship.
    d. decrease the security of the parent-child relationship.

20. A father brings his 12-month-old son in for the child's regular well-infant examination. The nurse knows that the best approach to the physical examination for this patient will be to
    a. have the infant sit on the parent's lap to complete as much of the examination as possible.
    b. place the infant on the examining table with parent out of view.
    c. perform examination in head-to-toe direction.
    d. completely undress the child and leave him undressed during the examination.

21. Of the following behaviors, the behavior that indicates to the nurse that a child may be reluctant to participate and cooperate during a physical examination is
    a. talking to the nurse.
    b. making eye contact with the nurse.
    c. allowing physical touching.
    d. sitting on parent's lap, playing with a doll.

22. The National Center for Health Statistics has revised the growth charts available for pediatric patients. The new charts include _____ (BMI) for age. The revised charts include all infants and children whatever their _____ or _____. Specialized charts exist to track growth of _____ infants.

23. The assessment method that provides the best information about the physical growth pattern of a preschool-age child is to:
    a. record height and weight measurements of the child on the standardized percentile growth chart.
    b. keep a flow sheet for height, weight, and head circumference increases.
    c. obtain a history of sibling growth patterns.
    d. measure the height, weight, and head circumference of the child.

24. T F Comparing children's growth trends with those of their parents is essential in evaluating adequate growth.

25. T F Breastfed infants grow faster than bottle-fed infants during the 6- to 18-month age period.

26. T F Growth is a continuous but uneven process, and the most reliable evaluation lies in comparison of growth measurements over a prolonged time.

27. T F Growth measurements during the physical examination should be age-specific and include length, height, weight, skinfold thickness, and arm and head circumference.

28. Head circumference is
    a. measured in all children up to the age of 24 months.
    b. equal to chest circumference at about 1 to 2 years of age.
    c. about 8 to 9 cm smaller than chest circumference during childhood.
    d. measured slightly below the eyebrows and pinna of the ears.

29. In infants and small children, the _____ pulse should be taken because it is the most reliable. This pulse should be counted for _____ because of the possibility of irregularities in rhythm.

30. Which of the following observations would *not* be recorded as part of the child's general appearance?
    a. Impression of child's nutritional status
    b. Behavior, interactions with parents
    c. Hygiene, cleanliness
    d. Vital signs

31. When assessing a 7-year-old child's lymph nodes, the nurse uses the distal portions of the fingers and gently but firmly presses in a circular motion along the occipital and postauricular node areas. The nurse records the findings as "tender, enlarged, warm lymph nodes." The nurse knows that the
    a. findings are within normal limits for the child's age.
    b. assessment technique was incorrect and should be repeated.
    c. findings suggest infection or inflammation in the scalp area or external ear canal.
    d. recording of the information is complete because it includes temperature and tenderness.

32. The nurse recognizes that an assessment finding of the head and neck that does *not* need referral is
    a. head lag before 6 months of age.
    b. hyperextension of the head with pain on flexion.
    c. palpable thyroid gland including isthmus and lobes.
    d. closure of the anterior fontanel at the age of 9 months.

33. Sinuses that are present soon after birth are the _____ and _____ sinuses.

34. Normal findings on examination of the pupil may be recorded as PERRLA, which means

    _____.

35. Which of the following assessments is an expected finding in the child's eye examination?
    a. Opaque red reflex of the eye
    b. Ophthalmoscopic examination reflecting veins that are darker in color and about one-fourth larger in size than the arteries
    c. Strabismus in the 12-month-old infant
    d. 5-year-old child who reads the Snellen eye chart at the 20/40 level

36. The test that measures the compliance of the tympanic membrane and the middle ear pressure is
    a. the Rinne test.
    b. the threshold acuity sweep test.
    c. vestibular testing.
    d. tympanometry.

37. Four-year-old Billy has been brought to the clinic by his parents because they have noticed a sudden foul odor in the mouth accompanied by a discharge from the right naris. The nurse knows that this is most likely to suggest:
    a. poor dental hygiene.
    b. foreign body in the nose.
    c. gingival disease.
    d. thumb-sucking.

38. The nurse asks 12-year-old Susan to repeat the word "99" several times while the palmar surfaces of the nurse's hands are placed on the child's chest. The nurse is palpating for conduction of sound through the respiratory tract. What is this called?
    a. Pleural friction rub
    b. Crepitation
    c. Normal respiratory movements
    d. Vocal fremitus

39. On auscultation of 8-year-old Tammie's lung fields, the nurse hears inspiratory sounds that are louder, longer, and higher pitched than on expiration. These sounds are heard over the chest, except over the scapula and sternum. These sounds are
    a. bronchovesicular breath sounds.
    b. vesicular breath sounds.
    c. bronchial breath sounds.
    d. adventitious breath sounds.

40. When the nurse is palpating for cardiac thrills, the nurse knows that thrills are
    a. vibrations caused by the flow of blood from one chamber to another through a narrowed opening.
    b. best felt with the dorsal surface of the hands.
    c. found at the point of maximum intensity.
    d. louder on inspiration than on expiration.

41. A heart sound that is the result of vibrations produced during ventricular filling and normally heard in some children is
    a. S_1.
    b. S_2.
    c. S_3.
    d. S_4.

42. In performing an examination for scoliosis, the nurse understands that which of the following is an incorrect method?
    a. The child should be examined in only his or her underpants (and bra, if an older girl).
    b. The child should stand erect with the nurse observing from behind.
    c. The child should squat down with hands extended forward so that the nurse can observe for asymmetry of the shoulder blades.
    d. The child should bend forward so that the back is parallel to the floor and the nurse can observe from behind.

43. During an examination, the female adolescent will likely
    a. prefer her parents to be present during the entire examination.
    b. desire to undress in private and will feel more comfortable when provided with a gown.
    c. prefer traumatic procedures such as ears and mouth examinations last.
    d. need to have heart and lungs auscultated first.

44. The nurse completes a physical examination on an adolescent and evaluates which of the following as an abnormal finding?
    a. Bowel sounds are stimulated by stroking the abdominal surface with the fingernail.
    b. No abdominal discomfort is experienced by the patient when supine with the legs flexed at the hips and knees.
    c. Eyes are open during palpation of the abdomen.
    d. When the nurse presses firmly over the area distal to the right side of the abdomen and quickly releases this pressure, pain is intensified in the lower right side.

45. Which of the following organs is located in the lower right quadrant of the abdomen?
    a. Bladder
    b. Liver
    c. Ovaries
    d. Appendix

III. THINKING CRITICALLY

1. Describe the differences between the ear canal of an infant and the ear canal of a school-age child.

2. Compare and contrast the differences in skin color changes between light-skinned and dark-skinned individuals.

3. The results of the Denver II screening on a child are abnormal. Describe an effective nursing approach to the initial explanation of the test results to the mother of the child.

The Infant and Family 36

I. LEARNING KEY TERMS

MATCHING: Match each term with its corresponding definition or description.

1. _____ Return of undigested food from the stomach, usually accompanied by burping.

2. _____ Vaccination; responsible for the decline of infectious diseases over the past 60 years.

3. _____ The unexpected and abrupt death of an infant under 1 year of age that remains unexplained after a complete postmortem examination; the leading cause of death in children between the ages of 1 month and 1 year.

4. _____ Dribbling of unswallowed formula from the infant's mouth immediately after a feeding.

5. _____ Cessation of breathing for 20 seconds or more.

6. _____ A major accomplishment of cognitive development that develops at approximately 9 to 10 months of age; the realization that objects continue to exist after they leave one's visual field.

7. _____ The process of giving up one method of feeding for another; usually refers to relinquishing the breast or bottle for a cup.

8. _____ Fusion of two ocular images that begins to develop at 6 weeks and should be well established by age 4 months.

9. _____ Paroxysmal abdominal pain manifested by a duration of more than 3 hours and by drawing up of the legs to the abdomen in an infant under the age of 3 months.

10. _____ Behaviors that demonstrate a preference for the mother and are a result of the 5- to 6-month-old infant developing the ability to distinguish the mother or other primary caregiver from other individuals; results from improving cognitive development and peaks at 8 months of age.

11. _____ A major intellectual achievement of infancy; the ability to use symbols.

12. _____ A characteristic behavior of social development that occurs in the second half of the first year of life; depends on the interaction rather than reflex.

a. Binocularity

b. Object permanence

c. Stranger fear

d. Attachment

e. Weaning

f. Immunization

g. Spitting up

h. Regurgitation

i. Colic

j. Sudden infant death (SIDS)

k. Apnea

l. Mental representation

II. REVIEWING KEY CONCEPTS AND CONTENT

13. If an infant weighs 9 kg at age 12 months, how many kilograms was the infant's probable birth weight?
    a. 1.5 kg
    b. 3 kg
    c. 4.5 kg
    d. 6 kg

14. If an infant's head circumference is 46 cm at 6 months, how many centimeters would you expect the infant's head circumference to be at 8 months?
    a. 46.5
    b. 47
    c. 47.5
    d. 49

15. The infant's posterior fontanel usually closes by
    a. 6 to 8 weeks.
    b. 3 to 6 months.
    c. 12 to 18 months.
    d. 9 to 12 months.

16. Which of the following characteristics of vision begins to develop by 6 weeks of age and should be well established by age 4 months?
    a. Corneal reflex
    b. Stereopsis
    c. Binocularity
    d. Strabismus

17. Which of the following assessment findings would be considered most abnormal?
    a. The infant who displays head lag at 3 months of age
    b. The infant who displays head lag at 6 months of age
    c. The infant who begins to roll from front to back at 4 months
    d. The infant who begins to roll from front to back at 6 months

18. Parenting
    a. is an instinctual ability.
    b. is a learned acquired process.
    c. begins shortly after birth.
    d. shapes the infant's environment positively.

19. Which one of the following play activities would be least appropriate to suggest to the mother for her 3-month-old infant to promote auditory and tactile stimulation?
    a. Playing music and singing along
    b. Using rattles
    c. Using an infant swing
    d. Placing toys a bit out of reach

20. Reactive attachment disorder stems from
    a. crying and vocalizing to the mother.
    b. clinging to the mother.
    c. crying when the mother leaves the room.
    d. maladaptive or absent attachment.

21. If a mother is concerned about the fact that her 14-month-old infant is not walking, the nurse would particularly want to evaluate whether the infant
    a. pulls up on the furniture.
    b. uses a pincer grasp.
    c. transfers objects.
    d. has developed object permanence.

22. If a mother is concerned about "spoiling" her child when crying and fussiness occurs, the nurse should encourage her to respond to her newborn's crying episodes with
    a. a delayed response of holding the infant.
    b. a prompt response of holding the infant.
    c. eliminating the use of the pacifier.
    d. feeding the infant.

23. Colic is more common in the infant who
    a. is between 3 and 6 months of age.
    b. has a difficult temperament.
    c. has other congenital abnormalities.
    d. has signs of failure to thrive.

24. The nurse should withhold the vaccine if the child
    a. has a low-grade fever.
    b. is currently taking antibiotics.
    c. has a moderately acute illness without fever.
    d. was born prematurely.

25. The nurse should withhold immunization with the oral polio vaccine if which of the following situations exists?
    a. The child had a temperature of 104° F 3 days after the previous immunization.
    b. The child has a cold with a temperature of 100° F.
    c. The child has had a kidney transplant.
    d. The child had a seizure a week after the previous immunization.

26. Which of the following techniques has been demonstrated by research to be most successful when two or more immunizations are given at one visit?
    a. Inject the less painful immunization first.
    b. Use an air bubble to clear the needle after the injection.
    c. Inject the immunizations simultaneously.
    d. Apply a topical anesthetic to the site for a minimum of 1 hour.

27. Which of the following types of injuries is a leading cause of death in infants?
    a. Poisoning
    b. Motor vehicle accidents
    c. Asphyxiation
    d. Falls

28. T   F   The incidence of SIDS is associated with diphtheria, tetanus, and pertussis vaccines.

29. T   F   Maternal smoking during and after pregnancy has been implicated as a contributor to SIDS.

30. T   F   Parents should be advised to position an infant on his or her abdomen to prevent SIDS.

31. T   F   The nurse should encourage the parents to sleep in the same bed as the infant being monitored for apnea of infancy in order to detect subtle clinical changes.

32. T   F   Parents should be advised to dress the infant in light clothing to avoid SIDS.

III. THINKING CRITICALLY

1. Describe the fine motor and gross motor, language, and social developmental milestones to assess in a 7-month-old infant who is coming to the well-child clinic.

2. Describe the interventions you would use with parents who have recently lost an infant to SIDS.

3. Describe the strategies to use when teaching parents of a child who is to be monitored at home for apnea of infancy.

37 The Toddler and Family

I. LEARNING KEY TERMS

MATCHING: Match each term with its corresponding description.

1. _____ The need to maintain sameness and reliability.

2. _____ The destruction of teeth resulting from the process of bathing the teeth in a cariogenic environment for a prolonged period; most often affects the maxillary incisor and the molars.

3. _____ The child's emergence from a symbiotic fusion with the mother.

4. _____ Soft bacterial deposits that adhere to the teeth and cause dental decay and periodontal disease.

5. _____ A necessary assertion of self-control in the toddler.

6. _____ Those achievements that mark children's assumption of their individual characteristics in the environment.

7. _____ The retreat from one's present pattern of functioning to past levels of behavior.

8. _____ Characterized by the child playing alongside, not with, other children.

9. _____ The developmental stage in which the toddler relinquishes dependence on others.

a. Autonomy

b. Negativism

c. Ritualism

d. Separation

e. Individuation

f. Parallel play

g. Regression

h. Plaque

i. Nursing caries (nursing bottle caries or bottle-mouth caries)

II. REVIEWING KEY CONCEPTS AND CONTENT

10. If the chest circumference of a toddler is 50 cm, what would you expect the head circumference to be?
    a. 25 cm
    b. 35 cm
    c. 50 cm
    d. 60 cm

11. Which of the following skills is *not* necessary for the toddler to acquire before separation and individuation can be achieved?
    a. Object permanence
    b. Lack of anxiety during separation from parents
    c. Delayed gratification
    d. Ability to tolerate a moderate amount of frustration

12. The usual number of words acquired by the age of 2 years is about
    a. 50.
    b. 100.
    c. 300.
    d. 500.

13. Which of the following types of play increases in frequency as the child moves through the toddler period?
    a. Parallel play
    b. Imitative play
    c. Tactile play
    d. Solitary play

14. Which of the following statements is false in regard to toilet training?
    a. Bowel training is usually accomplished after bladder training.
    b. Nighttime bladder training is usually accomplished after bowel training.
    c. The toddler who is impatient with soiled diapers is demonstrating readiness for toilet training.
    d. Fewer wet diapers signal that the toddler is physically ready for toilet training.

15. Which of the following strategies is appropriate for parents to use to prepare a toddler for the birth of a sibling?
    a. Explain the upcoming birth as early in the pregnancy as possible.
    b. Move the toddler to his or her own new room.
    c. Provide a doll for the toddler to imitate parenting.
    d. Tell the toddler that a new playmate will come home soon.

16. The best approach for extinguishing a toddler's attention-seeking behavior of a tantrum with head banging is to
    a. ignore the behavior.
    b. provide time-out.
    c. offer a toy to calm the child.
    d. protect the child from injury.

17. Which of the following statements about stress in toddlers is true?
    a. Toddlers are rarely exposed to stress or the results of stress.
    b. Any stress is destructive because toddlers have a limited ability to cope.
    c. Most children are exposed to a stress-free environment.
    d. Small amounts of stress help toddlers develop effective coping skills.

18. Regression in toddlers occurs when there is
    a. stress.
    b. a threat to their autonomy.
    c. a need to revert to dependency.
    d. all of the above.

19. Which of the following statements is true in regard to nutritional changes from the infant to the toddler years?
    a. Caloric requirements increase from 102 kcal/kg to 108 kcal/kg.
    b. Caloric requirements decrease from 108 kcal/kg to 102 kcal/kg.
    c. Protein requirements decrease from 2.2 kcal/kg to 1.5 kcal/kg.
    d. Protein requirements increase from 1.2 kcal/kg to 2.2 kcal/kg.

20. Which of the following methods is most effective for plaque removal?
    a. Brushing and flossing
    b. Annual fluoride treatments
    c. Allowing the child to brush his or her own teeth
    d. Using a large stiff toothbrush

21. Which of the following nutritional requirements increases during the toddler years?
    a. Calories
    b. Proteins
    c. Minerals
    d. Fluids

22. Physiologic anorexia in toddlers is characterized by
    a. strong taste preferences.
    b. extreme changes in appetite from day to day.
    c. heightened awareness of social aspects of meals.
    d. all of the above.

23. Healthy ways of serving food to toddlers include
    a. requiring a pattern of sitting at a table for meals.
    b. permitting nutritious nibbling.
    c. discouraging between-meal snacking.
    d. all of the above.

24. Which of the following strategies is least appropriate for the parent to use to help the toddler adjust to the initial dental visit?
    a. Explain to the child that a checkup won't hurt.
    b. Have the child observe his or her brother's examination.
    c. Have the child perform a checkup on a doll.
    d. Ask the dentist to reserve a thorough examination for another visit.

25. Children should be placed in convertible car restraints until
    a. they weigh 40 pounds.
    b. they reach 40 inches in height.
    c. the midpoint of the child's head is higher than the vehicle seat back.
    d. all of the above.

26. The parents should consider moving the toddler from the crib to a bed after the toddler
    a. reaches the age of 2 years.
    b. will stay in bed all night.
    c. reaches a height of 35 inches.
    d. is able to sleep through the night.

27. Give an example of an item that could cause
    aspiration or suffocation for each of the following
    categories of items hazardous to the toddler (e.g.,
    foods: hard candy).
    a. Foods
    b. Play objects
    c. Common household objects
    d. Electrical items

III. THINKING CRITICALLY

1. Describe four areas that the nurse should assess to obtain the information necessary to give adequate
   anticipatory guidance to the parents of a 12-month-old toddler.

2. Describe three gross motor developmental milestones that a 2-year-old toddler should have accomplished.

3. Describe three fine motor developmental milestones that a 2-year-old toddler should have accomplished.

4. Describe three language developmental milestones that a 2-year-old toddler should have accomplished.

5. Describe how negativism contributes to the toddler's acquisition of a sense of autonomy.

The Preschooler and Family

38

I. LEARNING KEY TERMS

MATCHING: Match each term with its corresponding definition or description.

1. _____ Activities that reproduce adult behavior; more typically seen at the end of the preschool period.

2. _____ Infectious disease that has declined greatly since the advent of immunizations and the use of antibiotics and antitoxins.

3. _____ Group activities that have no rigid organization or rules; typical of the preschool period.

4. _____ Partial arousal from a deep, nondreaming sleep.

5. _____ The deliberate attempt to destroy or significantly impair a child's self-esteem.

6. _____ The infliction of harm on a child caused by a parent or other person who fabricates or induces illness in the child.

7. _____ Sentences of about three or four words including only the most essential words to convey meaning.

8. _____ Scary dreams that are followed by full waking.

9. _____ The result of a preschooler's transductive reasoning; the belief that thoughts are all powerful.

10. _____ Failure to meet the child's need for affection, attention, and emotional nurturance.

11. _____ Articulation problems that occur when children are pressured to produce sounds ahead of their developmental level.

12. _____ The preschooler's way of understanding, adjusting to, and working out life's experiences.

13. _____ A type of speech pattern that occurs normally in children during the preschool period.

14. _____ The use, persuasion, or coercion of any child to engage in sexually explicit conduct.

15. _____ Deliberate infliction of bodily injury on a child usually by the child's caregiver.

a. Sense of initiative

b. Conscience

c. Intuitive thought

d. Play

e. Magical thinking

f. Telegraphic speech

g. Associative play

h. Imitative play

i. Imaginary playmates

j. Desensitization period

k. Aggression

l. Stuttering (stammering)

m. Dyslalia

n. Nightmares

o. Sleep terrors

p. Communicable disease

q. Prodromal symptoms

r. Child maltreatment

s. Physical neglect

t. Emotional neglect

u. Emotional abuse

v. Physical abuse

w. Munchausen syndrome by proxy

x. Sexual abuse

16. _____ The second stage of Piaget's preoperational phase; the transition to social awareness and the ability to consider other viewpoints.

17. _____ The deprivation of necessities such as food, clothing, shelter, supervision, medical care, and education.

18. _____ Behavior that attempts to hurt a person or destroys property; differs from anger.

19. _____ The superego; development in this area is a major task for the preschooler.

20. _____ Intentional bodily injury or neglect, emotional abuse or neglect, and/or sexual abuse of children, usually by adults.

21. _____ A type of conditioning that involves gradual introduction to an intimidating experience to help the child overcome apprehension.

22. _____ A feeling of accomplishment in one's activities; a psychosocial developmental task of the preschool period.

23. _____ Occur between early manifestations of a disease and its overt clinical syndrome.

24. _____ An invented companion that serves many purposes in the preschooler's development.

II. REVIEWING KEY CONCEPTS AND CONTENT

25. The approximate age range for the preschool period begins at age _____ years and ends at age _____ years.

26. The average annual weight gain during the preschool years is _____ kg/lb.

27. Which of the following statements about the average preschooler's physical proportions is true?
    a. Preschoolers have a squat and potbellied frame.
    b. Preschoolers have a slender but sturdy frame.
    c. The muscle and bones of the preschooler have matured.
    d. Sexual characteristics can be differentiated in the preschooler.

28. During the preschool years, anticipatory guidance shifts to a focus on
    a. protection rather than education.
    b. education and correcting dysfluency in speech patterns.
    c. education with an emphasis on reasoning.
    d. protection and safeguarding the immediate environment.

29. The moral and spiritual development of the preschooler is characterized by
    a. concern for why something is wrong.
    b. actions that are directed toward satisfying the needs of others.
    c. thoughts of loyalty and gratitude.
    d. a very concrete sense of justice.

30. T F Sleep terrors can be described as a partial arousal from a very deep nondreaming sleep.

31. T F Nightmares usually occur in the second half of the night.

32. T F   With sleep terrors, crying and fright persist even after the child is awake.

33. T F   With nightmares, the child is not very aware of another's presence.

34. When educating the preschool child about injury prevention, the parents should
    a. set a good example.
    b. help children establish good habits.
    c. be aware that pedestrian/motor vehicle injuries increase in this age group.
    d. all of the above.

35. A common finding in abused children's parents is that they
    a. were physically punished by their own parents.
    b. were physically abused by their parents.
    c. had inadequate knowledge of childrearing.
    d. are always members of a low socioeconomic population.

36. Which of the following statements is incorrect?
    a. The position of the child in the family has little effect on the abusive situation.
    b. One child is usually the victim in an abusive family, and removal of this child often places the other children at risk.

    c. The abusive family environment is one of chronic stress, including problems of divorce, poverty, unemployment, and poor housing.
    d. Child abuse is a problem of all social groups.

37. The nurse is talking with a 13-year-old child who has revealed that she is being sexually abused. Which of the following is a correct guideline for the nurse to utilize?
    a. Promise not to tell what the child reveals to you.
    b. Assure the child that she will not need to report the abuse.
    c. Avoid using leading statements that can distort the child's reporting of the problem.
    d. It is okay for the nurse to express anger and shock and to criticize the child's family.

III. THINKING CRITICALLY

Use the following scenario to respond to questions 1 through 4.

Imagine that you are a nurse on the staff of a pediatric group practice. A mother comes in to discuss her son, who is not quite 3 years old. He will attend the preschool program at a local private school this year. He has attended a home day care program since he was a baby, while his mother worked in her own interior decorating business.

An older woman runs the day care that the child has attended until now. The woman and her helper both treat the 12 children in her program as if they were family. The program is very structured in regard to schedule and routines.

The child's mother tells you that she is looking forward to Jacob's new environment. His teacher is very creative and approaches the classroom from the perspective of the child's development. There will be a lot of choices for activities during the day.

1. Based on the information above, analyze the data presented in relation to the child's needs and the concerns for a smooth transition.

2. Develop an expected outcome that is reasonable to establish for this mother and her child.

3. Describe interventions and strategies that are appropriate for you to suggest to this mother and her child.

4. Explain to the mother the characteristics that indicate the child is ready for preschool.

The School-Age Child and Family ⟨39⟩

I. LEARNING KEY TERMS

MATCHING: Match each term with its corresponding definition.

1. _____ Developmentally inappropriate degrees of inattention and impulsiveness.

2. _____ Commonly observed after an overwhelming stimulus such as physical abuse; characterized by a feeling of foreboding regarding the future and sense of hopelessness.

3. _____ The heterogeneous group of disorders manifested by significant difficulties in the acquisition and use of listening, speaking, reading, writing, reasoning, mathematic, or social skills.

4. _____ The repeated voluntary or involuntary passage of feces of normal or near-normal consistency into places not appropriate for that purpose according to the individual's own sociocultural setting.

5. _____ A slower development of pubertal growth than is physiologically normal.

6. _____ The principal oral problem in children and adolescents; if untreated can result in total destruction of the involved teeth.

7. _____ The period in which the secondary sex characteristics begin to develop, typically occurring during preadolescence.

8. _____ The beginning of the development of secondary sex characteristics.

9. _____ Exarticulated; "knocked out."

10. _____ One of the numerous psychologic symptoms that may become apparent in the third phase (coping) of posttraumatic stress syndrome.

11. _____ Elementary school children who are left to care for themselves before or after school without supervision of an adult.

12. _____ The common and troublesome disorder of bed-wetting; difficult to define because of the variable ages at which children achieve bladder control.

a. Prepubescence

b. Puberty

c. Latchkey children

d. Dental caries

e. Tooth evulsion

f. Constitutional delay

g. Attention deficit hyperactivity disorder

h. Learning disability

i. Enuresis

j. Encopresis

k. Posttraumatic stress disorder

l. Conversion reaction

II. REVIEWING KEY CONCEPTS AND CONTENT

13. The middle childhood is also referred to as "school-age" or the "school years." What ages does this period represent?
    a. Ages 5 to 13 years
    b. Ages 4 to 14 years
    c. Ages 6 to 12 years
    d. Ages 6 to 16 years

14. Physiologically, the middle years begin with _____ and end at _____.

15. T   F   In middle childhood there are fewer stomach upsets, better maintenance of blood sugar levels, and an increased stomach capacity.

16. T   F   Caloric needs are higher in relation to stomach size compared with the needs during preschool years.

17. T   F   The heart is smaller in relation to the rest of the body during the middle years.

18. T   F   During the middle years, the immune system develops little immunity to pathogenic microorganisms.

19. T   F   Backpacks are preferred to other book totes during middle years.

20. T   F   Physical maturity correlates well with emotional and social maturity during the middle years.

21. Generally, the earliest age at which puberty begins is age _____ for girls and age _____ for boys.

22. Middle childhood is the time when children:
    I.   learn the value of doing things with others.
    II. learn the benefits derived from division of labor in accomplishing goals.
    III. achieve a sense of industry and accomplishment.
    IV. expand interests and engage in tasks that can be carried to completion.
        a. I, II, III, and IV
        b. I, III, and IV
        c. I and IV
        d. II and III

23. A 6-year-old boy is starting in a new neighborhood school. On the first day of school he complains of a headache and tearfully tells his mother he does not want to go. His mother takes him to school, and the nurse is consulted. The nurse recognizes that this is a slow-to-warm-up child and suggests which of the following?
    a. Put him in the classroom with the other children and leave him alone.
    b. Insist that he join and lead the class song.
    c. Include him in activities without assigning him tasks until he willingly participates in activities.
    d. Send him home with his mother because he has a headache.

24. During the school-age years, children learn valuable lessons from age-mates. How is this accomplished?
    a. The child learns to appreciate the varied points of view that are within the peer group.
    b. The child becomes sensitive to the social norms and pressures of the group.
    c. The child's interactions among peers lead to the formation of intimate friendships between same-sex peers.
    d. all of the above.

25. Children's self-concepts are composed of their
    a. own critical self-assessment.
    b. interpretations of family members' opinions.
    c. interpretations of opinions of social contacts outside the family structure.
    d. all of the above.

26. Team membership characteristics that promote child development during the middle years include which of the following?
    a. Children learn to subordinate personal goals to group goals.
    b. Children learn about division of labor as an effective strategy for the attainment of a goal.
    c. Team play helps children learn about the nature of competition and the importance of winning.
    d. all of the above.

27. The factor that most influences the amount and manner of discipline and limit setting imposed on school-age children is
    a. the age of the parent.
    b. the education of the parent.
    c. response of the child to rewards and punishments.
    d. the ability of the parent to communicate with the school system.

28. To assist school-age children in coping with stress in their lives, the nurse should
    - I. be able to recognize signs that indicate the child is undergoing stress.
    - II. teach the child how to recognize signs of stress in herself or himself.
    - III. help the child plan a means for dealing with any stress through problem solving.
    - IV. reassure the child that the stress is only temporary.
      - a. I, II, III, and IV
      - b. I, II, and III
      - c. I, II, and IV
      - d. I and III

29. By the end of middle childhood, children should be able to assume personal responsibility for self-care in the areas of _____, _____, _____, _____, _____, and _____.

III. THINKING CRITICALLY

A 9-year-old boy is brought to the clinic by his mother for a school physical examination. His mother is concerned, because the child wants to join the school soccer team this year. On physical examination, the nurse discovers that since last year there has been an increase of 2 inches in height and a 10-pound weight gain. Health history is unchanged from the previous year. The young boy tells the nurse that he rides his bike more now than last year because he has a new "best friend" to go riding with.

1. Describe the areas of assessment that the nurse should expand upon.

2. Describe an appropriate response to the mother's concern about her son playing soccer.

3. Describe an educational session that would most benefit this child and his mother.

4. Describe how the mother of this 9-year-old boy can foster his development.

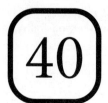 # The Adolescent and Family

I. LEARNING KEY TERMS

MATCHING: Match each term with its corresponding definition.

1. _____ The masculinizing hormones; secreted in small and gradually increasing amounts up to about 7 or 9 years of age, then followed by a rapid increase in both sexes, the level of androgens in males increasing over that in females with the onset of testicular function.

2. _____ Regular use of drugs for other than the accepted medical purposes; use of drugs resulting in physical or psychologic harm to the user and/or detrimental effects to society.

3. _____ The hormone that increases with the onset of testicular function.

4. _____ Behavior associated with drug use that is voluntary and culturally defined.

5. _____ Behaviors, associated with drug use that are physiologic and involuntary; not culturally defined.

6. _____ The initial appearance of menstruation; occurs about 2 years after the appearance of the first pubescent changes.

7. _____ The feminizing hormone; found in low quantities during childhood; secreted in slowly increasing amounts until about age 11 years in both males and females, then followed by a distinction in its secretion between the male and the female.

8. _____ Temporary breast enlargement and tenderness; common during mid-puberty in boys.

9. _____ Eating disorder characterized by binge eating and purging followed by self-deprecating thoughts, a depressed mood, and awareness that the eating pattern is abnormal.

10. _____ A period of transition between childhood and adulthood, beginning with the gradual appearance of secondary sex characteristics at about 11 or 12 years of age and ending with cessation of body growth at 18 to 20 years.

11. _____ The first period of puberty; occurs about 2 years immediately before puberty, when the child is developing preliminary physical changes that herald sexual maturity.

12. _____ Eating disorder characterized by a refusal to maintain a minimally normal body weight; severe weight loss in the absence of obvious physical causes.

13. _____ Occurs in males toward the end of the growth spurt of adolescence.

a. Puberty

b. Pubescence

c. Adolescence

d. Estrogen

e. Androgens

f. Testosterone

g. Menarche

h. Gynecomastia

i. Nocturnal emission

j. Amenorrhea

k. Dysmenorrhea

l. Obesity

m. Anorexia nervosa

n. Bulimia

o. Drug abuse

p. Drug tolerance

q. Addiction

258

14. _____ The maturational, hormonal, and growth process that occurs when the reproductive organs begin to function and the secondary sex characteristics develop.

15. _____ Absence of menstruation.

16. _____ Occurs when a child's actual body weight is greater than 120% of the ideal.

17. _____ Painful menses.

II. REVIEWING KEY CONCEPTS AND CONTENT

18. The normal age range for menarche is usually _____ to _____ years, with the average age being _____ years and _____ months for North American girls.

19. The hormone in the female that causes growth and development of the vagina, uterus, and fallopian tubes, as well as breast enlargement is
    a. estrogen.
    b. progesterone.
    c. follicle-stimulating hormone.
    d. luteinizing hormone.

20. The adolescent growth spurt is characterized as beginning
    a. sooner in boys
    b. between ages 9½ and 14½ in boys.
    c. sooner in girls.
    d. between the ages of 10½ and 16 years in girls.

21. Girls may be considered to have _____ if breast development has not occurred by age 13 or if menarche has not occurred by age 13.

22. The first pubescent change in boys is
    a. appearance of pubic hair.
    b. testicular enlargement with thinning, reddening, and increased looseness of the scrotum.
    c. penile enlargement.
    d. temporary breast enlargement and tenderness.

23. Which one of the following statements about pattern of growth during adolescence is true?
    a. Knowing the correct sequence of the growth pattern is useful only when assessing abnormal growth patterns versus normal growth patterns.
    b. Boys start an increase of muscle mass during early puberty that lasts throughout adolescence.
    c. Boys usually begin puberty and reach maturity about 2 years earlier than girls.
    d. Girls and boys have an increase in linear growth that begins for both during mid-puberty.

24. On the average, girls gain _____ to _____ inches in height and _____ to _____ pounds during adolescence, whereas boys gain _____ to _____ inches and _____ to _____ pounds.

25. Which of the following best describes the formal operational thinking that occurs between the ages of 11 and 14 years?
    a. Thought process includes thinking in concrete terms.
    b. Thought process includes information obtained from the environment and peers.
    c. Thought process includes thinking in abstract terms, possibilities, and hypotheses.
    d. All of the above.

26. Jimmy, a 13-year-old, is sent to the school nurse because he and some of his peers were caught chewing tobacco while playing baseball. The nurse knows that the best way to influence Jimmy's behavior for health promotion is which of the following?
    a. Tell Jimmy that he will be suspended from school if he continues to chew the tobacco.
    b. Show Jimmy pictures of oral cancers caused by chewing tobacco.
    c. Tell Jimmy about the dangers of chewing tobacco and stress the fact that girls do not like boys who chew tobacco.
    d. Arrange for a local baseball hero to talk with Jimmy and his friends to stress that he does not use chewing tobacco, his friends do not chew tobacco, and chewing tobacco causes ugly teeth.

27. According to Erikson, a key to identity achievement in adolescence is best described as
    a. related to the adolescent's interactions with others, serving as a mirror and reflecting information back to the adolescent.
    b. linked to the role he or she plays within the family.
    c. related to the adolescent's acceptance of parental guidelines.
    d. related to the adolescent's ability to finalize his or her plans for future accomplishments.

28. The formation of sexual identity development during adolescence usually involves which of the following?
   a. Forming close friendships with same-sex peers during early adolescence
   b. Developing intimate relationships with members of the opposite sex during the later part of adolescence
   c. Developing emotional and social identities separate from those of families
   d. All of the above

29. During adolescence, advances in cognitive development bring which of the following changes?
   a. Their beliefs become more concrete and less rooted in general ideologic principles.
   b. They show an increasing emotional understanding and acceptance of parents' beliefs as their own.
   c. They encounter few new situations or opportunities for decisions because of their past experiences.
   d. They develop a personal value system distinct from that of significant adults in their lives.

30. Compared with school-age children, adolescent peer groups are
   a. more likely to include peers of the opposite sex.
   b. less autonomous.
   c. less likely to influence members' socialization roles.
   d. more likely to require parental supervision.

31. The major causes of morbidity and mortality during adolescence are
   a. drownings.
   b. cancers.
   c. infectious diseases.
   d. health-damaging behaviors.

32. Of the following male reproductive problems, the one most likely to be identified in an adolescent male is
   a. hypospadias.
   b. cryptorchidism.
   c. testicular tumor.
   d. urethritis.

33. The adolescent with testicular cancer is most likely to present with which of the following signs and symptoms?
   a. Tender, painful swelling of the testes
   b. A mass in the posterior aspect of the scrotum that transilluminates
   c. A heavy, hard, painless mass palpable on the anterior or lateral surface of the testicle
   d. Asymptomatic scrotal mass that aches, especially after exercise or penile erection

34. In teaching the adolescent male how to perform testicular self-examination, the nurse includes which of the following instructions?
   a. Perform the procedure once a month after a warm shower.
   b. A raised swelling palpated on the superior aspect of the testicle indicates an abnormality.
   c. Use the second and third fingers on each hand, holding each testicle between the fingers while palpating it with the other fingers.
   d. Testicular tumors, although common in adolescents, are usually benign.

35. The nurse knows that which of the following adolescent females should be scheduled for her first pelvic examination?
   a. The 18-year-old who has not become sexually active
   b. The adolescent who has been menstruating for 2 years and has severe dysmenorrhea that is unrelieved by medication
   c. The adolescent who wants to start birth control pills
   d. All of the above

MATCHING: Match each term with its corresponding description. Terms may be used more than once.

36. _____ Breast enlargement that occurs during puberty.

37. _____ Palpated as a wormlike mass above the testicle that becomes smaller in size when the adolescent lies down.

38. _____ Treatment includes assurance to the adolescent that the disease is benign and temporary and occurs in about 50% of his peers.

39. _____ Inflammation that is a result of either infection or local trauma.

40. _____ Occurs when the testis hangs free from its vascular structure; results in partial or complete venous occlusion.

a. Varicocele

b. Epididymitis

c. Testicular torsion

d. Gynecomastia

41. _____ Presents with unilateral scrotal pain, redness, and swelling; may have urethral discharge, dysuria, fever, and pyuria; treated with antibiotics.

42. _____ Presents with scrotum that is swollen, painful, red, and warm; marked in adolescents by pain radiating to groin, with nausea, vomiting, and abdominal pain; fever and urinary symptoms usually not present; treated by immediate surgery.

43. _____ is defined as an absence of menses by age 16 when there are normal secondary sex characteristics.

44. _____ is defined as an absence of menses for 3 to 6 months in a previously menstruating female when pregnancy has been excluded.

45. The treatment of choice for an adolescent with dysmenorrhea is
   a. acetaminophen.
   b. oral contraceptives.
   c. nonsteroidal antiinflammatory drugs.
   d. estrogen suppression drugs.

46. It is important to assess adverse effects of exercise on the reproductive cycle in an adolescent with anorexia nervosa. The signs of adverse effects of exercise on an adolescent's reproductive cycle may include
   a. dysmenorrhea.
   b. weight loss.
   c. decreased appetite.
   d. amenorrhea.

III. THINKING CRITICALLY

1. Explain the principles of physical growth that are important for adolescent girls to understand if they are concerned about their weight.

2. Explain how a peer group contributes to the development of a sense of identity in the adolescent and why peer groups are an important influence during the adolescent years.

3. Describe three guiding principles to offer to parents of adolescents to help them better communicate with their adolescent child.

4. Explain how an adolescent can benefit from participating in sports.

5. Explain why there has been a recent increased incidence of anorexia and bulimia.

6. Identify the essential aspects of multidisciplinary treatment for anorexia nervosa and bulimia.

7. Describe the characteristics typically seen with adolescent suicide.

Chronic Illness, Disability, and End-of-Life Care ⟨41⟩

I. LEARNING KEY TERMS

MATCHING: Match each term with its corresponding description.

1. _____ A principle in the care of children with special needs that refers to establishing a normal pattern of living.

2. _____ Actions carried out by a person other than the patient to end the life of the patient suffering from a terminal illness.

3. _____ A child between the ages of birth to 21 years with a chronic disability that requires the routine use of a medical device to compensate for the loss of a life-sustaining bodily function; daily ongoing care and/or monitoring required by trained personnel.

4. _____ Coping mechanisms that result in movement away from adjustment; maladaptation to the crisis.

5. _____ A loss or abnormality of structure or function.

6. _____ The active total care of a patient whose disease is not responsive to curative treatment.

7. _____ Integration of children with special needs into regular classrooms.

8. _____ The concept of providing palliative care for the child with no reasonable expectation of cure so that he or she can live to the fullest without pain, with choices and dignity, and with family support.

9. _____ A condition or barrier imposed by society, the environment, or one's self.

10. _____ A functional limitation that interferes with a person's ability to walk, lift, hear, or learn.

11. _____ Coping mechanisms that result in movement toward adjustment and resolution of the crisis.

12. _____ Any mental and/or physical disability of obvious physical causes that is manifested before age 22 years and is likely to continue indefinitely.

13. _____ A syndrome that occurs within a few hours to days after a death, characterized by somatic distress, preoccupation with the image of the deceased, feelings of guilt and hostility, and loss of usual pattern of conduct.

14. _____ A condition that interferes with daily functioning for 3 months in a year, causes hospitalization of more than 1 month in a year, or (at time of diagnosis) is likely to do either of these.

a. Chronic illness

b. Congenital disability

c. Developmental delay

d. Developmental disability

e. Disability

f. Handicap

g. Impairment

h. Technology-dependent

i. Normalization

j. Mainstreaming

k. Approach behaviors

l. Chronic sorrow

m. Avoidance behaviors

n. Anticipatory grief

o. Acute grief

p. Palliative care

q. Euthanasia

r. Hospice

15. _____ An emotional response that is manifested through the life span of the parent-child interaction; acceptance interspersed with periods of intensified sorrow for losses, especially at certain landmarks of the child's development (e.g., entry into school, the onset of puberty).

16. _____ A maturational lag—an abnormal, slower rate of development in a child that demonstrates a functioning level below that observed in normal children of the same age.

17. _____ The behavioral reaction that occurs when death is the expected or possible outcome of a disorder.

18. _____ A disability that has existed since birth but is not necessarily hereditary.

II. REVIEWING KEY CONCEPTS AND CONTENT

19. Technologic advancements have inadvertently increased the incidence of
    a. deaths.
    b. disabilities.
    c. AIDS cases.
    d. asthma.

20. A goal that is considered inappropriate for family-centered care is to
    a. maintain the integrity of the family.
    b. empower the family members.
    c. support the family during stressful times.
    d. maintain a high level of control.

21. Parents in the _____ category usually have a high level of trust in the nurse and often want the nurse to make decisions.

22. Parents who fit in the _____ category use little verbal communication and may not accompany the child into the examination room.

23. If parents are in control of health-related decisions and use the nurses for consultation and direct care, the parents can be said to follow the pattern of _____.

24. Parents who keep track of the staff and seek detailed information are referred to as

    _____.

25. A major goal in working with the family of a child with special needs is to _____.

26. Identify one strategy to use to help break patterns of unproductive interaction in parents of a child with special needs.

27. Which of the following factors is more characteristic of a father's pattern than a mother's pattern of adjusting to a chronically ill child? The father is more likely to
    a. feel a threat to his self-esteem.
    b. report a periodic crisis pattern.
    c. forfeit personal goals.
    d. seek immediate professional counseling.

28. Describe the adaptive tasks of parents who have a child with a chronic condition.

29. The sibling of a child with a chronic disabling condition may feel
    a. left out and unimportant.
    b. concern for his or her own health.
    c. physical symptoms similar to his or her sibling's.
    d. all of the above.

30. Grandparents of a disabled child often have feelings of
    a. resentment.
    b. ambivalence.
    c. embarrassment.
    d. shame.

31. When the parents of a child with special needs experience chronic sorrow, the process
    a. of grief is pronounced and self-limiting.
    b. involves social reintegration after grieving.
    c. is characterized by realistic expectations.
    d. is interspersed with periods of intensified grief.

32. Which of the following stressors can usually be anticipated in a child with special needs?
    a. The approximate cost of the yearly medical bills
    b. The future needs for residential care
    c. The types of schooling and vocational training that will be needed
    d. The developmental milestones and the start of school causing stress of some kind

33. List the three common phases of families' responses to the diagnosis of a chronic illness or disability.

34. Which of the following strategies would enhance compliance in adolescents?
    a. Include the adolescent in the treatment discussions.
    b. Help the family set clear expectations.
    c. Clarify roles and provide written instructions.
    d. Do all of the above.

35. Fear of the unknown is one of the greatest threats to seriously ill children of which age group?
    a. Toddlers
    b. Preschoolers
    c. School-age children
    d. Adolescents

36. Immobilization is one of the greatest threats to seriously ill children of which age group?
    a. Toddlers
    b. Preschoolers
    c. School-age children
    d. Adolescents

37. Fear of punishment is one of the greatest threats to seriously ill children of which age group?
    a. Toddlers
    b. Preschoolers
    c. School-age children
    d. Adolescents

38. Inability to use their parents for emotional support is one of the greatest threats to seriously ill children of which age group?
    a. Toddlers
    b. Preschoolers
    c. School-age children
    d. Adolescents

39. When the parent of a child who is dying tells the nurse the child is in pain even when the child appears comfortable, the nurse should be sure that
    a. as needed (prn) pain control measures are instituted.
    b. pain control is administered on a preventive schedule.
    c. parents understand that pain is a physical process.
    d. parents understand that the child is probably in less pain than he or she appears.

40. Pain control is often a concern of dying children and their parents. Which of the following strategies should the nurse use to help them deal with this fear?
    a. Assure the parents that the pain will be relieved.
    b. Use heavy sedation to help them cope with this phase.
    c. Adopt a medication schedule that will prevent the pain from escalating.
    d. Give pain medications intravenously only when the child is near death.

41. List at least five physical signs of approaching death.

42. A family's reaction during the terminal stage of illness involves a period of intense anticipatory grieving characterized by
    a. depression.
    b. loss of hope.
    c. intensification of fears.
    d. all of the above.

43. The extended phase of mourning:
    a. usually takes about a year.
    b. is accompanied by support of the family at the funeral.
    c. may extend over years.
    d. can be eliminated if the family is well prepared.

44. Which of the following symptoms is considered normal acute grief behavior?
    a. Feeling the need to have friends and relatives around
    b. Feeling an emotional closeness to friends and relatives
    c. Hearing the dead person's voice
    d. All of the above

45. Which of the following approaches is best for the nurse to use with parents of a leukemic child to help them cope with their feeling about the child's impending death?
    a. Begin with an assessment.
    b. Reinforce the idea that repeat relapses and remissions are associated with a better prognosis.
    c. Begin to help the parents work through their depression.
    d. Use heavy sedation to help the child and the parents cope.

46. After a child's death, which of the following evaluation strategies is most likely to support and guide the family members through the resolution of their loss?
    a. A written questionnaire
    b. A telephone call placed 2 days after the death
    c. Meeting with the family at the time of death
    d. A telephone call placed 6 weeks after the death

47. Which of the following techniques is considered an example of the most therapeutic communication to use with the bereaved family?
    a. Cheerfulness
    b. Interpretation
    c. Validating loss
    d. Reassurance

III. THINKING CRITICALLY

1. Describe how the changes that have occurred in the provision of services have improved the care of children with special needs.

2. Describe why it is necessary for the nurse to assess the family's specific perceptions concerning their child's illness or disability.

3. Describe how children between the ages of 3 and 5 years view death.

4. Describe how a preschooler who becomes seriously ill is likely to perceive his or her illness.

5. Describe why adolescents, more than any other age group, have more difficulty coping with death, particularly their own.

Cognitive and Sensory Impairment

42

I. LEARNING KEY TERMS

MATCHING: Match each term with its corresponding description.

1. _____ Also referred to as partially sighted; refers to visual acuity between 20/70 and 20/200; usually allows child to obtain an education in the standard public school system with the use of normal-sized print.

2. _____ Refers to a person whose hearing disability precludes successful processing of linguistic information through audition, with or without a hearing aid.

3. _____ Visual loss that cannot be corrected with regular prescription lenses.

4. _____ Refers to a person who, generally with the use of a hearing aid, has residual hearing sufficient to enable successful processing of linguistic information through audition.

5. _____ A disability that may range in severity from mild to profound and includes the subsets of deaf and hard-of-hearing; one of the most common disabilities in the United States.

6. _____ Inability to express ideas in any form, either written or verbally.

7. _____ A region found in chromosome analysis that fails to condense during mitosis and is characterized by a nonstaining gap or narrowing.

8. _____ The inability to interpret sound correctly.

9. _____ The facial muscle coordination part of speech.

10. _____ Difficulty in processing details or discrimination among sounds.

11. _____ Technique in which the transmission of the audio portion of a television program is translated into subtitles that appear on the screen.

12. _____ The hearing and interpretation skills of speech.

13. _____ A unit of loudness measured at various frequencies; used to express the degree of hearing impairment.

a. Cognitive impairment

b. Mental retardation

c. Educable mentally retarded

d. Trainable mentally retarded

e. Task analysis

f. Receptive skills

g. Expressive skills

h. Fragile site

i. Hearing impairment

j. Deaf

k. Hard-of-hearing

l. Aphasia

m. Agnosia

n. Dysacusis

o. Decibel

p. Hearing threshold level

q. American sign language (ASL)/British sign language (BSL)

r. Refraction

s. Teletypewriters/telecommunications devises for the deaf (TDD)

t. Closed captioning

u. Visual impairment

v. School vision

w. Legal blindness

14. _____ Learning through a step-by-step process in which each step of a skill is taught completely before proceeding to the next activity.

15. _____ Equipment used to help deaf people communicate with each other over the telephone.

16. _____ Generally equivalent to children with moderate levels of cognitive impairment; accounts for approximately 10% of the mentally retarded population.

17. _____ The measurement of an individual's hearing impairment by means of an audiometer.

18. _____ Corresponds to the mildly retarded group, which constitutes approximately 85% of all people with mental retardation.

19. _____ Characterized by subaverage intellectual function, deficits in adaptive behavior, and onset before 18 years of age.

20. _____ A visual-gestural language using hand signals that roughly correspond to specific words and concepts in the English language.

21. _____ Visual acuity of 20/100 or less and/or a visual field of 20 degrees or less in the better eye; not a medical diagnosis; a legal definition that allows special considerations with regard to taxes, entrance into special school, eligibility for aid, and other benefits.

22. _____ A general term for any type of mental difficulty or deficiency.

23. _____ Refers to the bending of light rays as they pass through the lens of the eye.

II. REVIEWING KEY CONCEPTS AND CONTENT

MATCHING: Match the level of mental retardation/IQ range with the appropriate example of a child's maturation and/or development.

24. _____ A preschool-age child with noticeable delays in motor development and in speech.

a. Mild retardation (IQ of 50-55 to about 70)

25. _____ An adult who may walk but who needs complete custodial care.

b. Moderate retardation (IQ of 35-40 to 50-55)

26. _____ A school-age child who is able to walk and who can profit from systematic habit training.

c. Severe retardation (IQ of 20-25 to 35-40)

27. _____ A preschool-age child who may not be noticed as retarded but is slow to walk, feed self, and talk.

d. Profound retardation (IQ below 20-25)

28. The classification system for mental retardation allows for
    a. achieving the same goals for each person.
    b. identification of needs in four care dimensions.
    c. only intelligence and no other criteria.
    d. an age limit of 12.

29. Acquiring social skills for the cognitively impaired child includes
    a. teaching acceptable sexual behavior.
    b. exposing the child to strangers.
    c. greeting visitors without being overly friendly.
    d. all of the above.

30. Define *task analysis* and describe its use when teaching a mentally retarded child.

31. Another acceptable name for trisomy 21 is
    a. phenylketonuria.
    b. Turner syndrome.
    c. Down syndrome.
    d. Mongolism.

32. Prenatal testing and genetic counseling for Down syndrome should be offered to all women
    a. regardless of family history.
    b. with a family history of the disorder and who are of advanced maternal age.
    c. with no family history of the disorder and who are of advanced maternal age.
    d. who become pregnant in their adolescent years.

33. Fragile X syndrome is
    a. the most common inherited cause of mental retardation.
    b. the most common inherited cause of mental retardation next to Down syndrome.
    c. caused by an abnormal gene on chromosome 21.
    d. caused by a missing gene on the X chromosome.

34. Genetic counseling for parents of a child with fragile X syndrome is
    a. recommended whenever there is permutation.
    b. recommended whenever there is translocation.
    c. always recommended.
    d. seldom recommended.

35. The correct term to use for a person who is able to process linguistic information only with the use of a hearing aid is
    a. deaf-mute.
    b. hard-of-hearing.
    c. deaf.
    d. deaf and dumb.

36. Conductive hearing loss in children is most often a result of
    a. use of tobramycin and gentamicin.
    b. high noise levels from ventilators.
    c. congenital defects.
    d. recurrent serous otitis media.

37. In the assessment of an infant to identify whether a hearing impairment has developed, the nurse would look for
    a. a monotone voice.
    b. consistent lack of the startle reflex.
    c. a louder than usual cry.
    d. inability to form the utterance "da-da" by 6 months.

38. In the assessment of a child to identify whether a hearing impairment has developed, the nurse would look for
    a. a loud monotone voice.
    b. consistent lack of the startle reflex.
    c. a high level of social activity.
    d. attentiveness, especially when someone is talking.

39. All of the following are strategies that will enhance communication with a child who is hearing-impaired except
    a. touching the child lightly to signal presence of a speaker.
    b. speaking at eye level or a 45-degree angle.
    c. using facial expressions to convey a message better.
    d. moving and using animated body language to communicate better.

MATCHING: Match each impairment with its corresponding description.

40. _____ Increased intraocular pressure.

41. _____ Squinted or crossed eyes.

42. _____ Different refractive strength in each eye.

43. _____ Unequal curvatures in refractive apparatus.

44. _____ Opacity of crystalline lens.

45. _____ Farsightedness.

46. _____ Lazy eye.

47. _____ Nearsightedness.

a. Myopia

b. Hyperopia

c. Astigmatism

d. Anisometropia

e. Amblyopia

f. Strabismus

g. Cataracts

h. Glaucoma

48. If a child has a penetrating injury to the eye, the nurse should:
   a. apply an eye patch.
   b. attempt to remove the object.
   c. irrigate the eye.
   d. use strict aseptic technique to examine the eye.

49. Which of the following situations would be considered abnormal?
   a. A newborn that does not consistently follow a bright toy with his eyes
   b. A toddler whose mother says she looks cross-eyed
   c. A 5-year-old who has hyperopia
   d. Presence of a red reflex in a 7-year-old

50. Define the term *blindism*.

51. List at least eight of the strategies that the nurse can use during hospitalization with a child who has lost his or her sight.

52. Which of the following statements is correct about eye care and sports?
   a. Glasses may interfere with the child's ability in sports.
   b. Face mask and helmet should be required gear for softball.
   c. Contact lenses provide less visual acuity than glasses for sports.
   d. It is usually very difficult to convince children to wear their glasses to play sports.

53. Which of the following examples would be most indicative of a language disorder?
   a. A 22-month-old child who has not uttered his first word
   b. A 36-month-old who has not formed his first sentence
   c. An 18-month-old who uses short "telegraphic" phrases
   d. A 4-year-old whose speech is not entirely understandable

III. THINKING CRITICALLY

1. Describe the nursing interventions that should be used when caring for a hospitalized child who is cognitively impaired.

2. Describe why the hearing-impaired child is at a great disadvantage for developing social relationships.

3. Explain why it is difficult to teach a deaf child to speak.

4. Describe the measures that parents should use to help their children preserve their sight.

Family-Centered Home Care

I. LEARNING KEY TERMS

MATCHING: Match each term with its corresponding description.

1. _____ Process of establishing a normal pattern of living while providing for the child with complex medical needs.

2. _____ Services with the primary goal of ensuring continuity for the child and family across hospital, home, education, therapeutic, and other settings; coordinated among multiple providers to reduce the complexity of care for the child, reduce fragmentation of care, and decrease the burden of care for the family; addresses medical, nursing, health maintenance, finances, psychosocial concerns, and educational needs of the child and family.

3. _____ A shift from the traditional unidirectional relationships between health care providers and families; essential in the home care setting; characterized by communication, dialogue, active listening, negotiation, and awareness and acceptance of differences.

4. _____ Services based on the philosophy that the family is constant in the child's life, whereas the service systems and personnel within those systems fluctuate.

5. _____ Refers to care provided in the family residence for children with complex health care needs and their families.

6. _____ A unique resource that promotes family strengths through shared experiences of other families who have children with chronic health problems.

7. _____ A program of palliative and supportive care services providing physical, psychological, social, and spiritual care for dying people, their families, and other loved ones; available both in the home and inpatient settings.

a. Home care

b. Hospice care

c. Collaborative relationships

d. Normalization

e. Care coordination/case management

f. Family-centered care

g. Family-to-family (parent-to-parent) support

II. REVIEWING KEY CONCEPTS AND CONTENT

8. For third-party payers, the cost of caring for a child at home who is dependent on medical technology is usually *more* or *less* (circle one) than it would be if the child were not at home.

9. The area of home health nursing implementation most commonly used is known as
   a. block nursing.
   b. direct provision.
   c. private-duty nursing.
   d. intermittent skilled nursing.

10. Most home visits to the home care patient are focused on
    a. assisting the patient/caregiver to achieve independence.
    b. caring for an individual patient for a predetermined amount of time.
    c. total patient care by the nurse.
    d. all of the above.

11. A basic communication principle used in pediatric home care involves the idea that
    a. the nurse is always more informed than the family.
    b. the meaning of words used does not vary from culture to culture.
    c. the nurse and the family set mutual goals.
    d. coping mechanisms do not change over time.

12. The concept of family empowerment is used in home care nursing because it promotes a central goal of
    a. molding families to take on accepted behaviors.
    b. shaping behaviors of the parents.
    c. building on family strengths.
    d. all of the above.

13. The nursing process in home care nursing practice integrates
    a. normalization.
    b. various disciplines.
    c. family priorities.
    d. all of the above.

14. In home nursing practice the nurse strives to help the family maintain control over their
    a. home.
    b. child's care.
    c. personal lives.
    d. all of the above.

15. Laws that ensure that children who are dependent on medical technology are mainstreamed into the school system always result in
    a. a free, appropriate public education.
    b. payment for health care services in the school setting.
    c. the need for educational planning and coordination.
    d. all of the above.

III. THINKING CRITICALLY

1. Describe the needs and issues that must be addressed through care coordination for a child with complex medical needs.

2. Describe the features of collaborative relationships that are essential in the home care setting.

3. Describe the strategies a nurse should use to help resolve conflict in the home care setting.

44 Reaction to Illness and Hospitalization

I. LEARNING KEY TERMS

MATCHING: Match each term with its corresponding description.

1. _____ The very effective, nondirective modality for helping children deal with their concerns and fears; often helpful to the nurse in gaining insights into children's needs and feelings. Not used as an interpretive method with emotionally disturbed children.

2. _____ The type of care that pediatric nurses aim to provide; therapeutic care that minimizes the psychologic and physical distress experienced by children and their families.

3. _____ A psychologic technique reserved for use by trained and qualified therapists as an interpretative method with emotionally disturbed children.

4. _____ The major stress from middle infancy throughout the preschool years, especially for children ages 6 to 30 months.

5. _____ Strategies for lessening the perception of pain; when used with analgesics, can enhance these drugs' effectiveness; can also produce a cooperative child who continues to "suffer in silence."

a. Separation anxiety

b. Atraumatic care

c. Nonpharmacologic pain

d. Play therapy

e. Therapeutic play

II. REVIEWING KEY CONCEPTS AND CONTENT

6. Separation anxiety would be most expected in the hospitalized child at age
   a. 3 to 6 months.
   b. 6 to 30 months.
   c. 30 months to 2 years.
   d. 2 to 4 years.

MATCHING: Match each phase of separation anxiety with the behaviors that are typical of that phase.

7. _____ Inactive; withdraws from others; uninterested in environment; uncommunicative; regression behaviors.

8. _____ Becomes more interested in surroundings; interacts with caregivers; resigned to the situation; rarely seen in hospitalized children; occurs in prolonged parental absences.

9. _____ Cries; screams; attacks stranger physically and verbally; attempts to escape; continuous crying.

a. Protest

b. Despair

c. Detachment

10. One difference between toddlers and school-age children in their reactions to hospitalization is that the school-age child
    a. does not experience separation anxiety.
    b. has coping mechanisms in place.
    c. relies on his or her family more than the toddler.
    d. experiences separation anxiety to a greater degree.

11. A toddler is most likely to react to short-term hospitalization with feelings of loss of control that result from altered routines; this is often manifested by
    a. regression.
    b. withdrawal.
    c. formation of new superficial relationships.
    d. self-assertion and anger.

12. Which of the following risk factors make a child more vulnerable to the stressors of hospitalization?
    a. Urban dweller
    b. Strong-willed personality
    c. Female gender
    d. Passive temperament

13. The pediatric population in the hospital today is different from the pediatric population of 10 years ago in that the usual length of stay has
    a. decreased and the acuity has increased.
    b. increased and the acuity has decreased.
    c. increased and the acuity has increased.
    d. decreased and the acuity has decreased.

14. Describe at least one of the possible psychologic benefits a child might gain from hospitalization.

15. Siblings who visit their brother or sister in the hospital have an increased tendency to exhibit which of the following behaviors?
    a. Nail biting
    b. Anger
    c. Increased concentration in school
    d. Decreased concentration in school

16. To help the parents deal with the issues related to separation while their child is hospitalized, the nurse should suggest that parents should
    a. quietly leave while the child is distracted or asleep.
    b. teach the child what the hospital routines are.
    c. use associations to help the child understand time frames.
    d. visit over one extended time if rooming-in is impossible.

17. One technique used during hospitalization that can minimize the disruption in the routine of the school-age child who is not critically ill is
    a. time structuring.
    b. anaclitic care.
    c. self-care.
    d. regulating television viewing.

18. Which of the following age groups is most affected by the hospitalization in regard to feelings of loss?
    a. Infants
    b. Toddlers
    c. Preschoolers
    d. School-age children

19. Preparing children for intrusive procedures usually increases their
    a. feelings of control.
    b. fear.
    c. stress.
    d. misconceptions.

20. Whenever performing a painful procedure on a child, the nurse should attempt to
    a. perform the procedure in the playroom.
    b. standardize techniques from one age to the next.
    c. perform the procedure quickly.
    d. have the parents leave during the procedure.

21. After administering an intramuscular injection, the nurse would best reassure the young child with poorly defined body boundaries by
    a. telling the child that the bleeding will stop after the needle is removed.
    b. using a large bandage to cover the injection site.
    c. using a small bandage to cover the injection site.
    d. using a bandage but removing it a few hours after the injection.

22. One way to evaluate whether a child fears mutilation of body parts is to
    a. explain the procedure.
    b. ask the child to draw a picture of what will happen.
    c. stress the reason for the procedure.
    d. investigate the child's individual concerns.

23. Which of the following reactions to surgery is most typical of an adolescent's reaction to fear of bodily injury?
    a. Concern about the pain
    b. Concern about the procedure itself
    c. Concern about the scar
    d. Understanding explanations literally

24. In regard to pain assessment, nurses tend to
    a. underestimate the existence of pain in children but not in adults.
    b. underestimate the existence of pain in both children and adults.
    c. overestimate the existence of pain in children but not in adults.
    d. overestimate the existence of pain in both children and adults.

25. T   F   Children may not realize how much they are hurting when they are in constant pain.

26. T   F   Narcotics are no more dangerous for children than they are for adults.

27. T   F   Children cannot tell you where they hurt.

28. T   F   A 3-year-old child can use a pain scale.

29. T   F   Children tolerate pain better than adults.

30. T   F   Children may not admit having pain in order to avoid an injection.

31. T   F   Infants do not feel pain.

32. T   F   Children may believe that the nurse knows how they feel.

33. List the six strategies used in the QUESTT approach to pain assessment.

    Q:

    U:

    E:

    S:

    T:

    T:

34. When using patient-controlled analgesia (PCA) with children, the
    a. drug of choice is meperidine.
    b. parent should control the dosing.
    c. nurse should control the dosing.
    d. drug of choice is morphine.

35. The anesthetic cream EMLA is applied
    a. before invasive procedures.
    b. as preoperative oral sedation.
    c. for chronic cancer pain.
    d. postoperatively.

36. For postoperative or cancer pain control, analgesics should be administered
    a. as needed.
    b. around the clock.
    c. before the pain escalates.
    d. after the pain peaks.

37. The most common side effect from opioid therapy is
    a. respiratory depression.
    b. pruritus.
    c. nausea and vomiting.
    d. constipation.

38. The advantages of a hospital unit specifically for adolescents include
    a. three large meals a day and no snacks.
    b. a regular routine.
    c. increased socialization with peers.
    d. all of the above.

39. One of the best ways to support the parents when they first visit the child in the intensive care unit is to
    a. accompany them to the bedside.
    b. use picture books of the unit in the waiting area.
    c. limit the visiting hours so that parents are encouraged to rest.
    d. expect parents to stay with their child continuously.

40. Transfer from the intensive care unit to the regular pediatric unit can be best facilitated by
    a. discussing the details of the transfer at the bedside where the child can listen.
    b. establishing a schedule that resembles the child's home schedule.
    c. assigning a primary nurse who visits regularly before the transfer.
    d. explaining to the family that there are fewer nurses on the general unit.

Use the following scenario to respond to questions 41 through 44.

An 8-year-old boy is admitted to the pediatric unit for an appendectomy. He is in the third grade and is very active in after-school activities. Recently he began taking karate lessons, and he also plays baseball. He loves school, particularly when he is able to read. He awakens every morning at 6 AM to read, and reading is the last thing he does before falling asleep.

The child's parents are with him during the admission interview. His mother works, but she has made arrangements to take some time off during his hospital stay and after the surgery to be available to him.

41. Based on the above information, the nurse should expect
    a. a normal response to hospitalization.
    b. more anxiety than would normally be seen.
    c. difficulty with the parents.
    d. cultural factors to take precedence.

42. The nurse identifies which of the following nursing diagnoses for this child?
    a. Diversional activity deficit and powerlessness
    b. Activity intolerance and high risk for injury
    c. Anxiety/fear and self-care deficit
    d. All of the above are possible

43. Which of the following expected outcomes is most reasonable for this child's diagnosis of powerlessness?
    a. The child will tolerate increasingly more activity.
    b. The child will remain injury free.
    c. The child will play and rest quietly.
    d. The child will help plan care and schedule.

44. Which of the following interventions is best for the nurse to incorporate into this child's plan?
    a. Organize activities for maximum sleep time.
    b. Keep side rails up.
    c. Choose an appropriate roommate.
    d. Assist with dressing and bathing.

III. THINKING CRITICALLY

1. Describe at least three nursing interventions to use to promote positive family relationships.

2. Considering developmental and safety needs, what types of toys should be recommended for a 4-year-old child who is hospitalized?

3. Describe the strategies a nurse should use to establish a trusting relationship with hospitalized school-age children.

4. Which pain assessment scales are most suitable to use to assess pain in a 6-year-old child?

45 Pediatric Variations of Nursing Interventions

I. LEARNING KEY TERMS

MATCHING: Match each term with its corresponding description.

1. _____ Provides for total alimentary needs when feeding by way of the gastrointestinal tract is impossible, inadequate, or hazardous; also known as hyperalimentation.

2. _____ Designed for patients documented or suspected to be infected or colonized with highly transmissible or epidemiologically important pathogens.

3. _____ A noninvasive method of providing continual monitoring of partial pressure of oxygen in arterial blood that uses an electrode that is attached to the skin.

4. _____ The primary strategy for successful nosocomial infection control; synthesizes the major features of universal (blood and body fluid) precautions (UP), designed to reduce the risk of transmission of blood-borne pathogens, and body substance isolation (BSI), designed to reduce the risk of transmission of pathogens from moist body substances; applies to blood, all body fluids, secretions, and excretions except sweat, regardless of whether or not blood is visible in the body substance.

5. _____ Designed to reduce the risk of transmission of droplets suspended in the air for long periods of time.

6. _____ Designed to reduce the risk of transmission of infectious agents generated from the source person primarily during coughing, sneezing, or talking and during the performance of certain procedures such as suctioning and bronchoscopy.

7. _____ One who is legally under the age of majority but is recognized as having the legal capacity of an adult under circumstances prescribed by state law, such as pregnancy, marriage, high school graduation, living independently, or military service.

8. _____ A simple, continuous, noninvasive method of determining oxygen saturation; used to guide oxygen therapy.

9. _____ Designed to reduce the risk of transmission of epidemiologically important microorganisms by physical transfer of microorganisms to a susceptible host from an infected or colonized person or from a contaminated intermediate object.

a. Informed consent

b. Mature minors' doctrine

c. Emancipated minor

d. Standard precautions (isolation)

e. Transmission-based precautions (isolation)

f. Airborne precautions (isolation)

g. Droplet precautions (isolation)

h. Contact precautions

i. Peripheral venous access devices

j. Central venous access devices

k. Oxygen-induced (carbon dioxide) narcosis

l. Pulse oximetry

m. Transcutuaneous monitoring

n. Total parenteral nutrition

10. _____ A physiologic hazard of oxygen therapy, where the respiratory center has adapted to the continuously higher arterial carbon dioxide levels; hypoxia becomes the more powerful stimulus for respiration; occurs when oxygen is administered and the hypoxic drive is removed, resulting in hypoventilation, increased arterial carbon dioxide levels, and unconsciousness.

11. _____ Permits minors to give consent (even though they are not technically adults) as long as they understand the consequences of their decisions (e.g., statutes in many states permit minors to give consent on their own behalf to certain treatments such as for sexually transmitted diseases, contraceptive services, pregnancy, or drug or alcohol abuse).

12. _____ A device that is an alternative to keeping an intravenous line intact for intermittent use; the device remains in place and is flushed after infusion of medication.

13. _____ Refers to the legal and ethical requirement that the patient clearly, fully, and completely understand the proposed medical treatment to be performed, including significant risks associated with the treatment.

14. _____ Used for frequent hyperalimentation, blood sampling, or antibiotic therapy and for the management of long-term chemotherapy.

II. REVIEWING KEY CONCEPTS AND CONTENT

15. When the parents are divorced, who must consent to medical treatment of the child?
    a. The child
    b. Either parent
    c. Both parents
    d. The legal guardian

16. Emancipated minors are usually recognized as having the legal capacity of an adult in all matters. Which of the following reasons would most likely be considered as a reason for emancipation?
    a. The minor, who lives with his parents, is seeking treatment for a sexually transmitted disease.
    b. The minor, who lives with her parents, is seeking a prescription for contraceptives.
    c. The minor, who lives with his parents, is seeking treatment for drugs or alcohol.
    d. The minor, who lives with her spouse, is seeking treatment for pregnancy.

17. If a child needs support during an invasive procedure, the nurse should
    a. inform the parents about how the child did after the procedure.
    b. ask the parents to stay in the room, where they can have eye contact with the child.
    c. decide whether parental presence will be beneficial and try to let the parents choose.
    d. encourage the parents to stay close by to console the child immediately following the procedure.

18. List at least five strategies the nurse can use to support the child during and after a procedure.

19. Describe at least one play activity for each of the following procedures.

    a. Ambulation

    b. Range of motion

    c. Injections

d. Deep breathing

e. Extending the environment

f. Soaks

g. Fluid intake

20. To prepare a breastfed infant physically for surgery, the nurse would expect to
    a. permit breastfeeding up to 4 hours before surgery.
    b. withhold breastfeeding as of midnight the night before surgery.
    c. withhold breastfeeding from 4 to 8 hours before surgery.
    d. replace breast milk with formula and permit feeding up to 2 hours before surgery.

21. The most atraumatic choice for a preanesthetic medication would be
    a. intramuscular morphine sulfate.
    b. intravenous morphine sulfate through an established site.
    c. intramuscular promethazine, chlorpromazine, and meperidine.
    d. oral promethazine, chlorpromazine, and meperidine.

22. Fear of induction of anesthesia by mask can be minimized by applying
    a. the mask quickly and with assurance.
    b. an opaque mask.
    c. the mask while the child is sitting.
    d. the mask while the child is supine.

23. An increased heart rate, increased respiratory rate, and increased blood pressure in the immediate postoperative period of a young child would most likely indicate
    a. pain.
    b. infection.
    c. increased intracranial pressure.
    d. advanced shock.

24. The strategies that would be considered an organizational attempt to improve compliance of the family with a young child would be to
    a. incorporate teaching principles that are known to enhance understanding.
    b. encourage the family to adapt to the hospital medication schedules.
    c. evaluate and reduce the time the family waits for their appointment.
    d. all of the above.

25. When bathing an uncircumcised male child under the age of 3, the nurse should:
    a. gently remind the child to clean his genital area.
    b. not retract the foreskin.
    c. always retract the foreskin.
    d. avoid cleansing between the skinfolds of the genital area.

26. Care for an African-American child's hair includes braiding the hair
    a. when it is damp.
    b. tightly.
    c. when it is dry.
    d. after petroleum jelly is applied.

27. Which of the following examples of a child's food intake is the best sample of adequate documentation?
    a. Child ate about a cup of cereal with ½ cup of milk.
    b. Child ate an adequate breakfast.
    c. Child ate 80% of the breakfast served.
    d. Parent states that child ate an adequate breakfast.

28. After mouth or lip surgery, the nurse should restrain the child using
    a. arm and leg restraints.
    b. elbow restraints.
    c. a jacket restraint.
    d. a mummy restraint.

29. The best positioning technique for a lumbar puncture in a neonate is a
    a. side-lying position with neck flexion.
    b. sitting position.
    c. side-lying position with modified neck extension.
    d. side-lying position with knees to chest.

30. The most frequently used site for bone marrow aspiration in children is the
    a. femur.
    b. sternum.
    c. tibia.
    d. iliac crest.

31. To avoid the complication of necrotizing oseteochondritis when performing infant heel puncture, the puncture should be
    a. no deeper than 4.2 mm and on the inner aspect of the heel.
    b. no deeper than 2.4 mm and on the outer aspect of the heel.
    c. no deeper than 2.4 mm and on the inner aspect of the heel.
    d. no deeper than 4.2 mm and on the outer aspect of the heel.

32. To obtain a sputum specimen for tuberculosis in an infant, the nurse may need to
    a. have the infant cough.
    b. obtain mucus from the throat.
    c. insert a suction catheter into the back of the throat.
    d. perform gastric lavage.

33. Of the following choices for measuring 1 teaspoon of medication at home, the best device for the nurse to instruct the parent to use is the
    a. household soup spoon.
    b. household measuring spoon.
    c. hospital's USP standard dropper.
    d. household teaspoon.

34. All of the following techniques for medication administration to an infant are acceptable *except*
    a. adding the medication to the infant's formula.
    b. allowing the infant to sit in the parent's lap during administration.
    c. allowing the infant to suck the medication from an empty nipple.
    d. inserting the needleless syringe into the side of the mouth while the infant nurses.

35. When determining the needle length for intramuscular injection of medication into a child, the nurse should
    a. choose a 1-inch needle for a 4-month-old infant.
    b. use a needle length that is too short rather than one that is too long.
    c. choose a half-inch needle for a 4-month-old infant.
    d. grasp the muscle between the thumb and forefinger, choosing a length that is less than half the distance.

36. The preferred site for intramuscular injection in an infant is the
    a. deltoid muscle.
    b. dorsogluteal.
    c. vastus lateralis.
    d. ventrogluteal.

37. Total parenteral nutrition (TPN) is infused by way of a central intravenous line because
    a. other medications need to be infused with the TPN.
    b. several attempts to administer it peripherally have probably occurred.
    c. there is less risk of infection.
    d. the glucose in the solution is irritating.

38. To instill eyedrops in an infant whose eyelids are clenched shut, the nurse should
    a. apply finger pressure to the lacrimal punctum.
    b. place the drops in the nasal corner where the lids meet and wait until the infant opens the lid.
    c. administer the eyedrops before nap time.
    d. all of the above.

39. During continuous enteral feedings, the nurse should
    a. use the same pole as the intravenous line.
    b. use a parenteral burette to calibrate the feeding times.
    c. give the infant a pacifier for sucking.
    d. all of the above.

40. In the small infant, a feeding tube is usually inserted through the
    a. nose.
    b. mouth.

41. One of the major advantages of the recently developed skin-level devices for feeding children is that the button device
    a. does not clog as easily as other devices.
    b. eliminates the need for frequent bubbling.
    c. is less expensive than the traditional devices.
    d. eliminates the need for clamping.

42. When administering an enema to a small child, it is advisable to use
    a. a pediatric Fleet enema.
    b. a commercially prepared solution.
    c. an isotonic solution.
    d. plain water.

43. A young child with an ostomy pouch may need to
    a. wear one-piece outfits.
    b. begin toilet training at a later than usual age.
    c. limit activity to avoid skin damage.
    d. use a rubber band to help the appliance fit.

III. THINKING CRITICALLY

1. Describe methods for the nurse to use to support parents when restraints must be used with their child.

2. Explain the rationale for checking restraints at least every 2 hours.

3. Describe how to perform manual percussion of the chest wall.

Respiratory Dysfunction

$$\boxed{46}$$

I. LEARNING KEY TERMS

MATCHING: Match each term with its corresponding description.

1. _____ A key measurement of pulmonary function; a measurement of the maximum flow of air that can be forcefully exhaled in 1 second.

2. _____ A worsening of symptoms, either abrupt or progressive.

3. _____ Cessation of breathing for more than 20 seconds *or* for a shorter period of time when associated with hypoxemia or bradycardia.

4. _____ Exposure to environmental tobacco smoke; a well-established danger to children.

5. _____ The cessation of respiration.

6. _____ Inability of the respiratory apparatus to maintain adequate oxygenation of the blood, with or without carbon dioxide retention.

7. _____ The term used to indicate infection in a person who has a positive tuberculin skin test (TST), no physical findings of disease, and normal chest radiograph findings.

8. _____ In general, applies to two conditions: increased work of breathing with near normal gas exchange function *or* the inability to maintain normal blood gas tensions that develops from carbon dioxide retention with subsequent hypoxemia and acidosis.

9. _____ Allows an assessment of tympanic membrane mobility.

10. _____ The earliest manifestation of cystic fibrosis where the small intestine is blocked with thick, puttylike, tenacious, mucilaginous meconium in the newborn.

11. _____ The tuberculin skin test that is the most important indicator of whether a child has been infected with the tubercle bacillus.

12. _____ Irritants such as house dust mites, whose prevention (or reduced exposure to) is the goal of nonpharmacologic therapy for asthma.

13. _____ A series of subdiaphragmatic abdominal thrusts used to create an artificial cough; forces air, and with it the foreign body, out of the airway; recommended for children over 1 year of age.

14. _____ Faucial tonsils; usually removed during a tonsillectomy

a. Palatine tonsils

b. Pneumatic otoscopy

c. Purified protein derivative (PPD)

d. Latent tuberculosis infection (LTBI)

e. Passive smoking

f. Exacerbation

g. Peak expiratory flow rate (PEFR)

h. Allergen

i. Meconium ileus

j. Respiratory insufficiency

k. Respiratory failure

l. Respiratory arrest

m. Apnea

n. Heimlich maneuver

II. REVIEWING KEY CONCEPTS AND CONTENT

15. Most respiratory infections in children are caused by
    a. pneumococci.
    b. viruses.
    c. streptococci.
    d. *Haemophilus influenzae.*

16. The most likely reason that the respiratory infection rate increases drastically in the age range from 3 to 6 months is that the
    a. infant's exposure to pathogens is greatly increased during this time.
    b. viral agents that are mild in older children are extremely severe in infants.
    c. maternal antibodies have decreased and the infant's own antibody production is immature.
    d. diameter of the airways is smaller in the infant than in the older child.

17. The primary concern of the nurse when giving tips for how to increase humidity in the home of a child with a respiratory infection should be to make sure the child has
    a. continuous contact with the humidification source.
    b. a warm humidification source.
    c. a humidification source that is safe.
    d. a cool humidification source.

18. Which of the following is the best choice for the child with a respiratory disorder who needs bed rest but who is not cooperating?
    a. Be sure the mother takes the advice seriously.
    b. Allow the child to play quietly on the floor.
    c. Insist that the child play quietly in bed.
    d. Allow the child to cry until he or she stays in bed.

19. The best technique to prevent spread of nasopharyngitis is
    a. prompt immunization.
    b. to avoid contact with infected people.
    c. mist evaporization.
    d. to ensure adequate fluid intake.

20. Group A β-hemolytic streptococcal (GABHS) infection is usually a
    a. serious infection of the upper airway.
    b. common cause of pharyngitis in children over the age of 15 years.
    c. brief illness that places the child at risk for serious sequelae.
    d. disease of the heart, lungs, joints, and central nervous system.

21. In the postoperative period following a tonsillectomy, the child should be
    a. placed in the Trendelenburg position.
    b. encouraged to cough and deep breathe.
    c. suctioned vigorously to clear the airway.
    d. placed on bed rest for the day of surgery.

22. The best pain medication administration regimen for a child in the initial postoperative period following a tonsillectomy is
    a. at regular intervals.
    b. as needed.

23. Of the foods listed, the most appropriate selection to offer first to an alert child who is in the postoperative period following a tonsillectomy is
    a. strawberry ice cream.
    b. red cherry-flavored gelatin.
    c. an apple-flavored ice pop.
    d. cold diluted orange juice.

24. Which of the following signs is an early indication of hemorrhage in a child who has had a tonsillectomy?
    a. Continuous swallowing
    b. Decreasing blood pressure
    c. Restlessness
    d. All of the above

25. During influenza epidemics, it is generally believed the age group that provides a major source of transmission is the
    a. infant.
    b. school-age child.
    c. adolescent.
    d. elderly.

26. The usual clinical manifestations of influenza usually include all of the following *except*
    a. nausea and vomiting.
    b. fever and chills.
    c. sore throat and dry mucous membranes.
    d. photophobia and myalgia.

27. The infant is predisposed to developing otitis media because the eustachian tubes
    a. are relatively short and open.
    b. have a limited amount of lymphoid tissue.
    c. are relatively long and narrow.
    d. are completely underdeveloped.

28. An abnormal otoscopic examination would reveal
    a. visible landmarks.
    b. a light reflex.
    c. an opaque tympanic membrane.
    d. a mobile tympanic membrane.

29. Children with croup syndrome and some mucosal swelling
    a. require hospitalization.
    b. will need to be intubated.
    c. can be cared for at home.
    d. are over 6 years old.

30. The nurse should prepare for an impending emergency situation to care for the child with suspected
    a. spasmodic croup.
    b. laryngotracheobronchitis.
    c. acute spasmodic laryngitis.
    d. epiglottitis.

31. The nurse should suspect epiglottitis if the child has
    a. cough, sore throat, and agitation.
    b. cough, drooling, and retractions.
    c. absence of cough in the presence of drooling and agitation.
    d. absence of cough, hoarseness, and retractions.

32. In the child who is suspected of having epiglottitis, the nurse should
    a. have intubation equipment available.
    b. prepare to immunize the child for *Haemophilus influenzae*.
    c. obtain a throat culture.
    d. all of the above.

33. Since the advent of immunization for *Haemophilus influenzae*, there has been a decrease in the incidence of
    a. laryngotracheobronchitis.
    b. epiglottitis.
    c. Reye's syndrome.
    d. croup syndrome.

34. Which one of the following children is most likely to be hospitalized for treatment of croup?
    a. The 2-year-old child whose croupy cough worsens at night
    b. The 5-year-old child whose croupy cough worsens at night
    c. The 2-year-old child using the accessory muscles to breathe
    d. The child with inspiratory stridor during the physical examination

35. The nurse should expect to intubate the child diagnosed with
    a. acute spasmodic laryngitis.
    b. bacterial tracheitis.
    c. acute laryngotracheobronchitis.
    d. acute laryngitis.

36. Respiratory syncytial virus (RSV) is
    a. an uncommon virus that causes severe bronchiolitis.
    b. an uncommon virus that usually does not require hospitalization.
    c. a common virus that usually causes severe bronchiolitis.
    d. a common virus that usually does not require hospitalization.

37. The use of the monoclonal antibody palivizumab for the prevention of RSV is preferred over the RSV immune globulin (RSV-IGIV) in most high-risk children because
    a. it is administered intravenously.
    b. of its ease of administration, safety, and effectiveness.
    c. only it is licensed for the prevention of RSV disease.
    d. it is an immune globulin that neutralizes antibodies.

38. Nurses caring for a child with RSV who is receiving Ribavirin should
    a. have a skin test every 6 months.
    b. wear gloves and a gown when entering the room.
    c. turn off the aerosol machine before opening the tent.
    d. not care for other children with RSV at the same time.

39. Because of the potential for empyema, closed chest drainage is most likely to be used in:
    a. *Haemophilus pneumoniae*.
    b. mycoplasmal pneumonia.
    c. streptococcal pneumonia.
    d. staphylococcal pneumonia.

40. In an 8-month-old infant admitted to the hospital with pertussis, the nurse should particularly assess the
    a. living conditions of the infant.
    b. labor and delivery history of the mother.
    c. immunization status of the infant.
    d. alcohol and drug intake of the mother.

41. The best test to screen for tuberculosis is the
    a. chest x-ray.
    b. purified protein derivative (PPD) test.
    c. sputum culture.
    d. multipuncture test (MPT) (e.g., tine test).

42. The child who has active tuberculosis is treated with
    a. isoniazid.
    b. rifampin.
    c. pyrazinamide.
    d. a combination of the above drugs.

43. Severity of a foreign body aspiration is determined by
    a. location.
    b. type of object aspirated.
    c. extent of obstruction.
    d. all of the above.

44. Parents may be taught to deal with the aspiration of a foreign body in an infant under 12 months old by using
    a. back blows and chest thrusts.
    b. back blows only.
    c. the Heimlich maneuver only.
    d. a blind finger sweep.

45. Which of the following questions would be most important for the nurse to ask the parents of a child admitted to the hospital with a diagnosis of reactive airway disease?
    a. "What brings you to the hospital?"
    b. "What is your ethnic background?"
    c. "Do you have a history of asthma in your family?"
    d. "Was your pregnancy and delivery uneventful?"

46. The nurse examines a child with asthma and finds that there is hyperresonance on percussion. Breath sounds are coarse and loud with sonorous crackles throughout the lung fields. Expiration is prolonged; rales can be heard. There is generalized inspiratory and expiratory wheezing. The child has these symptoms two times a week with nighttime episodes a few times per month. The child's peak expiratory flow varies from 20% to 30%. Based on these findings, the nurse suspects that there is
    a. severe persistent asthma.
    b. moderate persistent asthma.
    c. mild persistent asthma.
    d. mild intermittent asthma.

47. When preparing for discharge, the nurse would most likely plan to teach the family of an asthmatic child to:
    a. keep the humidity at home above 50%.
    b. use only feather pillows.
    c. limit animal dander by removing cats and/or dogs.
    d. launder sheets and blankets regularly in cold water.

48. Which of the following principles should be a part of the home self-management program for a child with asthma?
    a. Individuals must learn not to abuse their medications so that they will not become addicted.
    b. It is easy to treat an asthmatic episode as long

as the child knows the symptoms.
    c. Although quite uncommon, asthma is very treatable.
    d. Children with asthma are usually able to participate in the same activities as nonasthmatic children.

49. The principal treatment for the insufficiency that occurs in cystic fibrosis is the administration of
    a. postural drainage.
    b. pancreatic enzymes.
    c. gentamicin.
    d. chest percussion.

50. Which of the following strategies would most likely be contraindicated for a child with cystic fibrosis to use?
    a. Forced expiration
    b. Aerobic exercise
    c. Chest physiotherapy
    d. Oxygen as desired

51. Supplements are given in cystic fibrosis in the form of
    a. only over-the-counter multivitamins.
    b. a water-miscible form of fat-soluble vitamins.
    c. limited amounts of pancreatic enzymes.
    d. all of the above.

52. List the four cardinal signs of impending respiratory failure.

53. Which of the following contains the early subtle signs of hypoxia?
    a. Peripheral cyanosis
    b. Central cyanosis
    c. Hypotension
    d. Mood changes and restlessness

54. Cardiac arrest in the pediatric population is most often a result of
    a. atherosclerosis.
    b. congenital heart disease.
    c. prolonged hypoxemia.
    d. undiagnosed cardiac conditions.

55. At what age range would the nurse place the bag-valve-mask over both the mouth and nose?
    a. Birth to 1 year
    b. 1 year to 3 years
    c. Birth to 3 years
    d. Birth to 2 years

56. The nurse would assess the carotid pulse in an emergency situation in a child who is
    a. 18 months old.
    b. 9 months old.
    c. 6 months old.
    d. 3 months old.

MATCHING: Match each drug used for pediatric emergency care with its appropriate use during resuscitation.

57. _____ Blocks vagal stimulation in the heart, resulting in an increase in cardiac output and heart rate.

58. _____ The first choice for shock-refractory ventricular tachycardia.

59. _____ Used for hypermagnesemia; needed for normal cardiac contractility.

60. _____ Causes vasoconstriction and increases cardiac output.

61. _____ Used for ventricular dysrhythmias.

62. _____ Acts on α- and β-adrenergic receptor sites, causing contraction, especially at the site of the heart, vascular, and other smooth muscle.

63. _____ Causes a temporary block through the atrioventricular node; must be administered rapidly.

64. _____ Used to buffer the pH.

a. Sodium bicarbonate

b. Calcium chloride

c. Amiodarone

d. Adenosine

e. Dopamine

f. Lidocaine

g. Epinephrine

h. Atropine

65. The Heimlich maneuver is recommended for children over the age of
    a. 4 years.
    b. 3 years.
    c. 2 years.
    d. 1 year.

III. THINKING CRITICALLY

1. Describe the parameters that should be assessed to establish respiratory status and detect any impending airway obstruction in a 20-month-old infant who is admitted to the hospital with a diagnosis of acute laryngotracheobronchitis.

2. Explain the rationale for the use of high humidity with cool mist to treat the croup syndromes.

3. Describe the parameters that the nurse should assess to recognize status asthmaticus.

4. Explain the rationale for each of the following clinical manifestations of cystic fibrosis.

   a. Respiratory symptoms

   b. Large, bulky, frothy, foul-smelling stools

   c. Voracious appetite

   d. Weight loss

   e. Anemia and bruising

5. Describe the instructions the nurse should give to a mother of a child with tuberculosis about returning to school.

Gastrointestinal Dysfunction 47

I. LEARNING KEY TERMS

MATCHING: Match each term with its corresponding description.

1. _____ Induction of IgE antibody formation—initial exposure resulting in an immune response and subsequent exposure inducing a much stronger response.

2. _____ Proteins that are capable of inducing IgE antibody formation.

3. _____ Characterized by extremely long intervals between defecation.

4. _____ The standard used to identify areas of nutritional concern; developed by the National Academy of Science's Food and Nutrition Board; intended to meet the physiologic needs of almost every healthy person.

5. _____ The infrequent passage of firm or hard stools or of small, hard masses with associated symptoms such as difficulty in expulsion, blood-streaked bowel movements, and abdominal discomfort; frequency not diagnostic.

6. _____ Lacking one or more of the essential amino acids.

7. _____ Stool normally passed within 24 to 36 hours after birth. (Newborns with irregularities in the passing of this stool should be evaluated further for congenital anomalies.)

8. _____ Dietary patterns that exclude meat.

9. _____ Used to successfully treat infants with isotonic, hypotonic, and hypertonic dehydration; the first line of treatment for diarrhea and dehydration.

10. _____ Trace elements with a daily requirement of less than 100 mg; exact role in nutrition unclear.

11. _____ Constipation with fecal soiling.

12. _____ Fluid compartment, 40% of which is lost when a child is dehydrated.

13. _____ Elements with daily requirements greater than 100 mg (e.g., calcium, phosphorus, magnesium, sodium, potassium, chloride, and sulfur).

14. _____ Fluid compartment that constitutes over half of the total body water at birth.

15. _____ Nutrients of which subclinical deficiencies are commonly seen in lower socioeconomic groups in the United States.

a. Vitamin

b. Macrominerals

c. Microminerals

d. Vegetarianism

e. Recommended Dietary Allowances

f. Incomplete protein

g. Allergens

h. Sensitization

i. Extracellular fluid

j. Intracellular fluid

k. Oral rehydration solution

l. Meconium

m. Constipation

n. Obstipation

o. Encopresis

II. REVIEWING KEY CONCEPTS AND CONTENT

MATCHING: Match each type of vegetarianism with its corresponding description.

16. _____ Eliminates any food of animal origin, including milk and eggs.

17. _____ Most restrictive of all types of vegetarianism, using brown rice as the mainstay of the diet.

18. _____ Excludes meat from the diet but allows milk, eggs, and sometimes fish (vegans).

19. _____ Excludes meat and eggs but allows milk.

a. Lactoovovegetarianism

b. Lactovegetarianism

c. Pure vegetarianism

d. Zen macrobiotics

20. Describe the major nutritional deficiencies that are most likely to occur in the diet of a family who follows a strict vegetarian diet.

21. Which of the following combinations of foods would ensure the most complete protein for a strictly vegetarian family if eaten together at the same meal?
    a. Milk and chicken
    b. Sunflower seeds and rice
    c. Rice and red beans
    d. Eggs and cheese

22. In the United States, protein and energy malnutrition (PEM) occurs when
    a. the food supply is inadequate.
    b. the food supply may be adequate.
    c. the adults eat first, leaving insufficient food for children.
    d. the diet consists mainly of starch grains.

23. Kwashiorkor results in populations in which
    a. the food supply is inadequate.
    b. the food supply is adequate for protein.
    c. the adults eat first, leaving insufficient food for children.
    d. the diet consists mainly of starch grains.

24. Nutritional marasmus usually results in populations in which
    a. the food supply is inadequate.
    b. the food supply is adequate for protein.
    c. the adults eat first, leaving insufficient food for children.
    d. the diet consists mainly of starch grains.

25. Which of the following diagnostic strategies is the most definitive for identifying a milk allergy?
    a. Stool analysis for blood
    b. Serum IgE levels
    c. A challenge of milk after elimination
    d. Skin testing

26. Treatment of cow's milk allergy in infants involves changing the formula to
    a. soy-based formula.
    b. goat's milk.
    c. casein/whey hydrolysate milk.
    d. breast milk.

27. Infants and young children are at high risk for fluid and electrolyte imbalances. Which of the following factors contributes to this vulnerability?
    a. Decreased body surface area
    b. Lower metabolic rate
    c. Mature kidney function
    d. Increased extracellular fluid volume

28. _____ dehydration occurs when electrolyte and water deficits are present in balanced proportion.

29. _____ dehydration occurs when the electrolyte deficit exceeds the water deficit. There is a greater loss of extracellular fluid, and plasma sodium concentration is usually _____ than 130 mEq/L.

30. _____ dehydration results from water loss in excess of electrolyte loss. This is often caused by a large _____ of water and/or a large _____ of electrolytes. Plasma sodium concentration is _____ than 150 mEq/L.

31. Of the following choices of describing dehydration or fluid loss in infants and young children, which describes the loss most accurately?
    a. As a percentage
    b. In milliliters per kilogram of body weight
    c. By the amount of edema present or absent
    d. By the degree of skin elasticity

32. An infant with moderate dehydration has what clinical signs?
    a. Mottled skin color, decreased pulse and respirations
    b. Decreased urine output, tachycardia, fever
    c. Dry mucous membranes, capillary filling >2 to 3 seconds
    d. Tachycardia, bulging fontanel, decreased blood pressure

33. A priority goal in the management of acute diarrhea is
    a. determining the cause of the diarrhea.
    b. preventing the spread of the infection.
    c. rehydrating of the child.
    d. managing the fever associated with the diarrhea.

34. A child, age 5, is started on a bowel habit retraining program for chronic constipation. Instructions to the family should include which of the following?
    a. Decrease the water and increase the milk in the child's diet.
    b. Establish a regular time when the child will sit on the toilet.
    c. Withhold playtime with friend if child does not have a daily bowel movement.
    d. Have child sit on the toilet each day until a bowel movement is produced.

35. To confirm the diagnosis of Hirschsprung disease, the nurse prepares the child for which of the following tests?
    a. Endoscopy
    b. Sonograms
    c. Rectal biopsy
    d. Esophagoscopy

36. The nurse would expect to see which of the following clinical manifestations in the child diagnosed with Hirschsprung disease?
    a. History of bloody diarrhea, fever, and vomiting
    b. Irritability, severe abdominal cramps, and fecal soiling
    c. Increased serum lipids and positive stool for O&P (ova and parasites)
    d. Constipation, visible peristalsis, and palpable fecal mass

37. It would be reasonable for the parents of a 2-month-old with gastroesophageal reflux to include which of the following in the infant's care?
    a. Stop breastfeeding because breast milk is too thin and easily leads to reflux.
    b. After feeding and burping, position the infant prone with the head and chest elevated 30 degrees.
    c. After feeding and burping, position the infant on his or her back with the head turned to the side.
    d. Try to increase feeding volume right before bedtime because this is the time when the stomach is more able to retain foods.

38. An 8-year-old has been diagnosed with giardiasis. The nurse should expect which of these signs and symptoms?
    a. Diarrhea with blood in the stools
    b. Nausea and vomiting with a mild fever
    c. Abdominal cramps with intermittent loose stools
    d. Weight loss of 5 lb over the last month

39. The nurse is teaching parents how to collect a specimen for enterobiasis using the test tape diagnostic procedure. Which of the following is included in the explanation?
    a. Use a flashlight to inspect the anal area while the child sleeps.
    b. Perform the test 2 days after the child has received the first dose of mebendazole.
    c. Test all members of the family at the same time using frosted tape.
    d. Collect the tape in the morning before the child has a bowel movement or bath.

40. Children with pinworm infections present with the principal symptom of
    a. perianal itching.
    b. diarrhea with blood.
    c. evidence of small ricelike worms in their stool and urine.
    d. abdominal pain.

41. Diagnostic evaluations for lead poisoning include
    a. blood levels for lead concentration, including screening done on finger and heel sticks with blood collected by venipuncture to confirm diagnosis.
    b. recommended universal screening for all children, with children ages 6 to 72 months given priority.
    c. radiographs of the long bones to reveal lead lines caused by deposition of lead.
    d. all of the above.

42. Reduction of poisonings in children and infants can be accomplished by
    a. use of child-resistant containers.
    b. educating parents and grandparents to place products out of reach of small children.
    c. educating parents to relocate plants out of reach of infants, toddlers, and small children.
    d. all of the above.

43. The first action parents should be taught to initiate in a poisoning is to
    a. induce vomiting.
    b. take the child to the family physician's office or emergency center.
    c. call the poison control center.
    d. follow the instructions on the label of the household product.

44. Gastric decontamination is aimed at removing ingested toxic products by _____

    _____

    _____

45. Which of the following would alert the nurse to possible peritonitis from a ruptured appendix in a child suspected of having appendicitis?
    a. Colicky abdominal pain with guarding of the abdomen
    b. Periumbilical pain that progresses to the lower right quadrant of the abdomen with an elevated WBC

c. Low-grade fever of 100.6° F with the child having difficulty walking and assuming a side-lying position with the knees flexed toward the chest
d. Temperature of 103° F, absent bowel sounds, and sudden relief from abdominal pain

46. The most common clinical manifestations expected with Meckel diverticulum include which of the following?
    a. Fever, vomiting, and constipation
    b. Weight loss, hypotension, and obstruction
    c. Painless rectal bleeding, abdominal pain, or intestinal obstruction
    d. Abdominal pain, bloody diarrhea, and foul-smelling stool

47. A common feature of inflammatory bowel disease is
    a. growth abnormalities.
    b. chronic constipation.
    c. obstruction.
    d. burning epigastric pain.

48. In the child with peptic ulcer disease, it would be unlikely to find
    a. *Helicobacter pylori*.
    b. a blood type O.
    c. a diet consisting of spicy foods.
    d. psychologic factors such as stressful life events.

49. The single most effective strategy to prevent and control hepatitis is _____.

MATCHING: Match each viral hepatitis type with its corresponding description. (Types may be used more than once.)

50. _____ The highest incidence of this type of hepatitis occurs in preschool and school-age children.

51. _____ Immunity by HBV vaccine is available.

52. _____ Non-A, non-B with transmission through the fecal-oral route or with contaminated water.

53. _____ Children with chronic HBV should be tested for this type of hepatitis.

54. _____ The major route of infection in children is mother-to-infant transmission.

55. _____ Incubation period 14 to 180 days; average 50 days.

a. Hepatitis A

b. Hepatitis B

c. Hepatitis C

d. Hepatitis D

e. Hepatitis E

56. Currently the 5-year survival rate for liver transplantation is
    a. 10%.
    b. 25%.
    c. 75%.
    d. 85%.

57. The best definition of *biliary atresia* is
    a. persistant jaundice with elevated direct bilirubin levels.
    b. progressive inflammatory process causing bile duct fibrosis.
    c. absence of bile pigment.
    d. hepatomegaly and palpable liver.

58. To detect a cleft palate, the nurse may need to
    a. assess the swallowing ability of the infant.
    b. assess color of lips.
    c. palpate the palate with a gloved finger.
    d. all of the above.

59. Which of the following options are best to use when feeding the infant with a cleft of the lip or palate?
    I. Use of "cleft palate" nipple or large, soft nipple with large hole, or breastfeeding
    II. Use of normal nipple
    III. Use of "gravity flow" nipple attached to a squeezable plastic bottle
    IV. Use of rubber-tipped Asepto syringe or Breck feeder
    a. I, II, III, and IV
    b. I, III, and IV
    c. I, II, and IV
    d. I and III

60. Postoperative care for the infant with a cleft of the lip or palate would *not* include the strategy of
    a. applying bilateral elbow restraints that are pinned to the infant's clothes.
    b. removing restraints one at a time at regular intervals.
    c. placing child in the upright infant seat position.
    d. vigorously suctioning the infant who is having difficulty breathing.

61. Feeding the infant with a cleft repair of either the lip or the palate postoperatively includes which of the following?
    I. If the infant had cleft lip repair, feeding begins with clear liquid.
    II. Feedings are resumed whenever tolerated after a cleft lip repair.
    III. Cleft palate repair feedings include the use of spoons and forks.
    IV. Cleft palate repair feedings include the use of cups and straws.
    a. I and II
    b. I, II, III, and IV
    c. I and III
    d. II and IV

62. An invagination of one portion of the intestine into another is called
    a. intussusception.
    b. pyloric stenosis.
    c. tracheoesophageal fistula.
    d. Hirschsprung disease.

63. A 5-month-old infant is suspected of having intussusception. What clinical manifestations would he most likely have?
    a. Crying with abdominal examination, vomiting, and currant-jelly-appearing stools
    b. Fever, diarrhea, vomiting, and lowered WBC
    c. Weight gain, constipation, and refusal to eat
    d. Abdominal distention, periodic pain, and hypotension

64. A 5-month-old infant's intussusception is treated with hydrostatic reduction. The nurse should expect care after the reduction to include
    a. administration of antibiotics.
    b. enema administration to remove remaining stool.
    c. observation of stools.
    d. rectal temperatures every 4 hours.

65. The nurse observes frothy saliva in the mouth and nose of the neonate and frequent drooling. When fed, the infant swallows normally, but suddenly the fluid returns through the nose and mouth of the infant. The nurse should suspect what medical condition?
    a. Esophageal atresia
    b. Cleft palate
    c. Anorectal malformation
    d. Biliary atresia

66. A 1-month-old infant is brought to the clinic by his mother. The nurse suspects pyloric stenosis, because the mother gives a history of
    a. diarrhea.
    b. projectile vomiting.
    c. fever and dehydration.
    d. abdominal distention.

67. The preoperative nursing plan for an infant with pyloric obstruction should include
    a. rehydration by intravenous fluids for fluid and electrolyte imbalance.
    b. nasogastric (NG) tube placement to decompress the stomach.
    c. parental support and reassurance.
    d. all of the above.

68. The assessment finding that is most likely to indicate anorectal malformation is
    a. a normal anal opening.
    b. a normal perineum.
    c. passage of meconium stool.
    d. absence of meconium or stool.

69. The most important therapeutic management for the child with celiac disease is
    a. eliminating corn, rice, and millet from the diet.
    b. adding iron, folic acid, and fat-soluble vitamins to the diet.
    c. eliminating wheat, rye, barley, and oats from the diet.
    d. educating the child's parents about the short-term effects of the disease and the necessity of reading all food labels for content until the disease is in remission.

70. The prognosis for children with short bowel syndrome has improved as a result of
    a. dietary supplemental vitamin B_{12} additions.
    b. improvement in surgical procedures to correct the deficiency.
    c. improved home care availability.
    d. total parenteral nutrition and enteral feeding.

71. Name the six major principles of emergency treatment for poisoning.

72. The nurse provides proper instructions to parents for ipecac syrup, including which of the following?
    a. Dispose of any ipecac; it is not recommended for immediate treatment.
    b. Administer the emetic within 3 hours of toxic ingestion.
    c. Have two doses of the emetic in the household for each child.
    d. Force fluids and encourage activity after the emetic is administered to facilitate its effectiveness.

73. T   F   Asymptomatic young children may have lead levels sufficiently elevated to cause neurologic and intellectual damage.

74. T   F   The greatest risk of lead poisoning is to poor African-American children under 6 years of age living in urban areas.

75. T   F   Lead-based paint from old housing remains the most frequent source of lead poisoning in children.

76. T   F   Lead-containing pottery or leaded dishes do not contribute to lead poisoning.

III. THINKING CRITICALLY

1. Describe the assessment parameters to use with a 3-year-old complaining of constipation.

2. Identify each stage of repair for Hirschsprung disease.

3. Describe what the parents of a child with gastroesophogeal reflux should be taught about positioning.

4. Differentiate between ulcerative colitis and Crohn's disease in regard to pathology, rectal bleeding, diarrhea, pain, anorexia, weight loss, and growth retardation.

48 Cardiovascular Dysfunction

I. LEARNING KEY TERMS

MATCHING: Match each term with its corresponding description.

1. _____ Abnormally fast heart rate.

2. _____ The consistent elevation of blood pressure beyond values considered to be the upper limits of normal.

3. _____ Removal of the recipient's heart to implant a new one from a donor.

4. _____ Abnormally slow heart rate.

5. _____ Refers to abnormalities of the myocardium in which the cardiac muscles' ability to contract is impaired; relatively rare in children.

6. _____ Refers to excessive cholesterol in the blood; believed to play an important role in atherosclerosis development.

7. _____ A general term for excessive lipids (fat) and fatlike substances; believed to play an important role in atherosclerosis development.

8. _____ Procedure leaving the recipient's own heart in place and implanting a new heart to act as an additional pump; rarely performed in children.

9. _____ The first treatment strategy to try for supraventricular tachycardia; performed by applying ice to the face, massaging one carotid artery, or having the child exhale against a closed glottis.

10. _____ A thickening and flattening of the tips of the fingers and toes; thought to be a result of chronic tissue hypoxemia and polycythemia.

11. _____ Cardiovascular efficiency diminished; microcirculatory perfusion marginal despite compensatory adjustments; tissue hypoxia, metabolic acidosis, and impairment of organ systems function.

12. _____ Procedure in which a radiopaque catheter is inserted through a peripheral blood vessel into the heart; contrast material injected; films taken of the dilution and circulation of the contrast material; used for diagnosis, treatment of valves/vessels, and electrophysiology studies.

13. _____ Slow heart rate.

a. Congenital heart disease

b. Acquired cardiac disorders

c. Tachycardia

d. Bradycardia

e. Cardiac catheterization

f. Congestive heart failure

g. Hypoxemia

h. Hypoxia

i. Cyanosis

j. Polycythemia

k. Clubbing

l. Hyperlipidemia

m. Hypercholesterolemia

n. Bradydysrhythmias

o. Tachydysrhythmias

p. Cardiomyopathy

q. Vagal maneuvers

r. Hypertension

s. Compensated shock

t. Uncompensated shock

u. Irreversible shock

v. Orthotopic heart transplantation

w. Heterotopic heart transplantation

14. _____ Condition in which actual damage to vital organs occurs and disruption/death occurs even if measurements return to normal with therapy.

15. _____ The inability of the heart to pump an adequate amount of blood to meet the metabolic demands of the body; not a disease; in children, most common in infants; usually secondary to increases in blood volume and pressure from anomalies; result of an excessive work load imposed on normal myocardium.

16. _____ Fast heart rate.

17. _____ An increased number of red blood cells; increases the oxygen carrying capacity of the blood.

18. _____ Includes primarily anatomic abnormalities present at birth that result in abnormal cardiac function, the consequences of which are hypoxemia and heart failure.

19. _____ Refers to an arterial oxygen tension (or pressure) that is less than normal and can be identified by a decreased arterial saturation or a decreased Pao_2.

20. _____ Vital organ function is maintained by intrinsic compensatory mechanism; blood flow is usually normal or increased, but generally uneven or maldistributed in the microcirculation.

21. _____ Disease processes or abnormalities that occur after birth and can be seen in the normal heart or in the presence of congenital heart defects; resulting from factors, such as infection, autoimmune responses, environmental factors, and familial tendencies.

22. _____ A reduction in tissue oxygenation that results from low oxygen saturation and Pao_2 and results in impaired cellular processes.

23. _____ A blue discoloration in the mucous membranes, skin, and nail beds of the child with reduced oxygen saturation; results from the presence of deoxygenated hemoglobin (hemoglobin not bound to oxygen); determined subjectively.

II. REVIEWING KEY CONCEPTS AND CONTENT

24. During fetal life, oxygenated blood travels into the left atrium through a structure known as the
    a. truncus arteriosus.
    b. foramen ovale.
    c. sinus venosus.
    d. ductus venosus.

25. In fetal circulation only a small amount of blood flows through the nonfunctioning
    a. lungs.
    b. foramen ovale.
    c. liver.
    d. coronary sinus.

26. Which disease in the mother during pregnancy is an important clue to the diagnosis of congenital heart disease?
    a. Rheumatoid arthritis
    b. Rheumatic fever
    c. Streptococcal infection
    d. Rubella

27. Coarctation of the aorta should be suspected when
    a. the blood pressure is higher in the arms than in the legs.
    b. the blood pressure in the right arm is different from the blood pressure in the left arm.
    c. the apical pulse is greater than the radial pulse.
    d. the point of maximum impulse is shifted to the left.

28. The test in which a transducer is placed behind the heart to obtain images of posterior heart structures is the
    a. electrocardiogram.
    b. echocardiogram.
    c. transesophageal echocardiogram.
    d. two-dimensional echocardiogram.

29. In children, the usual approach to the left ventricle of the heart in a cardiac catheterization is through the
    a. left side of the heart.
    b. right side of the heart.

30. List five of the most significant complications following a cardiac catheterization in an infant or young child.

31. If bleeding occurs at the insertion site after a cardiac catheterization, the nurse should apply
    a. warmth to the unaffected extremity.
    b. pressure below the insertion site.
    c. warmth to the affected extremity.
    d. pressure above the insertion site.

32. A 12-month-old would be classified as significantly hypertensive with a blood pressure that
    a. falls above the 99th percentile one time.
    b. persistently falls between the 95th and 99th percentiles.
    c. falls between the 95th and 99th percentiles one time.
    d. falls below the 99th percentile one time.

33. As a general rule, digoxin should not be administered to the older child whose pulse is
    a. 108.
    b. 98.
    c. 78.
    d. 68.

34. Infants with congestive heart failure are positioned with the head elevated to promote
    a. improved digestion.
    b. maximum chest expansion.
    c. an increase in afterload.
    d. improved hydration.

35. Fluid and nutritional guidelines for an infant with congestive heart failure rarely include
    a. sodium restriction.
    b. sodium supplements.
    c. fluid restriction.
    d. decreased caloric intake.

36. The two main angiotensin-converting enzyme (ACE) inhibitors most commonly used for children with congestive heart failure are
    a. digoxin and captopril.
    b. enalapril and captopril.
    c. enalapril and furosemide.
    d. spironolactone and captopril.

37. The electrolyte usually depleted with diuretic therapy is
    a. sodium.
    b. chloride.
    c. potassium.
    d. magnesium.

38. The nutritional needs of the infant with congestive heart failure are usually
    a. the same as an adult's.
    b. less than a healthy infant's.
    c. the same as a healthy infant's.
    d. greater than a healthy infant's.

39. The calories are usually increased for an infant with congestive heart failure by
    a. feeding every 2 hours.
    b. increasing the volume of each feeding.
    c. increasing the caloric density of the formula.
    d. increasing the feeding duration to 1 hour.

40. Which of the following clinical manifestations is a sign of chronic hypoxemia?
    a. Squatting
    b. Polycythemia
    c. Clubbing
    d. All of the above

41. Prostaglandin is administered to the newborn with a congenital heart defect to
    a. keep the ductus arteriosus open.
    b. close the patent ductus arteriosus.
    c. keep the foramen ovale open.
    d. close the foramen ovale.

42. Dehydration must be prevented in children who are hypoxemic because dehydration places the child at risk for
    a. infection.
    b. cerebral vascular accident.
    c. fever.
    d. air embolism.

MATCHING: Match each specific disorder with its corresponding type of defect. (Defects may be used more than once.)

43. _____ Patent ductus arteriosus.

44. _____ Coarctation of the aorta.

45. _____ Ventricular septal defect.

46. _____ Subvalvular aortic stenosis.

47. _____ Hypoplastic left heart syndrome.

48. _____ Atrioventricular canal defect.

49. _____ Pulmonic stenosis.

50. _____ Tetralogy of Fallot.

51. _____ Aortic stenosis.

52. _____ Tricuspid atresia.

53. _____ Valvular aortic stenosis.

54. _____ Truncus arteriosus.

55. _____ Atrial septal defect.

56. _____ Transposition of the great vessels.

a. Defects with decreased pulmonary blood flow

b. Mixed defects

c. Defects with increased pulmonary blood flow

d. Obstructive defects

57. Which of the following congenital heart defects usually has the best prognosis?
   a. Tetralogy of Fallot
   b. Ventricular septal defect
   c. Atrial septal defect
   d. Hypoplastic left heart syndrome

58. Which of the following sets of assessment findings are the most frequent clinical manifestations of an atrial septal defect in an infant or child?
   a. Decreased cardiac output and low blood pressure
   b. Congestive heart failure and a murmur
   c. Increased blood pressure and pulse
   d. Dyspnea and bradycardia

59. Parents of the child with a congenital heart defect should know the signs of congestive heart failure, which include
   a. poor feeding.
   b. sudden weight gain.
   c. increased efforts to breathe.
   d. all of the above.

60. A visit to the intensive care unit before open-heart surgery should take place
   a. several days before the surgery.
   b. at a busy time with a lot to see and hear.
   c. the day before surgery.
   d. several weeks before the surgery.

61. Describe the nursing care management to consider while suctioning an infant after cardiac surgery.

62. Because an incision is made through muscle, most children consider the most painful part of cardiac surgery to be the
   a. thoracotomy incision site.
   b. graft site on the leg.
   c. sternotomy incision site.
   d. intravenous insertion sites.

63. An infant who weighs 7 kg has just returned to the intensive care unit following cardiac surgery. The chest tube has drained 40 ml in the past hour. In this situation, what is the first action for the nurse to take?
   a. Notify the surgeon.
   b. Identify any other signs of hemorrhage.
   c. Suction the patient.
   d. Identify any other signs of renal failure.

64. An infant who weighs 7 kg has just returned to the intensive care unit following cardiac surgery. The urine output has been 5 ml in the past hour. In this situation, what is the first action for the nurse to take?
   a. Notify the surgeon.
   b. Identify any other signs of hypervolemia.
   c. Suction the patient.
   d. Identify any other signs of renal failure.

65. Following cardiac surgery, fluid intake calculations for a child would include
   a. intravenous fluids.
   b. arterial and CVP line flushes.
   c. fluid used to dilute medications.
   d. all of the above.

66. Following cardiac surgery, in addition to hourly recordings of urine, fluid output calculations in a child should include
   a. nasogastric secretions.
   b. blood drawn for analysis.
   c. chest tube drainage.
   d. all of the above.

67. List at least five complications of cardiac surgery in children.

68. One of the most important factors in preventing bacterial endocarditis is
   a. administration of prophylactic antibiotic therapy.
   b. surgical repair of the defect.
   c. administration of prostaglandin to maintain patent ductus arteriosus.
   d. administration of antibiotics after dental work.

69. The test that provides the most reliable evidence of recent streptococcal infection is the
   a. throat culture.
   b. Mantoux test.
   c. elevation of liver enzymes.
   d. antistreptolysis O test.

70. The peak age for the incidence of Kawasaki disease is in the
   a. infant age group.
   b. toddler age group.
   c. school-age group.
   d. adolescent age group.

71. Discharge teaching for a child with Kawasaki disease who received gamma globulin should include which of the following instructions?
   a. Peeling of the hands and feet should be reported immediately.
   b. Arthritis, especially in the weight-bearing joints, should be reported immediately.
   c. Defer measles, mumps, and rubella vaccine for 11 months.
   d. All of the above should be included in the instructions.

72. Most cases of hypertension in children are a result of
   a. essential hypertension.
   b. secondary hypertension.
   c. primary hypertension.
   d. congenital heart defects.

73. Elevated cholesterol
   a. can predict the long-term risk of heart disease for the individual.
   b. can predict the risk of hypertension in adulthood.
   c. plays an important role in producing atherosclerosis.
   d. plays an important role in producing congestive heart failure.

74. The heart transplant procedure that is used most often in children is the
   a. heterotopic heart transplantation.
   b. orthotopic heart transplantation.

III.   THINKING CRITICALLY

1. Identify the clinical manifestations that could indicate the presence of a congenital heart defect in an infant or young child.

2. List the components of a child's history that could indicate a high risk for congenital heart disease.

3. Explain why a child with congestive heart failure should be placed on a regimen of oral digitalis and diuretics.

4. Describe how to help families decrease their fear and anxiety and increase their coping behaviors when facing their child's surgery to correct a congenital heart defect.

49 Hematologic and Immunologic Dysfunction

I. LEARNING KEY TERMS

MATCHING: Match each term with its corresponding definition or description.

1. _____ Nosebleed.

2. _____ Heterozygous people who have hemoglobin containing HbA as well as abnormal HbS (sickle hemoglobin).

3. _____ The process that stops bleeding when a blood system vessel is injured.

4. _____ The single unit of inheritance.

5. _____ A condition in which the number of red blood cells and/or hemoglobin concentration is reduced below normal; oxygen-carrying capacity of the blood is diminished; less oxygen is available to the tissues.

6. _____ People who are homozygous with predominantly HbS (sickle hemoglobin).

a. Hemostasis

b. Anemia

c. Sickle cell trait

d. Sickle cell anemia

e. Epistaxis

f. Haplotype

II. REVIEWING KEY CONCEPTS AND CONTENT

7. The common childhood anemia that occurs more frequently in toddlers between the ages of 12 and 36 months is _____.

8. At birth the normal full-term newborn has maternal stores of iron sufficient to last how long?
   a. The first 5 to 6 months of life
   b. The first 2 to 3 months of life
   c. The first 8 months of life
   d. Less than 1 month of life

9. A 5-year-old with sickle cell anemia is admitted because of diminished RBC production triggered by a viral infection. The episode is characterized by distal ischemia and pain. The sickle cell crisis the child is most likely to be experiencing is
   a. vasoocclusive crisis.
   b. splenic sequestration crisis.
   c. aplastic crisis.
   d. hyperhemolytic crisis.

10. Therapeutic management of sickle cell crisis generally includes which one of the following?
    a. Long-term oxygen use to enable the oxygen to reach the sickled RBCs
    b. Increase in activity to promote circulation in the affected area
    c. Diet high in iron to decrease anemia
    d. Hydration for hemodilution through oral and IV therapy

11. In controlling severe pain related to vasoocclusive sickle cell crisis, the plan of care will most likely use
    a. administration of long-term oxygen.
    b. application of cold compresses to the area.
    c. intramuscular meperidine (Demerol).
    d. intravenous or oral opioids.

12. A 2-year-old child is to begin therapy for a-thalassemia. Educational sessions with the parents will most likely need to include the information that
    a. the child will need only occasional blood transfusions.
    b. an iron-chelating agent will be administered.
    c. the child will probably not live to adulthood.
    d. bone marrow transplant is the usual treatment.

13. Treatment for the child with aplastic anemia will most likely include
    a. administration of testosterone.
    b. administration of iron-chelating agents.
    c. irradiation.
    d. bone marrow transplant.

14. Primary prophylaxis in hemophilia patients involves the infusion of factor VIII
    a. regularly at the emergency room before joint damage occurs.
    b. regularly at home before the onset of joint damage.
    c. whenever bleeding into a joint occurs.
    d. when bleeding begins to impair joint function.

15. A 5-year-old boy previously diagnosed with hemophilia A is being admitted with hemarthrosis. The nurse knows that which of the following would most likely be included in the plan of care?
    I.   Ice packs to the affected area
    II.   Application of a splint or sling to immobilize the area
    III. Administration of factor VIII concentrate intramuscularly
    IV.   Administration of aspirin or aspirin-containing compounds
    V.   Administration of factor VII concentrate intravenously
    VI.   Active range-of-motion exercises
    VII. Teaching him how to administer AHF to himself
        a. I, III, and VI
        b. II, III, IV, and VI
        c. I, V, and VII
        d. I, II, V, and VI

16. An acquired hemorrhagic disorder characterized by excessive destruction of platelets and a discoloration caused by petechiae beneath the skin with normal bone marrow is called

    _____.

17. The cancer that occurs with the most frequency in children is
    a. lymphoma.
    b. neuroblastoma.
    c. leukemia.
    d. melanoma.

18. In young children, treatments for mouth ulcers may include
    a. viscous lidocaine.
    b. lemon glycerin swabs.
    c. chlorhexidine gluconate.
    d. hydrogen peroxide.

19. Children who develop moon face from short-term steroid therapy used to treat cancer may experience symptoms of
    a. acute toxicities.
    b. decreased appetite.
    c. permanent facial change.
    d. altered body image.

20. Typically the measures used to control the transmission of infection in the immunocompromised child during hospitalization include
    a. use of any semiprivate room.
    b. prophylactic antibiotics.
    c. chemotherapy.
    d. handwashing.

21. Hodgkin's disease increases in incidence in children
    a. under the age of 5 years.
    b. between the ages of 5 and 10 years.
    c. between the ages of 11 and 14 years.
    d. between the ages of 15 and 19 years.

22. The Reed-Sternberg cell is a significant finding because it
    a. is characteristic of leukemia.
    b. eliminates the need for a lymph node biopsy for staging.
    c. eliminates the need for laparotomy for staging.
    d. is characteristic of Hodgkin's disease.

23. In children and adolescents, HIV is likely to be transmitted
    a. perinatally from the mother.
    b. through blood products before 1985.
    c. to adolescents engaged in IV drug use.
    d. all of the above.

24. The American Academy of Pediatrics recommends that all children infected with HIV receive their immunizations, but the nurse recognizes that children with HIV who are receiving intravenous gamma globulin prophylaxis may not respond to the
    a. varicella vaccine.
    b. oral poliovirus vaccine.
    c. measles-mumps-rubella vaccine.
    d. all of the above.

25. Diagnosis of severe combined immunodeficiency disease (SCID) is primarily based on
    a. failure to thrive.
    b. delayed development.
    c. feeding problems.
    d. susceptibility to infections.

26. In Wiskott-Aldrich syndrome, the most notable effect of the disease at birth is which of the following?
    a. Bleeding
    b. Infection
    c. Eczema
    d. Malignancy

III. THINKING CRITICALLY

1. Describe the best way to manage pain during a sickle cell crisis that will help avoid clock watching and undermedicating.

2. Identify the emergency measures (with rationales) that are used when a child with hemophilia starts to bleed.

3. Describe the interventions (with rationales) that the nurse should use to maintain skin integrity in a child with a diagnosis of leukemia.

4. List the precautions necessary for parents of a 4-month-old infant with AIDS to use when coming into contact with the infant's body fluids.

Genitourinary Dysfunction

$\boxed{50}$

I. LEARNING KEY TERMS

MATCHING: Match each term with its corresponding description.

1. _____ Procedure of separating colloids and crystalline substances by circulating a blood filtrate outside the body and exerting hydrostatic pressure across a semi-permeable membrane with simultaneous infusion of a replacement solution.

2. _____ Presence of bacteria in the urine.

3. _____ Fluid accumulation in the abdominal cavity.

4. _____ Accumulation of body fluid in the interstitial spaces and body cavities.

5. _____ Accumulation of nitrogenous waste within the blood, resulting in elevated blood urea nitrogen and creatinine levels.

6. _____ A reduction in the serum albumin level.

7. _____ Inflammation of the bladder.

8. _____ Procedure in which colloids and crystalline substances are separated by using the abdominal cavity as a semi-permeable membrane through which water and solute of small molecular size move by osmosis and diffusion based on concentrations on either side of the membrane.

9. _____ Shift of fluid from the plasma to the interstitial spaces, resulting in a reduction in the vascular fluid volume.

10. _____ Inflammation of the urethra.

11. _____ Procedure in which colloids and crystalline substance are separated by circulating the blood outside the body through artificial membranes, which permits a similar passage of water and solutes.

12. _____ Dilation of the renal pelvis from distention caused by a backup of urine above an obstruction.

13. _____ Inflammation of the upper urinary tract and kidneys.

14. _____ The most immediate threat to the life of a child with acute renal failure; excess potassium in the blood; treated with Kayexalate and dialysis.

15. _____ Condition in which albumin is lost into the urine because of glomerular permeability.

a. Bacteriuria

b. Cystitis

c. Urethritis

d. Pyelonephritis

e. Urosepsis

f. Hydronephrosis

g. Hyperalbuminuria

h. Hypoalbuminemia

i. Edema

j. Ascites

k. Hypovolemia

l. Azotemia

m. Uremia

n. Hyperkalemia

o. Hemodialysis

p. Peritoneal dialysis

q. Hemofiltration

16. _____ The retention of nitrogenous products that produces toxic symptoms; a serious condition that often involves body systems other than the renal system.

17. _____ Febrile urinary tract infection coexisting with systemic signs of bacterial illness; blood culture reveals presence of urinary pathogen.

II. REVIEWING KEY CONCEPTS AND CONTENT

18. Which of the following does *not* predispose the child to urinary tract infections?
    a. The short urethra in the young female
    b. The presence of urinary stasis
    c. Urinary reflux
    d. Lower urine pH

19. For the child with nephrosis, one aim of the therapy is to reduce
    a. excretion of urinary protein.
    b. excretion of fluids.
    c. serum albumin levels.
    d. urinary output.

20. Acute glomerulonephritis would most likely be suspected if the child presented with the clinical manifestations of
    a. normal blood pressure, generalized edema, and oliguria.
    b. periorbital edema, tea-colored urine, and anorexia.
    c. fatigue, elevated serum lipid levels, and elevated serum protein levels.
    d. temperature elevation, circulatory congestion, and normal creatinine serum levels.

21. The nurse caring for the child with acute glomerulonephritis would expect to
    a. enforce complete bed rest.
    b. weigh the child daily.
    c. perform peritoneal dialysis.
    d. ensure a diet low in protein.

22. Clinical manifestations of nephrotic syndrome include
    a. hyperlipidemia, hypoalbuminemia, edema, and proteinuria.
    b. hematuria, hypertension, periorbital edema, and flank pain.
    c. oliguria, hypocholesterolemia, and hyperalbuminemia.
    d. hematuria, generalized edema, hypertension, and proteinuria.

23. When teaching the family of a child with nephrotic syndrome about prednisone therapy, the nurse includes the information that
    a. corticosteroid therapy begins after BUN and serum creatinine elevation.
    b. prednisone is administered orally in a dosage of 4 mg/kg of body weight.
    c. after proteinuria and edema resolve, the dose is gradually tapered.
    d. the drug is discontinued as soon as the urine is free from protein.

24. Renal injury, acquired hemolytic anemia, central nervous system symptoms, and thrombocytopenia are characteristic clinical manifestations of the disorder known as
    a. minimal-change nephrotic syndrome.
    b. Wilms' tumor.
    c. hemolytic-uremic syndrome.
    d. vesicoureteral reflux.

25. The most frequent cause of transient acute renal failure in infants and children is
    a. nephrotoxic agents.
    b. obstructive uropathy.
    c. dehydration.
    d. burn shock.

26. The primary manifestation of acute renal failure is
    a. edema.
    b. oliguria.
    c. metabolic acidosis.
    d. weight gain and proteinuria.

27. The most immediate threat to the life of the child with acute renal failure is
    a. hyperkalemia.
    b. anemia.
    c. hypertensive crisis.
    d. cardiac failure from hypovolemia.

28. Drug therapy used for the removal of potassium is
    a. furosemide.
    b. glucose 50% and insulin.
    c. Kayexalate.
    d. calcium gluconate.

29. The manifestation of chronic renal failure that would probably have the most detrimental social consequences for the developing child is
    a. anemia.
    b. growth retardation.
    c. bone demineralization.
    d. septicemia.

30. Which of the following is included in dietary regulation of the child with chronic renal failure?
    a. Restricting protein intake below the recommended daily allowance
    b. Including protein in the diet that has high biologic value
    c. Restricting potassium when creatinine clearance falls below 50 ml/min
    d. Giving vitamin A, E, and K supplements

31. Methods of dialysis for management of renal failure are _____, _____, and _____.

32. _____ is the preferred method of dialysis for children with life-threatening hyperkalemia that needs to be rapidly corrected.

33. _____ dialysis is usually recommended for small children.

34. The major complication associated with peritoneal dialysis is _____.

35. Continuous arteriovenous hemofiltration is an ideal form of dialysis for children with _____ from _____.

36. A child, age 12, had a renal transplant 5 months ago. He now presents to the hospital outpatient clinic with fever, tenderness over the graft area, decreased urinary output, and a slightly elevated blood pressure. The nurse's priority at this time is to
    a. recognize that the child is probably undergoing acute rejection and to notify the physician immediately.
    b. recognize that this is an episode of increased inflammation within the donor kidney because the child has probably been noncompliant with his immunosuppressant drugs.
    c. obtain urine for culture and sensitivity and a blood count to quickly identify the child's infection before alerting the physician.
    d. recognize the child is in chronic rejection and that no present therapy can halt the progressive process.

III. THINKING CRITICALLY

1. Describe the nursing interventions to use to provide proper nutrition for the child who has minimal-change nephrotic syndrome.

2. Explain how the nurse might help a small child conserve energy in order to recover from minimal-change nephrotic syndrome.

3. Explain how the nurse might help provide diversional activities for a school-age child admitted for acute glomerulonephritis.

4. Explain why a child with glomerulonephritis is placed on a low-protein diet while in acute renal failure.

5. Describe the nursing interventions to use to promote optimum home care for a 15-year-old child who is to perform home peritoneal dialysis.

Cerebral Dysfunction (51)

I. LEARNING KEY TERMS

MATCHING: Match each term with its corresponding definition or description.

1. _____ Occurring within the anterior two thirds of the brain, mainly the cerebrum; location of a small number (less than 40%) of brain tumors in children.

2. _____ A sign of severe dysfunction of the cerebral cortex characterized by adduction of the arm at the shoulders, flexion of the arm on the chest with the wrist flexed and hands fisted, and extension and adduction of the lower extremities.

3. _____ Brief malfunctions of the brain's electrical system resulting from cortical neuronal discharges; most frequently observed neurologic dysfunction in children; clinical manifestations determined by the site of origin and may include unconsciousness or altered consciousness, involuntary movements, and changes in perception, behaviors, sensations, and posture.

4. _____ A sign of dysfunction at the level of the midbrain; characterized by rigid extension and pronation of the arms and legs; may not be evident when the child is quiet, but can usually be elicited by applying painful stimuli such as pressure of a blunt object on the base of the nail.

5. _____ The most common head injury; a transient and reversible neuronal dysfunction, with instantaneous loss of awareness and responsiveness resulting from trauma to the head and persisting for a relatively short time, usually minutes or hours, followed by amnesia; not always marked by loss of consciousness.

6. _____ Determined by observations of the child's responses to the environment; the earliest indicator of improvement or deterioration in neurologic status.

7. _____ Required whenever children undergo a procedure while sedated even if the child remains conscious (conscious sedation).

8. _____ Below the tentorium cerebelli; the location of the majority of tumors (about 60%) in children.

9. _____ The ability to process stimuli and produce verbal and motor responses; one of the two components of consciousness.

10. _____ State of unconsciousness from which the patient cannot be aroused even with powerful stimuli.

11. _____ An arousal-waking state that includes the ability to respond to stimuli; one of the two components of consciousness.

12. _____ Depressed cerebral function; the inability to respond to sensory stimuli and to have subjective experiences.

a. Alertness

b. Cognitive power

c. Unconsciousness

d. Coma

e. Level of consciousness

f. Decorticate posturing

g. Decerebrate posturing

h. Postanesthesia care

i. Concussion

j. Infratentorial

k. Supratentorial

l. Seizure

II. REVIEWING KEY CONCEPTS AND CONTENT

13. The sign that can be used to indicate increased intracranial pressure in the infant but not in the older child is:
    a. projectile vomiting.
    b. headache.
    c. bulging fontanel.
    d. pulsating fontanel.

14. The best indicators to use to determine the depth of the comatose state is
    a. motor activity.
    b. level of consciousness.
    c. reflexes.
    d. vital signs.

15. Using the Glasgow Coma Scale, the nurse knows that children older than 3 years should
    a. be able to state their name.
    b. always be assessed without parents present.
    c. not have a response to painful stimuli.
    d. be able to state clearly the place and time.

16. The nurse's priority when caring for a child during a seizure is to
    a. intervene to halt the seizure.
    b. restrain the child.
    c. protect the child from injury.
    d. place a solid object between the teeth.

17. The reflex pattern that would be considered most healthy in young infants is a
    a. negative Moro reflex and a positive tonic neck reflex.
    b. negative Moro reflex and a negative tonic neck reflex.
    c. positive Moro reflex, and a positive tonic neck reflex.
    d. positive Moro reflex and a negative tonic neck reflex.

18. Which of the following nursing observations would usually indicate pain in a comatose child?
    a. Increased flaccidity
    b. Increased oxygen saturation
    c. Decreased blood pressure
    d. Increased agitation

19. The activity that has been shown to increase intracranial pressure is
    a. using earplugs to eliminate noise.
    b. range-of-motion exercises.
    c. suctioning.
    d. osmotherapy.

20. Which of the following neurologic conditions occurs more often in children with a head injury than in adults with a head injury?
    a. Cerebral hyperemia
    b. Hypoxic brain damage
    c. Cerebral edema
    d. Subdural hemorrhage

21. Epidural hemorrhage is less common in children under 2 years of age than in adults because
    a. the middle meningeal artery is embedded in the bone surface of the skull until approximately 2 years of age.
    b. fractures are less likely to lacerate the middle meningeal artery in children under 2 years of age.
    c. separation of the dura from bleeding is more likely to occur in children than in adults.
    d. there is an increased tendency for the skull to fracture in children under 2 years of age.

22. After craniocerebral trauma, children usually have a
    a. lower frequency of psychologic disturbances than adults.
    b. higher mortality rate than adults.
    c. less favorable prognosis than adults.
    d. higher frequency of psychologic disturbances than adults.

23. The epidemiology of bacterial meningitis has changed in recent years because of the
    a. increased surveillance of tuberculosis.
    b. increased awareness of rubella vaccines.
    c. routine use of *H. influenzae* type B vaccine.
    d. routine use of hepatitis B vaccine.

24. The most common mode of transmission for bacterial meningitis is
    a. vascular dissemination of an infection elsewhere.
    b. direct implantation from an invasive procedure.
    c. direct extension from an infection in the mastoid sinuses.
    d. direct extension from an infection in the nasal sinuses.

25. Secondary problems from bacterial meningitis are most likely to occur in the
    a. child with meningococcal meningitis.
    b. infant under 2 months of age.
    c. infant over 2 months of age.
    d. child with *H. influenzae* type B meningitis.

26. Which of the following types of meningitis is self-limiting and least serious?
    a. Meningococcal meningitis
    b. Tuberculous meningitis
    c. *H. influenzae* meningitis
    d. Nonbacterial (aseptic) meningitis

27. Which of the following domestic animals should be the target of a community rabies vaccination program?
    a. Dogs
    b. Hamsters
    c. Cats
    d. Parakeets

28. The link between aspirin and Reye's syndrome
    a. is firmly established.
    b. is a cause-and-effect relationship.
    c. precludes the use of aspirin in children.
    d. all of the above.

29. The type of seizure, also known as a *petit mal seizure*, that occurs more often in children between the ages of 4 and 12 years is the
    a. generalized seizure.
    b. absence seizure.
    c. atonic seizure.
    d. jackknife seizure.

30. The antiepileptic drug that is controversial because it has the side effects of aplastic anemia or hepatic failure is
    a. felbamate.
    b. valproic acid.
    c. ethosuximide.
    d. adrenocorticotropic hormone.

31. The risk factors associated with recurrence of epilepsy include
    a. polytherapy.
    b. abnormal electroencephalogram (EEG).
    c. frequent seizures on antiepileptic medication.
    d. all of the above.

32. In most children who have a febrile seizure, the temperature factor that triggers the seizure tends to be the
    a. rapidity of the temperature elevation.
    b. duration of the temperature elevation.
    c. severity of the temperature elevation.
    d. any of the above.

33. When a child has a febrile seizure, it is important for the parents to know that the child will
    a. probably not develop epilepsy.
    b. most likely develop epilepsy.
    c. most likely develop neurologic damage.
    d. usually need tepid sponge baths to control fever.

III. THINKING CRITICALLY

1. Describe the parameters to assess and the interventions to use to maintain a stable intracranial pressure in an 8-year-old child who has been unconscious for 3 days.

2. Describe what interventions would help comfort the parents of a 3-year-old who comes to the emergency room after being rescued from a swimming pool.

3. Describe the assessment data that would be most helpful to obtain from a 4-year-old child who is admitted for possible seizure disorder.

4. Describe nursing interventions for the newborn with hydrocephalus.

Endocrine Dysfunction ⑤②

I. LEARNING KEY TERMS

MATCHING: Match each term with its corresponding definition or description.

1. _____ Protruding eyeballs; occurs in hyperthyroidism.

2. _____ Ketone bodies in the urine.

3. _____ Insatiable thirst.

4. _____ Elevation of the blood glucose; usually caused by illness, growth, or emotional upset.

5. _____ Occurs when serum glucose level exceeds the renal threshold (180 mg/dl) and glucose "spills" into the urine.

6. _____ Insulin reaction; usually caused by bursts of physical activity without additional food or delayed, omitted, or incompletely consumed meals.

7. _____ The condition produced by the presence in the blood of ketone bodies; strong acids lower serum pH.

8. _____ Excessive urination.

9. _____ Hyperventilation that is characteristic of metabolic acidosis; occurs as a result of the respiratory system attempting to eliminate excess carbon dioxide by increased depth and rate of respirations.

10. _____ Carpal spasm elicited by pressure applied to nerves of the upper arm.

11. _____ Premature activation of the hypothalamic pituitary-gonadal axis; early maturation of gonads, secretion of sex hormones and development of secondary sex characteristics.

12. _____ Carpopedal spasm, muscle twitching, cramps, seizures, and sometimes stridor; indicative of disorders of the parathyroid function.

13. _____ Excess growth hormone after epiphyseal closure; characterized by facial features such as overgrowth of the head, lips, nose, tongue, jaw, and paranasal and mastoid sinuses.

14. _____ Facial muscle spasm elicited by tapping the facial nerve in the region of the parotid gland.

a. Acromegaly

b. Precocious puberty

c. Polyuria

d. Polydipsia

e. Exophthalmos

f. Chvostek's sign

g. Trousseau's sign

h. Tetany

i. Glycosuria

j. Ketonuria

k. Ketoacidosis

l. Kussmaul respirations

m. Hypoglycemia

n. Hyperglycemia

II. REVIEWING KEY CONCEPTS AND CONTENT

15. List the three components of the endocrine system. _____, _____, _____.

MATCHING: Match each hormone or gland with its corresponding effect.

16. _____ Prepares uterus for fertilized ovum.

17. _____ Influences development of secondary sex characteristics.

18. _____ Promotes secondary sex characteristics (breast development) during puberty in females.

19. _____ Stimulates the liver and other cells to release stored glucose (glycogenolysis).

20. _____ Promote metabolism; mobilize body defenses during stress; suppress inflammatory reaction.

21. _____ Produces the same effects on various organs as those caused by direct sympathetic stimulation; vasoconstriction and raises blood pressure.

22. _____ Regulates sodium retention and excretion.

23. _____ Stimulates testes to produce spermatozoa.

24. _____ Regulates metabolic rate.

25. _____ Promotes glucose transport into the cells.

a. Parathyroid

b. Glucocorticoids

c. Aldosterone

d. Thyroid

e. Androgen

f. Glucagon

g. Epinephrine

h. Progesterone

i. Insulin

j. Estrogen

k. Testosterone

26. _____ with vitamin D, maintains homeostasis of blood calcium concentration.

27. In a child with hypopituitarism, the growth hormone levels are usually
   a. elevated after 20 minutes of strenuous exercise.
   b. elevated 45 to 90 minutes after the onset of sleep.
   c. below normal after being stimulated pharmacologically.
   d. below normal at birth.

28. The appropriate treatment of choice for the child with idiopathic hypopituitarism may be
   a. biosynthetic growth hormone.
   b. human growth hormone.
   c. surgical removal of the tumor.
   d. any of the above.

29. Which of the following statements about growth hormone replacement therapy in the child with idiopathic hypopituitarism is true?
   a. Therapy will continue for life.
   b. Therapy will not result in achievement of a normal familial height.
   c. Therapy requires subcutaneous injection.
   d. Therapy requires intramuscular injection.

30. The best time to administer grown hormone replacement injections is
   a. in the morning.
   b. exactly at 7 AM
   c. at bedtime.
   d. exactly at 7 PM

31. Explain the difference between acromegaly and pituitary hyperfunction that would not be considered acromegaly.

32. Parents of the child with precocious puberty need to know that
    a. dress and activities should be aligned with the child's sexual development.
    b. heterosexual interest will usually be advanced.
    c. the child's mental age is congruent with the chronologic age.
    d. overt manifestations of affection represent sexual advances.

33. The most common cause of thyroid disease in children and adolescents is
    a. Hashimoto disease.
    b. Graves disease.
    c. goiter.
    d. thyrotoxicosis.

34. When a thyroidectomy is planned, the nurse should explain to the child that
    a. iodine preparations will be mixed with flavored foods and then eaten.
    b. the child will need to hyperextend his or her neck postoperatively.
    c. the skin, not the throat, will be cut.
    d. laryngospasm can be a life-threatening complication.

35. A common cause of secondary hyperparathyroidism is
    a. maternal hyperparathyroidism.
    b. chronic renal disease.
    c. an adenoma.
    d. renal rickets.

36. Pheochromocytoma is a tumor characterized by
    a. secretion of insulin.
    b. secretion of catecholamines.
    c. adrenal crisis.
    d. myxedema.

37. The parents of a child who has Addison disease should be instructed to
    a. use extra hydrocortisone only for crises.
    b. discontinue the child's cortisone if side effects develop.
    c. decrease the cortisone dose during times of stress.
    d. report signs of adrenal insufficiency to the physician.

38. Which of the following tests, which yields immediate results, is particularly useful in diagnosing congenital adrenogenital hyperplasia?
    a. Chromosome typing
    b. Pelvic ultrasound
    c. Pelvic x-ray
    d. Testosterone levels

39. Definitive treatment for pheochromocytoma consists of
    a. surgical removal of the thyroid.
    b. administration of potassium.
    c. surgical removal of the tumor.
    d. administration of beta blockers.

40. Most children with diabetes mellitus tend to exhibit characteristics of
    a. maturity-onset diabetes of youth.
    b. gestational diabetes.
    c. type 2 diabetes.
    d. type 1 diabetes.

41. The currently accepted etiology of type 1 diabetes takes into account
    a. genetic factors.
    b. autoimmune mechanisms.
    c. environment factors.
    d. all of the above.

42. Glycosylated hemoglobin is an acceptable method to use to
    a. diagnose diabetes mellitus.
    b. assess the control of diabetes.
    c. assess oxygen saturation of the hemoglobin.
    d. determine blood glucose levels most accurately.

43. The most common acute complication of diabetes that a young child encounters is
    a. retinopathy.
    b. ketoacidosis.
    c. hypoglycemia.
    d. hyperosmolar nonketotic coma.

44. In regard to insulin administration
    a. insulin should never be premixed.
    b. insulin syringes should never be reused.
    c. insulin doses under 2 units should be diluted.
    d. an air bubble in the syringe is insignificant.

45. Exercise for the child with diabetes mellitus
    a. is restricted to noncontact sports.
    b. may require a decreased intake of food.
    c. may necessitate an increased insulin dose.
    d. may require an increased intake of food.

46. Problems of adjustment to diabetes are most
    likely to occur when diabetes is diagnosed in
    a. infancy.
    b. adolescence.
    c. the toddler years.
    d. the school-age years.

III. THINKING CRITICALLY

1. Describe the clinical manifestations usually seen in a child with hypopituitarism.

2. Describe the clinical manifestations usually seen in a child with diabetes insipidus.

3. Identify what symptoms would be expected in a child with type 1 diabetes mellitus who is experiencing hypoglycemia.

4. Describe what interventions are indicated to treat hypoglycemia in the child with type 1 diabetes mellitus.

5. List the nursing goals that should be included in a teaching plan for a child with type 1 diabetes mellitus.

Integumentary Dysfunction

53

I. LEARNING KEY TERMS

MATCHING: Match each term with its corresponding definition or description.

1. _____ Flat, circumscribed, nonpalpable lesion; less than 1 cm in diameter.

2. _____ Elevated, circumscribed, palpable, encapsulated lesion filled with liquid or semisolid material.

3. _____ Pinpoint, tiny, and sharp circumscribed spots in the superficial layers of the epidermis.

4. _____ Elevated, superficial lesion filled with purulent fluid (e.g., impetigo).

5. _____ Bruises; localized red or purple discoloration caused by extravasation of blood into dermis and subcutaneous tissues.

6. _____ Dried serum, blood, or purulent exudate; slightly elevated; size varies; brown, red, black, tan, or straw in color (e.g., eczema).

7. _____ Elevated, firm, circumscribed palpable lesion; deeper in dermis than a papule; 1 to 2 cm in diameter.

8. _____ Reddened area caused by increased amounts of oxygenated blood in the dermal vasculature.

9. _____ Absence of sensation.

10. _____ Vesicle greater than 1 cm in diameter.

11. _____ Abnormal sensation; prickling.

12. _____ Loss of all or part of epidermis; depressed, moist, and glistening; follows rupture of vesicle or bulla.

13. _____ Elevated, circumscribed, superficial lesion filled with serous fluid; less than 2 cm in diameter (e.g., blister, varicella).

14. _____ Diminished sensation.

15. _____ Elevated, palpable, firm, circumscribed lesion less than 1 cm in diameter; brown, red, pink, tan, or bluish-red in color (e.g., wart).

16. _____ Excessive sensitiveness.

17. _____ Heaped-up keratinized cells, flaky exfoliation; irregular; thick or thin; dry or oily; varied size; silver, white, or tan in color (e.g., psoriasis).

a. Pruritis

b. Anesthesia

c. Hyperesthesia

d. Hypoesthesia

e. Paresthesia

f. Erythema

g. Ecchymoses

h. Petechiae

i. Macule

j. Patch

k. Plaque

l. Wheal

m. Papule

n. Vesicle

o. Bulla

p. Nodule

q. Pustule

r. Cyst

s. Crust

t. Scale

u. Lichenification

v. Scar

w. Keloid

18. _____ Loss of epidermis; linear or hollowed-out crusted area, dermis exposed.

19. _____ Elevated, irregular-shaped area of cutaneous edema; solid, transient, and changing; variable in diameter; pale pink with lighter center (e.g., urticaria, insect bite).

20. _____ Fibrous tissue replacing injured dermis; irregular; pink, red, or white; may be atrophic or hypertrophic.

21. _____ Itching.

22. _____ Elevated, flat-topped, firm, rough, superficial lesion greater than 1 cm in diameter.

23. _____ Rough, thickened epidermis; accentuated skin markings caused by rubbing or irritation; often involves flexor aspect of extremity (e.g., chronic dermatitis).

24. _____ Irregularly shaped, elevated, progressively enlarging scar; grows beyond boundaries of the wound; caused by excessive collagen formation during healing.

25. _____ Flat; nonpalpable lesion; irregular in shape; greater than 1 cm in diameter.

26. _____ Regeneration of capillaries; the process in which angiocytes regenerate the outer layers of capillaries and endothelial cells producing the lining.

27. _____ Skin is removed from the donor site; tiny grid lock slits are cut into the skin that allow the skin to cover a greater area; results in less desirable cosmetic and functional outcome.

28. _____ The stage of wound healing in which platelets act to seal off the damaged blood vessels and begin to form a stable clot; normally occurs within minutes of the initial injury to the skin.

29. _____ Painful procedure to remove devitalized tissue in order to promote healing.

30. _____ Loss of epidermis and dermis; concave; varies in size; exudative; red or reddish blue (e.g., decubiti).

31. _____ The "beefy" pebbled red tissue usually found in the base of healing wounds.

32. _____ Linear crack or break from epidermis to dermis; small, deep, and red (e.g., athlete's foot).

33. _____ Procedure in which skin is removed from the donor site and placed intact over the recipient site and sutured in place; used in areas where cosmetic results are most visible.

34. _____ Healing that includes granulation and contracture; characterized clinically by the presence of granulation tissue.

35. _____ Allergy with a hereditary tendency.

x. Excoriation

y. Erosion

z. Fissure

aa. Ulcer

bb. Hemostasis

cc. Angiogenesis

dd. Proliferation phase

ee. Urushiol

ff. Nits

gg. Arthropods

hh. Atopy

ii. Granulation

jj. Debridement

kk. Allograft (homograft)

ll. Xenograft

mm. Sheet graft

nn. Mesh graft

36. _____ The oil that is the offending substance in poisonous plants (ivy, oak, and sumac).

37. _____ Procedure in which skin for graft is obtained from a variety of species, most notably pigs.

38. _____ Insects, arachnids (mites), ticks, spiders, and scorpions.

39. _____ Procedure in which skin for graft is obtained from human cadavers that are screened for communicable diseases.

40. _____ Pediculosis capitis eggs.

II. REVIEWING KEY CONCEPTS AND CONTENT

41. The nurse recognizes that in the care of a wound to promote healing, it would be *unlikely* to use a treatment plan that included
    a. nutritional management with sufficient protein, calories, vitamin C, and zinc.
    b. irrigation of wounds with normal saline.
    c. application of povidone-iodine daily.
    d. application of an occlusive dressing.

42. Care of bacterial skin infections in children may include all of the following *except:*
    a. good handwashing.
    b. keeping the fingernails short.
    c. puncturing the surface of the pustule.
    d. application of topical antibiotics.

43. A type of fungal infection of the skin is:
    a. tinea corporis.
    b. herpes simplex type 1.
    c. scabies.
    d. warts.

44. Which of the following statements about scabies is *false?*
    a. Clinical manifestations include intense pruritus—especially at night—and papules, burrows, or vesicles on interdigital surfaces.
    b. Treatment is the application of permethrin 5% with 1% lindane cream or 10% crotamiton as alternatives.
    c. There is great variability in the type of lesions that are formed.
    d. The rash and itching will occur only where mites are present.

45. When the nurse teaches parents about pediculosis capitis, instructions should include the fact that lice are likely to
    a. infest black girls with curly hair.
    b. infest white girls with straight hair.
    c. jump or fly from one person to another.
    d. be invisible to the naked eye.

46. Treatment for a child with Lyme disease who is under the age of 8 usually includes
    a. doxycycline.
    b. amoxicillin.
    c. cefuroxime.
    d. erythromycin.

47. A school-age child has come in contact with poison ivy at a picnic. The best intervention for the nurse to implement at this time is
    a. washing the area with a strong soap and water solution.
    b. applying Calamine lotion to the area.
    c. preventing spread by instructing the child not to scratch the lesions.
    d. to flush the area with cold running water for 15 minutes.

48. Skin disorders related to drug sensitivity include
    a. erythema multiforme.
    b. Stevens-Johnson syndrome.
    c. generalized epidermal necrosis.
    d. all of the above.

49. The most effective method for tick removal in a child is to
    a. use a tweezers or forceps and pull straight up with a steady, even pressure.
    b. apply mineral oil to the back of the tick and wait for it to back out.
    c. use the fingers to pull the tick out with a straight, steady, even pressure.
    d. remove the stinger as quickly as possible.

50. Dog bites in children
    a. occur most often in girls over 4 years of age.
    b. occur most often in children less than 5 years of age.
    c. occur most often from stray dogs.
    d. occur most often in the legs and lower body.

51. T   F   The incidence of diaper dermatitis is generally reported as greater in bottle-fed infants than in breastfed infants.

52. The best strategy for the nurse to recommend to the parents of an infant with diaper dermatitis is to
    a. apply 0.1% tacrolimus ointment sparingly.
    b. avoid cornstarch because it promotes yeast growth.
    c. use a hand-held dryer on the open lesions.
    d. use diapers impregnated with petrolatum.

53. The cause of atopic dermatitis appears to be related to
    a. inadequate parenting.
    b. congenital heat intolerance.
    c. abnormal function of the skin.
    d. all of the above.

54. The type of lesions seen in acne that are more prone to cause scarring are
    a. noninflamed lesions.
    b. closed comedones.
    c. inflamed lesions.
    d. blackheads.

55. A 16-year-old girl presents to the nurse because of acne on her face, shoulders, and neck areas. After talking with her, the nurse makes a nursing diagnosis of deficient knowledge related to proper skin care. The best strategy for the nurse to include in her plan of care is to
    a. wash the areas vigorously with antibacterial soap.
    b. brush the hair down on the forehead to conceal the acne areas.
    c. avoid the use of all cosmetics.
    d. gently wash the areas with a mild soap once or twice daily.

56. The practitioner has prescribed isotretinoin for acne for a 16-year-old sexually active girl, and the adolescent returns for a follow-up visit after 1 month of treatment. The follow-up assessment should include
    a. screening for depression.
    b. cholesterol and triglyceride levels.
    c. a discussion about adequate contraception.
    d. all of the above.

57. Burns are caused by _____, _____, and _____ agents.

58. _____ burns are the most common cause of burn injuries in toddlers.

59. Burn wounds that require a circumferential dressing should be wrapped
    a. from distal to proximal.
    b. from proximal to distal.
    c. very loosely.
    d. tight enough to immobilize the body part.

60. Burns involving the epidermis and varying degrees of the dermis that are painful, moist, red, and blistered are known as
    a. superficial first-degree burns.
    b. partial-thickness (second-degree) burns.
    c. full-thickness third-degree burns.
    d. fourth-degree burns.

61. The severity of burn injury is determined by
    a. the body area involved.
    b. the causative agent.
    c. the age of the victim.
    d. all of the above.

62. The nurse recognizes that which of the following pediatric patients is at higher risk of complications from burn injury?
    a. The 12-month-old infant
    b. The 3-year-old toddler
    c. The 10-year old school-age child
    d. The 15-year-old adolescent

63. Initial emergency care of the burned child should include which of the following?
    a. Stop the burning process for burns with ice packs.
    b. Apply ointments to the burned area before transfer of the child.
    c. Remove jewelry and metal.
    d. Apply neutralizing agents to the skin of chemical burn areas.

64. Which instruction should *not* be included in the teaching plan for the parents of a 2-year-old child who has suffered a minor burn injury?
    a. Wash the wound twice daily with mild soap and tepid water.
    b. Soak the dressing in tepid water before removal to reduce discomfort.
    c. Administer acetaminophen immediately after each dressing change.
    d. Watch the wound margins for redness, edema, or purulent drainage.

65. If fluid replacement for a burned child weighing less than 30 kg is adequate, the nurse should expect the child to
    a. maintain an hourly urinary output of 30 ml per hour.
    b. maintain an hourly urinary output of 1 to 2 ml/kg per hour.
    c. have an increasing hematocrit.
    d. exhibit normal capillary refill.

66. The child with a major burn injury requires which of the following nutrition plans?
    a. High-protein, high-caloric diet
    b. Vitamin A and C supplements
    c. Supplements of zinc
    d. All of the above

67. An 8-year-old child suffered partial second-degree burns of his chest, abdomen, and upper legs while on a recent camping trip. He is scheduled for hydrotherapy each morning for 20 minutes followed by debridement of the wounds. The best nursing action to assist the child at this time would be to
    a. ensure that pain medication is given before hydrotherapy.
    b. hold breakfast until the child returns from treatment.
    c. offer sedation after the procedure to promote rest.
    d. reassure the child that hydrotherapy is not painful.

Use the following scenario to respond to questions 68 through 72.

A 5-year-old child is brought to the emergency center after his clothes caught on fire while he was playing in the family garage with matches. He has partial-thickness second-degree burns and full-thickness third-degree burns of his anterior chest, anterior abdomen, upper right arm, both shoulders, and right hand. There is singed nasal hair apparent on physical examination and some minor burns apparent on his face. A Foley catheter is inserted, and a small amount of clear urine is obtained. Two IV routes are established for fluid replacement.

68. In conducting the physical examination of the 5-year-old child's burns, the nurse calculates the extent of body surface area involvement. How does the nurse best assess to see whether circulation to the area is intact?
    a. Touch the area to see whether the child feels pain.
    b. Test injured surfaces for blanching and capillary refill.
    c. Inspect the burns for eschar formation.
    d. Watch for edema of the affected part.

69. Based on the information given, the nurse should be careful to observe the child for
    a. inhalation injury.
    b. facial deformities.
    c. sepsis.
    d. renal failure related to formation of myoglobin.

70. The child has normal bowel sounds 24 hours following admission and is placed on a high-caloric, high-protein diet, of which he eats very little. His hydrotherapy sessions are scheduled right after breakfast and before supper. To increase the child's dietary intake, the best action for the nurse to take is to
    a. show him a feeding tube and explain to him that if he does not eat more, the tube will need to be inserted.
    b. maintain the current meal schedule and stay with him until he eats all of his meal.
    c. rearrange his meal and hydrotherapy schedule to prevent conflicts.
    d. insist that he stop snacking between meals.

71. Considering the extent and distribution of the child's burns, the nursing diagnosis with the highest priority during the management phase of this child's illness is
    a. impaired gas exchange related to inhalation injury.
    b. high risk for altered nutrition: less than body requirements related to loss of appetite.
    c. fluid volume deficit related to edema associated with burn injury.
    d. high risk for infection related to denuded skin, presence of pathogenic organisms, and altered immune response.

72. The child progressed well with skin grafts and healing and is now ready for discharge. The nurse will know that his parents understand discharge instructions by which of the following statements?
    a. "He will need to wear this elastic support bandage for only 1 month."
    b. "He will not be able to participate in any sports until the grafts have taken hold firmly."
    c. "We will visit the teacher and his peers before he returns to school to prepare them for his appearance."
    d. "We will need to protect him from normal activities until he requires no further surgery."

73. When advising parents about the use of sunscreen for their children, the nurse should tell them that
    a. a waterproof sunscreen with a minimum 15 SPF is recommended for children.
    b. the lower the number of SPF, the higher the protection.
    c. sunscreens are not as effective as sun blockers.
    d. the sunscreen should be applied 1 hour before the child is allowed in the sun.

74. In caring for the child with frostbite, the nurse remembers that
    a. slow thawing is associated with less tissue necrosis.
    b. the frostbitten part appears white or blanched, feels solid, and is without sensation.
    c. rewarming produces a small return of sensation with a small amount of pain.
    d. rewarming is accomplished by rubbing the injured tissue.

III. THINKING CRITICALLY

1. Describe at least three strategies (with rationales) that may be used in the care of the child with a skin disorder.

2. Formulate at least three nursing diagnoses for a child who has atopic dermatitis.

3. Describe the interventions to suggest to the mother of a 2-month-old infant to prevent diaper rash and to treat it if it occurs.

4. Explain why school-age children are highly susceptible to infestations of head lice.

5. Explain the rationale for wearing sterile gowns, masks, and gloves while in the room of a child who has sustained a thermal injury.

Musculoskeletal or Articular Dysfunction (54)

I. LEARNING KEY TERMS

MATCHING: Match each term with its corresponding definition or description.

1. _____ Produced by compression of porous bone; appears as a raised or bulging projection at the fracture site; occurs in the most porous portion of the bone; more common in young children.

2. _____ The process of separating opposing bone to encourage regeneration of new bones in the created space; may be used when limbs are of unequal length and new bone is needed to elongate the shorter limb.

3. _____ Occurs when the bone is bent but not broken; a child's flexible bone can be bent 45 degrees or more before breaking.

4. _____ Occurs when a bone is angulated beyond the limits of bending, one side bending and the other side breaking.

5. _____ Used when significant pull must be applied to achieve realignment and immobilization; pins or wires may be used to ensure that the stress is placed on the bone and not on the surrounding tissue.

6. _____ Fractures in which small fragments of bone break off from the fractured shaft and lie in the surrounding tissue.

7. _____ A fracture in which bone fragments cause damage to other organs or tissues such as the lung or bladder.

8. _____ Divides the bone fragments.

9. _____ Applied when there are minimal displacements and little muscle spasticity; contraindicated when there is skin damage.

10. _____ Fracture with an open wound through which the bone is protruding or has protruded.

11. _____ Used in uncomplicated arm or leg fractures; used to realign bone fragments for immediate cast application.

12. _____ Produced by attaching weight to the distal bone fragment.

13. _____ Black and blue discoloration; the escape of blood into the tissues.

14. _____ Backward force; provided by the body's weight.

15. _____ A fracture that does not produce a break in the skin.

a. Ecchymosis

b. Simple or closed fracture

c. Compound or open fracture

d. Complicated fracture

e. Comminuted fracture

f. Bend fracture

g. Buckle or torus fracture

h. Greenstick fracture

i. Complete fracture

j. Traction

k. Countertraction

l. Manual traction

m. Skin traction

n. Skeletal traction

o. Distraction

II. REVIEWING KEY CONCEPTS AND CONTENT

16. An appropriate nursing intervention for the care of a child with an extremity in a new plaster cast is
    a. keeping the cast covered with a sheet.
    b. using the fingertips when handling the cast to prevent pressure areas.
    c. using heated fans or dryers to circulate air and speed the cast-drying process.
    d. turning the child at least every 2 hours to help dry the cast evenly.

17. Bone healing is characteristically more rapid in children because
    a. children have less constant muscle contraction associated with the fracture.
    b. children's fractures are less severe than adult's.
    c. children have an active growth plate that helps speed repair with deformity less likely to occur.
    d. children have thickened periosteum and more generous blood supply.

18. When caring for a 7-year-old child after insertion of skeletal traction, it would be contraindicated for the nurse to
    a. gently massage over pressure areas to stimulate circulation.
    b. release the traction when repositioning the child in bed.
    c. inspect pin sites for bleeding or infection.
    d. assess for alterations in neurovascular status.

MATCHING: Match each type of traction with its corresponding description.

19. _____ A type of upper extremity traction in which the arm, bent at the elbow, is suspended vertically by skin or skeletal attachment and traction is applied to the distal end of the humerus.

20. _____ A type of running traction in which the pull is only in one direction; it is used to reduce fractures of the femur to realign bone fragments for cast application.

21. _____ Uses a system of wires, rings, and telescoping rods that permits limb lengthening to occur.

22. _____ Treatment of fractures of the humerus in which the arm is suspended horizontally.

23. _____ Inserted through burr holes in the skull to provide cervical traction.

24. _____ Uses skin traction on the lower leg and a padded sling under the knee.

25. _____ A type of skin traction with the leg in an extended position; used primarily for short-term immobilization.

26. _____ Skeletal traction in which the lower leg is supported by a boot cast or a calf sling and a pin or wire is placed in the distal fragment of the femur.

27. _____ Used with or without skin or skeletal traction; suspends the leg in a flexed position to relax the hip and hamstring muscles.

28. _____ Extends from the groin to midair above the foot.

a. Dunlop traction

b. Crutchfield or Barton tongs

c. Buck extension

d. Russell traction

e. 90-degree-90-degree traction

f. Balance suspension traction

g. Thomas splint

h. Pearson attachment

i. Cervical traction

j. Bryant traction

k. Ilizarov external fixator (IEF)

l. Overhead suspension traction

29. _____ Supports the lower leg.

30. _____ May be accomplished by insertion of Crutchfield tongs through burr holes in the skull.

31. A 7-year-old boy is diagnosed with Legg-Calvé-Perthes disease. The manifestation that is *not* consistent with this diagnosis is
    a. intermittent appearance of a limp on the affected side.
    b. hip soreness, ache, or stiffness that can be constant or intermittent.
    c. pain and limp most evident on arising and at the end of a long day of activities.
    d. specific history of injury to the area.

32. Slipped femoral capital epiphysis is suspected when an adolescent or preadolescent
    a. begins to limp and complains of pain in the hip continuously or intermittently.
    b. has pain without restriction of abduction and internal rotation.
    c. complains of referred pain in the chest region.
    d. all of the above.

33. An accentuation of the lumbar curvature beyond physiologic limits is termed _____.
    An abnormally increased convex angulation in the curvature of the thoracic spine is termed

    _____.

34. Diagnostic evaluation is important for early recognition of scoliosis. The correct procedure for the school nurse conducting this examination would be to view the child
    a. standing and walking fully clothed to look for uneven hanging of clothing.
    b. from the front to evaluate bone maturity.
    c. from the left and right side while the child is completely undressed.
    d. from behind, when bending forward while the child is wearing only underpants.

35. Nursing implementation directed toward nonsurgical management in a teenager with scoliosis primarily includes
    a. promoting self-esteem and positive body image.
    b. promoting immobilization of the legs.
    c. promoting adequate nutrition.
    d. preventing infection.

36. The plan of care for the child during the acute phase of osteomyelitis always includes
    a. performing wound irrigations.
    b. maintaining IV infusion site.
    c. isolation of the child.
    d. weight-bearing exercises for the affected area.

37. Nursing considerations for the patient diagnosed with osteogenesis imperfecta include
    a. preventing fractures by careful handling.
    b. providing nonjudgmental support as evaluation of abuse occurs.
    c. providing guidelines to the parents to promote optimum development.
    d. all of the above.

38. The goal that is most appropriate for the child with juvenile idiopathic arthritis is for the child to be able to exhibit signs of
    a. adequate joint function.
    b. improved skin integrity.
    c. weight loss and improved nutritional status.
    d. adequate respiratory function.

39. The majority of children with clinical manifestations of systemic lupus erythematosus present with
    a. Raynaud phenomenon, especially of the feet and legs.
    b. development of herpes simplex in dry, cracked skin areas.
    c. cutaneous involvement including skin disease as the chief complaint.
    d. patchy areas of alopecia without remission.

40. To promote adequate joint function in the child with juvenile idiopathic arthritis, the most appropriate nursing intervention would be to
    a. incorporate therapeutic exercises in play activities.
    b. provide heat to affected joints by use of tub baths.
    c. provide written information for all treatments ordered.
    d. explore and develop activities in which the child can succeed.

III. THINKING CRITICALLY

1. Describe the instructions parents should receive to limit the swelling under a cast and to maintain the integrity of the cast.

2. Identify the strategies to use to maintain 90-degree–90-degree traction for the treatment of a 13-year-old child's fractured femur.

3. List the clinical signs that indicate congenital hip dysplasia in the newborn.

4. Describe the strategies that will promote development of a positive self-image in a 14-year-old girl who is admitted for a Harrington rod procedure for scoliosis.

Neuromuscular or Muscular Dysfunction $\boxed{55}$

I. LEARNING KEY TERMS

MATCHING: Match each term with its corresponding definition or description.

1. _____ Congenital condition in which brain is totally exposed or extruded through an associated skull defect; usually spontaneously aborted.

2. _____ A visible defect with an external saclike protrusion that contains meninges, spinal fluid, and nerves.

3. _____ Characterized by a spongiform mass for a brain; incompatible with life usually beyond a few days.

4. _____ Characterized by wide-based gait; rapid repetitive movements, performed poorly; disintegration of movements of the upper extremities when the child reaches for objects.

5. _____ Visible defect with an external saclike protrusion that encases meninges and spinal fluid; but no neural elements.

6. _____ Combination of spasticity and athetosis.

7. _____ Characterized by abnormal involuntary movement such as athetosis, slow, wormlike, writhing movements that usually involve the extremities, trunk, neck, facial muscles, and tongue.

8. _____ Herniation of brain and meninges through a defect in the skull producing a fluid-filled sac.

9. _____ May involve one or both sides; hypertonicity with poor control of posture, balance, and coordinated motion; impairment of fine and gross motor skills; abnormal postures and overflow of movement to other parts of the body increased by active attempts at motion.

10. _____ Class of defects involving failure of the osseous spine to close.

11. _____ Skull defect through which various tissues protrude.

a. Spastic cerebral palsy

b. Dyskinetic cerebral palsy

c. Ataxic cerebral palsy

d. Mixed-type cerebral palsy

e. Cranioschisis

f. Exancephaly

g. Anencephaly

h. Encephalocele

i. Spina bifida

j. Meningocele

k. Myelomeningocele

II. REVIEWING KEY CONCEPTS AND CONTENT

12. The etiology of cerebral palsy is most commonly related to
    a. existing prenatal brain abnormalities.
    b. maternal asphyxia.
    c. childhood meningitis.
    d. preeclampsia.

13. A child is suspected of having cerebral palsy because he has clinical manifestations of wide-based gait and rapid repetitive movements of the upper extremities when he reaches for an object. Based on this information, the clinical classification of cerebral palsy this child might have is
    a. spastic.
    b. dyskinetic.
    c. ataxic.
    d. mixed-type.

14. Disabilities and problems associated with cerebral palsy usually include
    a. intelligence testing in the abnormal range.
    b. eye cataracts that will need surgical correction.
    c. seizures with athetosis and diplegia.
    d. coughing and choking while eating.

15. While performing a physical examination on a 6-month-old infant, the nurse suspects cerebral palsy, because the infant
    a. is able to hold on to the nurse's hands while being pulled to a sitting position.
    b. has no Moro reflex.
    c. has no tonic neck reflex.
    d. has an obligatory tonic neck reflex.

16. The goal of therapeutic management for the child with cerebral palsy is
    a. assisting with motor control of voluntary muscle.
    b. maximizing the capabilities of the child.
    c. delaying the development of sensory deprivation.
    d. surgical correction of deformities.

17. A condition commonly seen in children with spina bifida, latex allergy, can be identified with a 90% to 95% sensitivity with a test called
    a. Skin prick testing.
    b. Allergy provocative testing.
    c. Radioallergosorbent test (RAST).
    d. Serum level of IgA.

18. The disease inherited only as an autosomal recessive trait and characterized by progressive weakness and wasting of skeletal muscles caused by degeneration of anterior horn cells is
    a. Werdnig-Hoffmann disease.
    b. cerebral palsy.
    c. Kugelberg-Welander disease.
    d. Guillain-Barré syndrome.

19. Major goals in the nursing care of children with muscular dystrophy include
    a. promoting strenuous activity and exercise.
    b. promoting large caloric intake.
    c. preventing respiratory tract infection.
    d. preventing mental retardation.

20. With the muscle wasting associated with the disease process of muscular dystrophy, the nurse should expect the serum levels of creatine phosphokinase to be
    a. normal.
    b. decreased.
    c. elevated.
    d. unable to be determined accurately with muscle wasting and incapacitation.

21. Findings that support the diagnosis of Guillain-Barré syndrome would include a laboratory test result of
    a. elevated CBC.
    b. cerebrospinal fluid high in protein.
    c. cerebrospinal fluid high in glucose.
    d. elevated CPK.

22. A priority nursing consideration for the child in the acute phase of Guillain-Barré syndrome is
    a. careful observation for difficulty in swallowing and respiratory involvement.
    b. prevention of contractures.
    c. prevention of bowel and bladder complications.
    d. prevention of sensory impairment.

23. Nursing implementations for the child with tetanus include
    a. controlling or eliminating stimulation from sound, light, and touch.
    b. observing for location and extent of muscle spasms.
    c. arranging for the child not to be left alone, because these children are not mentally alert.
    d. all of the above.

24. Infant botulism usually presents with symptoms of
    a. diarrhea and vomiting.
    b. constipation and generalized weakness.
    c. high fever and seizure activity.
    d. failure to thrive.

25. Nursing considerations for the pediatric patient with botulism include
    a. teaching the parents the importance of administering enemas and cathartics for bowel function.
    b. preparing the parents for the fact that the child will have muscular disability after the illness.
    c. using honey as a formula sweetener to increase oral intake.
    d. teaching parents that boiling is not always an adequate prevention.

26. Children with neurogenic bladder should receive
    a. regular urologic care.
    b. regular bladder emptying.
    c. medications to improve bladder storage and continence.
    d. all of the above.

III. THINKING CRITICALLY

1. Identify the nursing goals that would help children with cerebral palsy and their parents.

2. Describe how you would intervene to assist a 5-year-old boy with muscular dystrophy and his parents in regard to avoiding the pitfalls of overprotection.

3. Describe nursing interventions aimed at preventing the complications of Guillain-Barré syndrome.

4. List the primary nursing goals for the initial stabilization in the acute phase of care for an adolescent who arrives at the hospital with paraplegia caused by a spinal cord injury.

Answer Key

CHAPTER 1: CONTEMPORARY MATERNITY NURSING

I. Reviewing Key Concepts and Content

1. c   2. h   3. d   4. i   5. f   6. a
7. g   8. b   9. e
10. Maternity nursing
11. Integrative health care
12. *Healthy People 2010*
13. Nursing Interventions Classification (NIC)
14. Outcomes of care
15. Best practice
16. Clinical benchmarking
17. Standards of practice
18. Evidence-based practice
19. *Factors contributing to infant mortality:* limited maternal education, young maternal age, unmarried, poverty, lack of prenatal care, poor nutrition, smoking, alcohol and drug use, poor maternal health habits
20. *Changes that have occurred in maternity care; how changes have affected health care:* see Childbirth Practices section; discuss the following: increase in nurse midwives as primary obstetric care providers, use of regional anesthesia, family-centered birthing, childbirth education classes, early discharge and discharge at 24 to 48 hours, activities of lactation consultants and doulas, emphasis on home care, neonatal security.
21. *The four predominant causes for maternal mortality* are embolism, hemorrhage, gestational hypertension, infection.
22. *Barriers to early and ongoing prenatal care:* see Limited Access to Care section for a discussion of several barriers.
23. F   24. F   25. F   26. T   27. T   28. F
29. T   30. F   31. T   32. F   33. T   34. F
35. F   36. F   37. F   38. T

II. Thinking Critically

1. *Nursing director of inner-city prenatal clinic:* see Trends in Fertility and Birth Rate, Incidence of Low Birth Weight, Infant and Maternal Mortality Trends, Increase in High Risk Pregnancy, and Limited Access to Care sections; answer should include the following:

- Biostatistics and contributing factors
- Factors associated with high risk pregnancy
- Benefits of prenatal care; impact of inadequate prenatal care
- Importance of self-care and consumer involvement; devise ways to encourage participation in prenatal care and overcome barriers

2. *High technology will not reduce rate of preterm birth and LBW infants:* see sections that cover the following topics to formulate your answer:
- Factors associated with LBW and IMR
- Factors that escalate rate of high risk pregnancy
- High-tech care: what it can and cannot do High-tech care is no longer the solution; answer should reflect factors associated with IMR, the high cost of care management for high risk pregnancies and compromised infants as compared with the cost and effectiveness of early, ongoing, comprehensive prenatal care.

3. *Three proposed changes in health care and its delivery including rationale:* changes proposed should reflect efforts toward improving access to care, using research-based approaches and standards to guide care, and creating health care services that address the factors associated with poor pregnancy outcomes.

4. *Incentives and services to overcome barriers to prenatal care:* see Limited Access to Care Problems section; address solutions to the following barriers: inability to pay, lack of transportation, dependent child care, minority status, cultural beliefs, young maternal age, homeless, unmarried.

5. *Value of prenatal HIV testing:* see HIV/AIDS in Pregnancy and the Newborn sections; emphasize that early diagnosis and treatment of the mother dramatically decrease the rate of transmission of the virus to the fetus.

6. *Facilitating health literacy:* see Health Literacy section; include therapeutic communication techniques and preparation of bilingual written materials in answer.

CHAPTER 2:   THE FAMILY AND CULTURE

I.   Reviewing Key Concepts and Content

1. b   2. e   3. d   4. c   5. f   6. a
7. b   8. e   9. c   10. d   11. a
12. Culture
13. Subculture
14. Cultural relativism
15. Acculturation
16. Assimilation
17. Ethnocentrism
18. Cultural competence
19. Future-oriented
20. Past-oriented
21. Present-oriented
22. Personal space
23. Family
24. Nuclear
25. Extended
26. Binuclear
27. Single parent, economically, socially
28. Reconstituted
29. Homosexual
30. Family functions, affective, socialization, reproductive, economic, health care
31. Affective
32. Socialization
33. Reproductive
34. Economic
35. Health care
36. Family dynamics, negotiation, boundaries, channels
37. Family systems theory
38. Family developmental theory
39. Family stress
40. T   41. F   42. F   43. F   44. T   45. T
46. T   47. T
48. *Discuss purpose of incorporating products of culture when providing care:* see Childbearing Beliefs and Practices section.
    a. *Communication:* consider language; need for a translator; dialect, style, and volume of speech; meaning of touch and gestures.
    b. *Personal space:* include feelings of territoriality; recognize that comfort zone must be established in terms of touch, proximity to others, and handling of possession; ensure that patient is in control of personal space to ensure a sense of autonomy and security.
    c. *Time orientation:* consider past, present, and future orientations and how this could affect meeting appointment times and health care practices, beliefs, and goals.
    d. *Family roles:* consider parent role; roles for grandparents and siblings; father's participation in pregnancy, childbirth, and childcare.

49. Choice a is correct; choices b, c, and d reflect the characteristics of families with closed boundaries; they are more prone to crises because they have a narrow network to help them in times of stress.
50. Choice c is correct; this is the stage of launching children and moving on; choice a is leaving home: single young adults; choice b is the family with young children; choice d is the family in later life.
51. Choice b is correct; providing explanations, especially when performing tasks that require close contact, can help to avoid misunderstandings; touching the patient, making eye contact, and taking away the right to make decisions can be interpreted by patients in some cultures as invading their personal space.
52. Choice d is correct; choices a, b, and c are incorrect interpretations based on the woman's culture and customs; Native-Americans often use cradle boards and avoid handling their newborn often; they should not be fed colostrum.

II.   Thinking Critically

1. *Imagine that you are a nurse working in a multicultural prenatal clinic:* use Table 2-3 to formulate your answer; consider components of communication, personal space, time orientation, family roles; identify the degree to which each woman/family adheres to their cultures, beliefs, and practices; do not stereotype.
2. *Pamela, a Native-American pregnant woman:*
    a. *Questions to ask:* see questions listed in the Cultural Awareness box.
    b. *Communication approach to use:* see Childbearing Beliefs and Practices section; include concepts of communication patterns, space, time, and family roles when formulating your answer.
    c. *Identify Native-American beliefs and practices:* see Table 2-3 to formulate your answer; remember to determine her individual beliefs and practices to avoid stereotyping.
3. *Family M—recent birth of twin girls:*
    a. *Identify family life stage:* family with young children stage; accepting new members into the family system (Table 2-1).
    b. *Developmental tasks of this stage:* see Table 2-1 for a full list of tasks that the family needs to accomplish.
    c. *Describe cultural beliefs and practices:* Table 2-3 outlines newborn care guidelines for several ethnic groups, including those Hispanic families are likely to follow.

4. *Sunni refugee couple from Iraq seeking prenatal care:*
   - Consider the process of working with a translator (see Box 2-1); show respect for this couple by addressing questions and comments to them and not to the translator.
   - Box 2-1 outlines the preparation measures, interaction during the interview, and consultation with translator after the interview.
   - Consult Chapter 3 for information regarding the stressors faced by refugees and the health care needs they present.
   - Research Iraq and become familiar with Sunni cultural/religious beliefs and practices and the current political and religious turmoil that led this couple to come to the United States at this time.

CHAPTER 3: COMMUNITY AND HOME CARE

I. Reviewing Key Concepts and Content

1. T   2. F   3. T   4. F   5. F   6. F
7. T   8. T   9. F   10. F   11. F   12. T
13. Geographically defined, residents, cultural, religious, ethnic, activities, functions
14. Walking
15. Participant observation
16. Census data, population, age, sex, ethnic, socioeconomic, educational, employment, housing
17. Aggregates
18. Primary prevention
19. Secondary prevention
20. Tertiary prevention
21. High risk, vulnerable populations, adolescent, minority, migrant homeless, immigrants, refugees
22. *Indicators to assess community health and well-being;* see Box 3-1 to formulate answer.
23. *Community-based health promotion activities for childbearing families:* see Community Health Promotion section to formulate answer.
24. *Cite problems faced by migrant laborers/families:* see Migrants section; include in answer such problems as financial instability, child labor, poor housing and education, cultural barriers, limited access to services, hazardous work conditions, domestic violence, health problems such as diabetes, hypertension, malnutrition, tuberculosis, and substance abuse.
25. *State three characteristics of refugees that increase their vulnerability:* see Refugees and Immigrants subsection; include in answer such characteristics as grief of leaving homeland and loss of family members; effects of surviving trauma of war and refugee camps including rape; experiencing multiple health problems such as infection, malnutrition, stress disorders; cultural differences including inexperience with Western medicine.

26. *Ways nurses can use of the telephone to provide health services:* see Telephonic Nursing Care section; include warm lines, advice lines, and telephonic nursing assessment, consultation, and education.

II. Thinking Critically

1. *Home care nurse must become familiar with neighborhoods and their resources:*
   a. *Walking survey:* a walking survey involves use of observation skills during a trip through a community.
   b. *Use of findings:* see Box 3-2, which discusses each of the survey's components; describe how each of these components could reflect a community's strengths and problems; strengths could be used to provide patients with needed support; nurse could mobilize community leaders to solve identified problems; try using the survey to assess your community and the community in which your college is located.
2. *Marie, a single parent of two children, is homeless:* (see Homeless Women and Implications for Nursing sections).
   a. *Basis for health problems to which she and her children are most vulnerable:* lack of preventive care and resources, limited to no access to primary care resulting in the use of ERs for health care
   b. *Marie's vulnerability for pregnancy:* victimization, economic survival, lack of access to health-care and birth control measures, need for closeness and intimacy, doubt fertility
   c. *Principles to guide nurse when providing care:* treat with respect and dignity, case management to coordinate care to meet multiple needs, flexible appointment times providing service when they come in, make each interaction count, be purposeful, keep her empowered, help her to reconnect with her support system if possible and appropriate.
3. *Consuelo, pregnant wife of a migrant worker and mother of two:* (see Migrant Women section).
   - Begin by confirming that she is pregnant.
   - Consider risks she faces including an increased risk for miscarriage, inadequate prenatal care, and infant mortality.
   - Evaluate exposure to teratogens.
   - Inadequate availability and use of contraceptives, increased rate of STIs including HIV, and poor nutrition are major concerns that need to be addressed.
   - Lack of trust and fear may be barriers to seeking and continuing with prenatal care.

4. *List questions for a postpartum follow-up telephone call:* see Telephonic Nursing Care section; include questions guided by expected postpartum physical and emotional changes; ask her how she is feeling and managing, condition of her newborn (eating, sleeping, eliminating), response of other family members to newborn, sources of happiness and stress, adequacy of help and support being received and need for additional support or referrals.

5. *Home visit to a postpartum woman at 36 hours after birth:* see Boxes 3-3 and 3-4, and Care Management, the first home care visit section to answer each component of this exercise, including the approach you would take to prepare, your actions during the visit, safety precautions and infection control measures you would follow, how you would end the visit, and the interventions you would follow after the visit, including documentation of assessments, actions, and responses.

6. *Angela, a pregnant woman with hyperemesis gravidarum:* see Health Care across the Perinatal Continuum of Care section for a and b and Care Management and Intervention subsection for c.
   a. *Criteria for discharge readiness:* include criteria related to Angela's health status and that of her fetus, availability of qualified home care professionals, family resources, and cost effectiveness of discharging her to home care.
   b. *Information needed to institute high-tech care in the home:* medical diagnosis and prognosis, treatment required, medication history, drug dosing information, and type of infusion access device that will be used.
   c. *Home environment criteria:* safe place to store medications and infusion supplies; do a walk-through inspection to determine temperature of the home, general cleanliness, adequacy of area to prepare and administer prescribed treatment.

7. *Importance and cost-effectiveness of home health care services for postpartum women and their families:* see Perinatal Services section; include the following in your answer:
   • Ability to observe first hand, the home environment and family dynamics; natural; adequacy of resources; safety.
   • Teaching can be tailored to the woman, her family, and her home.
   • Services are less expensive than hospital.
   • Prevention, early detection, and treatment measures can be offered.
   • Services may lead to long-term positive effects on parenting and child health.
   • Use research findings and recommendations of professional organizations to validate proposal.
   • Investigate insurance reimbursement for home care.

CHAPTER 4: HEALTH PROMOTION AND PREVENTION

I. Reviewing Key Concepts and Content

1. T	2. F	3. F	4. T	5. F	6. F
7. T	8. T	9. T	10. F	11. T	12. F
13. T	14. F	15. F	16. T	17. F	18. F
19. T	20. F	21. T	22. F	23. T	24. T
25. F					

26. Preconception counseling
27. Safer sex practices
28. Ask, assess, advise, assist
29. Intimate partner violence (IPV), wife battering, spouse abuse, domestic, family
30. Repeated, increasing tension, battery, calm, remorse, honeymoon
31. Rape, sexual assault, penetration, force, physical coercion, date or acquaintance, marital, gang, stranger, psychic
32. Sexual harassment
33. Female genital mutilation, infection, hemorrhage, urinary, maternal, infant, labor
34. *Risks for gynecologic cancers:*
    a. *Risks for cervical cancer:* see Evidence-Based Practice box for list of risks.
    b. *Measures to reduce risk for cervical cancer:* use risk factors identified as the basis for recommended preventive measures, including the following:
       • Encourage young women to wait to become sexually active until their bodies are mature.
       • Use safer sex practices (Box 4-6).
       • Avoid multiple sexual partners.
       • Avoid smoking.
       • Encourage sexually active women to seek regular health care.
35. *Pamphlet to alert adolescents to dangers of STIs*
    a. *Safer sex:* see Safer Sexual Practices section and Box 4-6; include meaning and importance of safer sex, description of practices; emphasize importance of both partners participating.
    b. *Consequences of STIs:* see Sexual Practices section; discuss effectiveness of currently available treatment methods, emphasizing that some STIs can be cured but can return if behavior does not change and that some STIs cannot be cured; describe consequences of STIs including infertility, ectopic pregnancy, genital cancer, AIDS, death, and neonatal morbidity and mortality.
36. *Why violent crimes against women are underreported:* see Sexual Assault section; answer should include such concepts as fear of retribution, lack of understanding, stigma surrounding violent situations, guilt and shame, embarrassment.

37. *Characteristics of battered women:* see Characteristics of Women in Abusive Relationships section for a discussion of battered women with the identification of several characteristics.

38. Choice d is correct; the blood cholesterol level should be checked every 5 years but more frequently if the woman is at risk for/or experiencing cardiac or lipid problems; endometrial biopsies are not recommended on a routine basis for most women but women at risk for endometrial cancer should have one done at menopause; fecal occult blood tests and mammograms should be done annually for women over 50 years of age.

39. Choice a is correct; all women, not just specific groups, should participate in preconception care 1 year before planning to get pregnant.

40. Choice a is correct; condoms, especially when used with spermicides, can prevent the transmission of STIs; other barrier methods also interfere with the transmission of STIs, thereby reducing the incidence of PID; combination OCPs offer some protection against development of ovarian and endometrial cancer; condoms, not diaphragms, offer the most protection from STIs.

41. Choice c is correct; smoking is associated with preterm birth not postterm pregnancies

42. Choice b is correct; multiple sexual partners as well as early age of first sexual intercourse, smoking, and human papillomavirus (HPV) are common risk factors for cervical cancer; nulliparity and early or late menopause are associated with endometrial cancer.

43. Choice b is correct; anxiety and depression can lead to use of alcohol, tobacco, and drugs as a means of coping; inadequate diet results in low maternal weight gain, increasing the risk for anemia and giving birth to a low-birth-weight newborn; the rate of miscarriage, preterm birth, and stillbirth is increased; abused women are more likely to experience infections, headaches, pain, and depression.

II. Thinking Critically

1. *Importance of preconception care:* see Preconception Counseling section and Box 4-1; this nurse should:
   - Define preconception counseling and what it entails and stress the importance of both partners participating.
   - Identify impact of a woman's health status and lifestyle habits on the developing fetus during the first trimester.
   - Describe how preconception counseling can help a couple choose the best time to begin a pregnancy.

2. *Woman requesting advice regarding diet and exercise to lose weight* (see Box 4-4 and Nutrition and Physical Fitness and Exercise sections):
   - Start with 24-hour to 3-day nutritional recall; based on analysis of woman's current nutritional habits suggest use of food pyramid, emphasize complex carbohydrates and foods high in iron and calcium, reduce fat intake, ensure adequate fluid intake, avoiding those high in sugar, alcohol, or caffeine; use weight changes and activity patterns to determine adequacy of caloric intake.
   - Aerobic exercise: discuss weight bearing vs. non–weight-bearing exercises as well as frequency and duration of exercise sessions for maximum benefit.

3. *Woman experiencing stress*
   a. *Physical and emotional manifestations of stress:* see Stress section and Box 4-5 for a listing of typical manifestations of stress, both physical and emotional.
   b. *Stress management:* see Stress Management section:
      - Help Alice identify and discuss her sources of stress and how she feels when experiencing stress.
      - Help Alice formulate her goals in life and set priorities; work on time management to allow for relaxing times.
      - Discuss her interests, hobbies to be incorporated into a stress management program designed for her; develop alternatives to alcohol and smoking for relaxation such as biofeedback, guided imagery, yoga.
      - Refer to support group for stress management.
   c. *Smoking cessation:* see Smoking Substance Use Cessation sections and Box 4-7.
      - Use the four *A's* formula of ask, assess, advise, assist.
      - Have Alice describe her smoking: how much, how long, triggers to smoking.
      - Discuss how she stopped before.
      - Suggest various strategies available to stop smoking, helping her to make a decision on a method that is right for her.

4. *Pregnant woman who smokes and does not appreciate danger of smoking during pregnancy:* see Smoking section of Health Behaviors and Box 4-4.
   - Discuss impact of smoking on pregnancy using statistics, illustrations, research, and case studies to convince her that smoking does have harmful effects on her, her pregnancy, and on the baby before and after it is born.
   - Help her change her behavior by referring her to smoking cessation programs; use motivation of pregnancy to at least limit smoking, if she cannot stop completely.

5. *Woman's concern regarding violence against women:* see Violence against Women and Health Protection sections.
   - Discuss woman's current circumstances and what she does now to protect herself.
   - Discuss how she changed her behavior based on the experiences of her friends and how she helped or did not help them, her evaluation of how the legal and health care system met the needs of her friends, and what could have and should have been done to help her friends.
   - Review the cycle of violence and measures found to be helpful when assisting a woman who is experiencing violence.
   - Discuss protective and legal services, including hot lines and emergency centers; facilitate access to services to promote assertiveness, self-defense techniques, self-help groups.
6. *Disproving myths regarding violence against women:* use Violence Against Women section and Table 4-3 to gather the information required to refute each myth.
7. *Cues indicative of physical abuse and suggested interventions* (see Assessment and Diagnoses sections and the Guidelines/Guías Box).
   a. *Identify target body areas:* injuries (minor bruising to serious injuries) to head, breasts, abdomen, and genitalia; fractures requiring significant force, multiple injuries at various stages of healing, patterns left by objects used in the abuse.
   b. *Suspicion that pregnant woman is being abused:*
      - Use appropriate communication techniques, including direct questions.
      - Perform interview and examination in a private setting; female health care provider might be helpful.
      - If injuries are noted, tell her that these are common in women who are abused; tell her she is not responsible for another person's abusive behavior.
      - Consider legal implications.
   c. *Abuse is confirmed:* see Plan of Care and Implementation section; formulating a plan and making referrals are important parts of the answer.
   d. *Why pregnancy leads to violence:*
      - Stress of pregnancy may strain relationship, decrease ability to cope; increasing frustration leads to violence
      - Jealous of fetus; seen as an intruder in their relationship
      - Angry with woman, fetus
      - Attempt to end pregnancy
   e. *Adverse effects of violence on pregnancy:*
      - Inadequate diet and rest with low maternal weight gain, anemia; increased risk for infections, headache, pain, depression
      - Use of alcohol, drugs, tobacco to cope with stress
      - Increased risk for low birth weight, miscarriage, preterm birth, stillbirth
      - Interference with attachment process with newborn
      - Delay in seeking prenatal care, missed appointments

CHAPTER 5: HEALTH ASSESSMENT

I. Reviewing Key Concepts and Content

1. Mons pubis
2. Labia majora
3. Labia minora
4. Prepuce
5. Frenulum
6. Fourchette
7. Clitoris
8. Vaginal vestibule
9. Perineum
10. Vagina, rugae, Skene's, Bartholin's
11. Fornices
12. Uterus, cul de sac of Douglas
13. Corpus
14. Isthmus
15. Fundus
16. Endometrium
17. Myometrium
18. Cervix
19. Endocervical, internal os, external os
20. Squamocolumnar junction, transformation
21. Uterine (fallopian) tubes
22. Ovaries, ovulation, estrogen, progesterone, androgen
23. Breasts
24. Tail of Spence
25. Nipple
26. Areola
27. Montgomery's glands (tubercles)
28. Acini
29. Lactiferous sinuses (ampulae)
30. **External female genitalia:** A. mons pubis; B. prepuce of clitoris; C. frenulum of clitoris; D. labia minora; E. vestibule; F. fourchette; G. perineum; H. anus; I. vaginal orifice; J. labia majora; K. vestibule; L. urethra; M. glans of clitoris
    Perineal body: A. posterior fornix of vagina; B. buttocks; C. rectum; D. anus; E. perineal body; F. vagina; G. urethra; H. symphysis pubis; I. bladder; J. anterior fornix of vagina; K. uterus; L. cul de sac of Douglas
    Cross section of uterus: A. fundus; B. body (corpus of the uterus); C. endometrium; D. myometrium; E. internal os of cervix; F. external os of cervix; G. vagina; H. endocervical

canal; I. lateral fornix of vagina; J. cardinal ligament; K. uterine blood vessels; L. broad ligament; M. ovary; N. fimbriae; O. infundibulum of uterine tube; P. ampulla of uterine tube; Q. ovarian ligament; R. isthmus of uterine tube; S. interstitial portion of uterine tube

Breast (sagittal section): A. clavicle; B. intercostal muscle; C. pectoralis major; D. alveolus; E. ductule; F. duct; G. lactiferous duct; H. lactiferous sinus; I. nipple pore; J. suspensory ligament of Cooper; K. sixth rib; L. second rib

Breast (anterior dissection): A. acini cluster; B. lactiferous (milk) duct; C. lactiferous sinus (ampulla); D. nipple pore; E. areola; F. Montgomery's gland (tubercle)

Female pelvis: A. seventh lumbar vertebra; B. iliac crest; C. sacral promontory; D. sacrum; E. acetabulum; F. obturator foramen; G. subpubic arch under symphysis pubis; H. ischium; I. pubis; J. ilium; K. sacroiliac joint

31. Menstrual cycle

    Diagram of menstrual cycle: A. gonadotropin-releasing hormone (GnRH); B. follicle-stimulating hormone (FSH); C. luteinizing hormone (LH); D. follicular phase; E. luteal phase; F. Graafian follicle; G. ovum; H. corpus luteum; I. estrogen; J. progesterone; K. menses; L. proliferative phase; M. secretory phase; N. ischemic phase; O. hypothalamic-pituitary Cycle; P. ovarian Cycle; Q. endometrial cycle

    Hormones of the menstrual cycle: see Endometrial Cycle, Hypothalamic-Pituitary Cycle, and Ovarian Cycle sections for a description of GnRH, FSH, LH, estrogen, and progesterone; see Prostaglandin section for a description of prostaglandins.

32. F	33. T	34. T	35. F	36. F	37. T
38. F	39. T	40. T	41. F	42. F	43. F
44. F	45. T	46. T	47. T	48. T	49. T

50. *Guidelines for performing a Pap smear:* guidelines for each component of the procedure are outlined in Box 5-3 Procedure: Papanicolaou Smear.

51. *Characteristics of a palpated lump:* location, size, mobility, consistency, tenderness, type of borders

52. *Breast self-examination technique:* see Guidelines box: BSE; A. –; B. –; C. +; D. +; E. +; F. –; G. +; H. +; I. +

53. Choice d is correct; clean gloves are required only if open lesions are present and when compressing the nipple if discharge is anticipated; fingers should not be lifted; two hands are used for women with large, pendulous breasts.

54. Choice c is correct; self-examination should not be used for self-diagnosis but rather to detect early changes and seek guidance of a health care provider if changes are noted.

55. Choice b is correct; do not ask questions during the examination because it may distract the patient, interfering with relaxation measures she

may be using; only offer explanations as needed during the examination.

56. Choice c is correct; women should not tub bathe, use vaginal medications or contraceptives, or douche for 24 hours before the test; OCPs can continue.

57. Choice a is correct; all women should be screened because abuse can happen to any woman; abuse often escalates during pregnancy; the most commonly injured sites are head, neck, chest, abdomen, breasts, and upper extremities. If abuse is suspected the nurse needs to assess further to encourage disclosure and then assist the woman to take action and formulate a plan.

II. Thinking Critically

1. *State how culture, disabilities, abuse, and age can influence health assessment of women:* see specific sections for each factor in the health assessment.

2. Nurse responses to concerns and questions of women.

   a. *Hymen:* hymen can be perforated with strenuous exercise, insertion of tampons, masturbation, GYN examination as well as during vaginal intercourse.

   b. *How to get ready for first GYN examination:* explain what will occur and each guideline to follow for preparation and why each is important for the accuracy of the test; tell her to avoid douching, vaginal medications, and intercourse for 24 hours before the examination; she should not be menstruating.

   c. *Signs indicating ovulation:* midcycle spotting and pain (mittelschmerz), breast swelling and tenderness, elevated basal body temperature, cervical mucous changes (Spinnbarkeit), and other changes in behavior and emotions individual to each woman (premenstrual signs).

   d. *Douching:* vaginal secretions are usually acidic and protect the reproductive tract from infection; a douche may alter this acidity and injure the mucosa, thereby increasing the risk for infection; gentle and regular front-to-back washing with mild soap and water is all that is necessary to be clean

3. *Woman anxious about first GYN examination* (see Box 5-1 and Pelvic Examination section).

   • Explain each component of the examination, how it is done, why it is performed, and how it will feel.

   • Show her the instruments that will be used.

   • Encourage her to verbalize what she is feeling, her concerns, and questions.

   • Teach her simple relaxation measures such as deep breathing.

   • Ensure her privacy and modesty and tell her how it will be maintained throughout the examination.

4. *Health history of a new patient at a Women's Health Clinic:*
   a. *Components:* see History section for a list and description of components.
   b. *Writing questions:* use components of health history as a guide; write questions that are open ended, clear, concise, address only one issue, and progress from general to specific.
   c. *Therapeutic communication techniques with examples* (see Interview section).
      • Use facilitation, reflection, clarification, empathetic responses, confrontation, interpretation.
      • Be sensitive and nonjudgmental in your approach; use a relaxed, confident, professional manner.
      • Use full name of patient; introduce yourself.
      • Consider comfort and privacy of the environment in which the interview will take place.
5. *Teaching self-examination techniques:* each technique involves cognitive, psychomotor, and affective learning; use a variety of methodologies including discussion (when, how often, why, expected and reportable findings, who to call, what will be done if abnormal findings are experienced); explore feelings regarding self-examination; provide literature with illustrations; demonstrate and have patient redemonstrate using practice models and then patient themselves as appropriate.
   Breast self-examination: see Guidelines box, BSE.
   Vulvar (genital) self-examination: see Vulvar Self-Examination section.
6. *Culturally sensitive approach to women's health care* (see Cultural Considerations and Communication Variations sections).
   • Approach woman in a respectful and calm manner.
   • Consider modifications in the examination to maintain her modesty.
   • Incorporate communication variations such as conversational style, pacing, spacing, eye contact, touch, time orientation.
   • Take time to learn about the woman's cultural beliefs and practices regarding well woman assessment and care.
7. *Screening for abuse when providing well woman care* (see Chapter 4 to help with answering these questions: Violence Against Women section, Box 4-8, and Guidelines/Guías box):
   a. *Adjusting the environment and communication style:* provide for comfort and privacy; assess the woman alone without her partner or adult children present.
   b. *Abuse indicators:* see Violence Against Women section, Box 4-8, and Guidelines/Guías box for identification of several indicators of possible abuse and areas of the body most commonly

injured, including during pregnancy, specific somatic complaints, and behaviors including a pattern of canceling health care appointments.
   c. *Questions to ask:* see Fig. 5-11, which lists the four questions that all women should be asked in a very direct manner.
   d. *Approach if abuse is confirmed:*
      • Acknowledge the abuse and affirm that it is unacceptable and common; tell her that you are concerned and that she does not deserve it.
      • Communicate that it can recur; cite the cycle of violence (see Chapter 4); tell her that help is available; empower her to use this help.
      • Help her formulate an escape plan; provide her with access to community resources, including shelters.
8. *Describe events in each cycle composing the menstrual cycle:* see Hypothalamic-Pituitary Cycle, Ovarian Cycle, and Endometrial Cycle sections of the Menstrual cycle for a description of the events and changes characteristic of each cycle.
9. *Assisting with a pelvic examination:* see Box 5-1 Procedure: Assisting with Pelvic Examination and Pelvic Examination section for your answer.
   a. *Patient preparation and support:* teach about what is to occur as part of the examination, assist to change clothes, tell her to empty her bladder, and assist her to get into the position required for the examination; tell her how to relax and provide privacy; inform and support her throughout the examination; assist her with cleansing, getting into an upright position, and dressing as needed after the examination; discuss any questions or concerns the woman may have related to the examination.
   b. *Assist the health care provider:* assist with preparing and supporting the patient, preparing equipment, taking care of specimens, including correct labeling, sending to the lab.

CHAPTER 6: COMMON HEALTH PROBLEMS

I. Reviewing Key Concepts and Content

1. Amenorrhea, pregnancy, anorexia nervosa, amenorrhea, stress, weight loss, eating, strenuous exercise, mental illness
2. Eating, amenorrhea, osteoporosis
3. Dysmenorrhea, during, shortly before, primary dysmenorrhea, 6 to 12, ovulation, estrogen, progesterone, secondary dysmenorrhea
4. Premenstrual syndrome (PMS), symptoms occur in the luteal phase and resolve within a few days of the onset of menses, symptom-free follicular phase, symptoms are recurrent

5. Endometriosis, proliferative, secretory, menstruation, inflammatory, fibrosis, adhesions, dysmenorrhea, dyspareunia, diarrhea, defecation, constipation, fertility
6. Abnormal uterine bleeding (AUB), dysfunctional uterine bleeding (DUB), anovulation

7. T	8. F	9. F	10. T	11. F	12. F
13. F	14. T	15. T	16. T	17. F	18. F
19. F	20. T	21. T			

22. Sexually transmitted infections (STIs) or sexually transmitted diseases (STDs), chlamydia, HPV, gonorrhea, HSV-2, syphilis, HIV
23. Safer sex practices, know partner, reduce number of partners, low risk sex, avoid exchange of body fluids
24. Condom (male, female)
25. Chlamydia
26. Gonorrhea
27. Syphilis, primary syphilis, chancre, 5 to 90, secondary syphilis, 6, 6, symmetric maculopapular rash, palms, soles, lymphadenopathy, fever, headache, malaise, condylomata lata, latent, tertiary syphilis
28. Pelvic inflammatory disease (PID), menses, abortion, pelvic surgery, childbirth
29. Human papillomavirus (HPV), condylomata acuminata
30. Herpes simplex virus type 2 (HSV-2), lesions, fever, chills, malaise, dysuria, 2 to 3
31. Hepatitis A virus (HAV), milk, shellfish, water, person to person
32. Hepatitis B virus (HBV)
33. Hepatitis C virus (HCV)
34. Human immunodeficiency virus (HIV), cellular immune
35. Group B streptococcus (GBS)
36. Bacterial vaginosis, fishy
37. Candidiasis, pruritus, dryness, dysuria, thick, white, lumpy, cottage–cheese-like, vaginal walls, cervix, labia
38. Trichomoniasis

39. T	40. F	41. F	42. F	43. F	44. T
45. F	46. T	47. F	48. F	49. T	50. F
51. T	52. T	53. T	54. F	55. T	56. F
57. T	58. T	59. F	60. T	61. F	

62. *Common risk factors for STIs:* Box 6-3 cites many common risk behaviors according to sexual, drug use–related, and blood-related risks.
63. *Infection control principles and practices:* see Box 6-5 for an explanation of Standard Precautions and precautions for invasive procedures.
64. *Reproductive tract infections table:* see specific infection sections for information related to typical clinical manifestations and management guidelines for each of the infections listed.

65. *Heterosexual transmission of HIV to women* (see HIV section)
    a. *Mode of transmission:* exchange of body fluids (semen, blood, vaginal)
    b. *Clinical manifestations during seroconversion:* viremic, influenza-type responses such as fever, headache, night sweats, malaise, lymphadenopathy, myalgia, nausea, diarrhea, weight loss, sore throat, rash
    c. *Management:* education related to disease process, measures to prevent transmission of infection and to maintain resistance to infection, healthy lifestyle practices, contraception, and signs of opportunistic infections; expert multidisciplinary care with a holistic focus; use of prophylactic medication; referrals (psychologic, legal, financial) as needed

66. F	67. T	68. F	69. F	70. T	71. T
72. T	73. F	74. T	75. F	76. F	77. T
78. F	79. T	80. b	81. d	82. a	83. e
84. c					

85. *Educating women about breast cancer* (see Malignant Conditions of the Breast section).
    a. *Information regarding risk factors:* see Etiology section and Box 6-6 to determine risk factors to teach women; identify factors, degree of risk they represent alone and in combination; include research findings; discuss how risk factors can influence health care, including suggestions for assessment methods and frequency, lifestyle changes, and prevention methods for very high risk women.
    b. *Manifestations suggestive of breast cancer:* often unilateral in the upper outer quadrant; lump or thickening of the breast, hard and fixed or soft and spongy, well defined or irregular borders, dimpling (fixed to integument), nipple discharge
    c. *Diagnostic tests:* mammography, ultrasound, MRI, biopsy of tumor tissue or fluid
86. *Definitions of treatment approaches:* see appropriate sections for a description of each treatment approach.
87. Choice b is correct; the 13-year-old reflects several of the risk factors associated with this menstrual disorder, namely: presently in a growth period, participating in a sport that is stressful, subjectively scored, requires contour revealing clothing, and success is favored by a prepubertal body shape.
88. Choice c is correct; choices a, b, and d all interfere with prostaglandin synthesis, whereas acetaminophen has no antiprostaglandin properties; prostaglandins are a recognized factor in the etiology of dysmenorrhea.
89. Choice a is correct; decreasing the ingestion of red meats and switching from a high-fat to a low-fat diet has been associated with symptom relief;

asparagus and cranberry juice have a natural diuretic effect that can reduce edema and related discomforts; simple refined sugars, not complex carbohydrates, should be avoided along with salt for 7 to 10 days before menstruation to reduce fluid retention.

90. Choice d is correct; alcohol, tobacco, and caffeine can worsen symptoms experienced, whereas exercise can provide relief as can peaches and watermelon both of which have a natural diuretic effect; current research suggests that vitamin B_6 is not an effective form of treatment, but calcium, magnesium, and vitamin E are safe and moderately effective with few side effects.

91. Choice c is correct; women taking danazol often experience masculinizing changes; amenorrhea is an outcome of taking this medication; ovulation may not be fully suppressed; therefore birth control is essential because this medication is teratogenic.

92. Choice a is correct; dysmenorrhea is painful menstruation; dysuria is painful urination; dyspnea is difficulty breathing.

93. Choice a is correct; because these infections are often asymptomatic, they can go undetected and untreated causing more damage including ascent of the pathogen into the uterus and pelvis, resulting in PID and infertility; many effective treatment measures are available, including for chlamydia.

94. Choice b is correct; choice a is indicative of candidiasis; choice c is indicative of HSV-2; choice d is indicative of trichomoniasis.

95. Choice b is correct; Flagyl is used to treat bacterial vaginosis and trichomoniasis; erythromycin is effective in the treatment of chlamydia; acyclovir is used to treat herpes.

96. Choice b is correct; choices a, c, and d are not used to treat GBS infection; acyclovir is used orally to treat herpes; there are no lesions with GBS.

97. Choice d is correct; recurrent infections commonly involve only local symptoms that are less severe; stress reduction, healthy lifestyle practices, and acyclovir can reduce recurrence rate; viral shedding can occur before lesions appear

98. Choice d is correct; breast cancer is more common among Caucasian women; it is most prevalent among women 40 years of age and older as menopause is approached; the majority of women do not exhibit the identified risk factors; two risk factors are obesity and high-fat diets.

99. Choice b is correct; the right arm should be used as much as possible to maintain mobility and prevent lymphedema; loose nonrestrictive clothing should be worn; tingling and numbness are expected findings for as long as a few months after surgery.

100. Choice a is correct; pain is a common finding; it usually begins a week before the onset of menses; leakage from nipples is not associated with this disorder; surgery is unlikely and is only attempted in a few selected cases; overall cancer risk is 5%.

101. Choice d is correct; fibroadenomas are generally small, unilateral, firm, nontender, moveable lumps located in the upper outer quadrant; borders are discrete and well defined; discharge is not associated with this disorder.

II. Thinking Critically

1. *Woman with hypogonadotropic amenorrhea* (see Hypogonadotropic Amenorrhea section).
   a. *Risk factors exhibited:* athletic competition subjectively scored, inappropriate body fat to lean ratio, nutritional deficits related to need to maintain body size, stress and vigorous exercise, need to wear body revealing clothing, prepubertal body shape favors success
   b. *Nursing diagnosis:* disturbed body image related to delayed onset of menstruation and development of secondary sexual characteristics
   c. *Expected outcomes:*
      • Marie will state the reason for the delayed onset of the pubertal changes she is experiencing.
      • Marie will participate in a therapeutic regimen that will favor age-appropriate physical development.
   d. *Care management:*
      • Initiate stress reduction measures.
      • Reduce exercise or gain weight through good nutrition to alter fat to lean body ratio.
      • Involve family and coach in treatment plan.
      • Discuss risk for osteoporosis.
      • Begin hormonal treatment or calcium supplementation if needed.
2. *Woman with primary dysmenorrhea* (see Dysmenorrhea section).
   a. *Compare and contrast primary and secondary dysmenorrhea:* see Dysmenorrhea section for description of each disorder.
   b. *Nursing diagnoses:* consider the areas of pain and ineffective role performance as the focus for nursing management of this woman's primary dysmenorrhea; use assessment data to determine which nursing diagnosis will take precedence.
   c. *Relief measures:* discuss basis of the problem and that it usually diminishes with age; suggest nonpharmacologic measures such as exercise, relaxation techniques, good nutrition, heating pad; pharmacologic measures such as NSAIDs and oral contraceptives may be prescribed.

3. *Woman experiencing PMS* (see PMS section).
   a. *Typical signs and symptoms:* clinical manifestations are usually related to effects of fluid retention, behavioral and emotional changes, cravings, headache, fatigue/energy level, and backache.
   b. *Nursing diagnosis:* nursing diagnoses could include pain, activity intolerance, disturbed sleep pattern, diarrhea, constipation, ineffective role performance; use assessment findings to determine those that would apply to a particular patient including those that are priority.
   c. *Nursing approach:*
      • Obtain a detailed history and encourage woman to keep a diary of physical and emotional manifestations (what occurs, when, contributing circumstances) from one cycle to another.
      • Individualize plan based on this woman's experiences.
      • Discuss nutrition, exercise, and lifestyle/career measures.
      • Refer to appropriate support group or for counseling if needed.

4. *Woman with endometriosis* (see Endometriosis section).
   a. *Clinical manifestations:* dysmenorrhea (secondary), pelvic pain and heaviness, thigh pain, GI symptoms, diarrhea, constipation dyspareunia, abnormal bleeding, metrorrhagia and menorrhagia.
   b. *Pathophysiology of the disorder:* growth of endometrial tissue outside uterus mainly in the pelvis; implants respond to cyclical changes in hormones; bleeding of implants leads to inflammatory response, formation of scar tissue, fibrosis, anemia.
   c. *Pharmacologic management:* each medication used is discussed in Management section; oral contraceptives are used to create a pseudopregnancy; GnRH antagonists and androgenic synthetic steroids are used to create a pseudomenopause; goal is cause implants to shrink and atrophy.
   d. *Support measures:* educate regarding disease process; discuss treatment options; refer to support groups and counseling as appropriate, work with couple together and separately to allow for expression of feelings and concerns; review options for pregnancy since infertility can be an outcome.

5. *Woman attending first visit at a women's health clinic*
   a. *Write one question for each STI risk factor category:* see Box 6-3; questions should reflect risks identified, and be open-ended, clear, concise, and nonjudgmental.
   b. *Major points to emphasize for STI prevention:* see Safer Sex Practices section, Table 6-4, and Guidelines box: Prevention of Genital Tract Infections in Women
      • Know partner: questions to ask, how to assess genitalia.
      • Avoid relations with many partners.
      • Insist on barrier method; be prepared.
      • Do not make decisions based on appearances and unfounded assumptions.
      • Know low risk sexual practices and those that are unsafe.
   c. *Measures to help patient develop assertiveness and communication skills related to safer sexual practices* (see Box 6-4).
      • Emphasize importance of discussing prevention measures, including condom use with partner at a time removed from sexual activity.
      • Role play using possible partner responses for woman to react to; rehearse how she will handle various situations so she can sort out her feelings and fears ahead of time.
      • Reassure that her reluctance is not unusual.

6. *Pregnant woman diagnosed as HIV positive at 4 weeks of gestation:* see HIV-counseling for HIV Testing section.
   • Oral zidovudine (AZT) at 14 to 34 weeks' gestation, IV during labor, and orally to newborn for 6 weeks after birth
   • Elective cesarean birth
   • Breastfeeding is contraindicated

7. *Woman with severe PID* (see Pelvic Inflammatory Disease section).
   a. *Risk factors:*
      • Menstrual history; pathogen ascent into uterus usually occurs at end of or just after menses.
      • Recent abortion, pelvic surgery, childbirth, D&C, purulent vaginal discharge, irregular bleeding or longer/heavier menstrual period
      • Sexual history for STIs, risky behaviors; history of sexual partner(s) if possible
   b. *Diagnostic criteria:* oral temperature greater than 38.3°C, abnormal cervical or vaginal discharge, increased erythrocyte sedimentation rate, lab documentation of cervical infection, lower abdominal tenderness, bilateral adnexal tenderness, cervical motion tenderness
   c. *Nursing diagnoses during acute phase:* pain, anxiety (effect on sexuality and future fertility), impaired physical mobility, diarrhea, constipation, urinary retention
   d. *Management guidelines:*
      • Position and activity: Encourage bed rest in the semi-Fowler position to keep pelvis in the dependent position; elevate legs slightly to prevent pulling on pelvis, which would increase discomfort.

- Comfort measures: Suggest analgesics, back rub, hygiene, relaxation techniques, diversional activities, proper positioning.
- Support measures: provide time for woman to express feelings; include partner in care as appropriate; help woman to deal with effects of the PID and the potential long-term effects; use a nonjudgmental, empathetic approach.
- Health education: Instruct how to comply with treatment regimen, including taking medications effectively, refraining from intercourse until fully healed, use of contraceptives and safer sex practices.

e. *Self-care during recovery phase:* see Home Care box—sexually Transmitted Infections and Guidelines box: Prevention of Genital Tract Infections in Women for self-care suggestions; emphasize activity restrictions, importance of rest, good nutrition, taking medications completely, and follow-up.

f. *Reproductive risks:* tubal obstructions and adhesions leading to ectopic pregnancy or infertility, chronic pelvic pain, and dyspareunia are possible.

8. *Woman diagnosed with gonorrhea* (see Gonorrhea section).

   a. *Nursing diagnosis:* anxiety related to potential effect of STI on future sexual function *or* risk for ineffective sexuality pattern related to recent diagnosis of STI.

   b. *Management:*
   - Educate Laura about STIs including gonorrhea; discuss cure, control, and recurrence factors.
   - Discuss self-care measures: Home Care box, Sexually Transmitted Infections; Guidelines box, Prevention of Genital Tract Infections in Women.
   - Discuss safer sex practices and practice assertiveness with partners.
   - Review genital self-examination technique.

9. *Reducing pain of condylomata associated with HPV infection:* see HPV section.
   - Bathe with oatmeal solution.
   - Keep area clean and dry; use a cool dryer.
   - Wearing cotton underwear, loose-fitting clothing.
   - Practice healthy lifestyle to enhance immune system and healing process.

10. *Woman diagnosed with herpes simplex virus 2* (see HSV section).

    a. *Measures to relieve pain and prevent secondary infection:*
    - Use antiviral medications correctly.
    - Cleanse lesions BID with saline; use a warm sitz bath with baking soda.
    - Keep dry with cool hair dryer or pat dry; use hydrogen peroxide, Burow's solution.

- Wear cotton underwear, loose clothing.
- Take oral analgesics; limit use of topicals to decrease discomfort.
- Modify diet and lifestyle to enhance healing.

    b. *Preventing/reducing recurrence:*
    - Educate regarding etiology, signs of recurrence, transmission, treatment, precipitating factors for reactivation of virus; self-assessment.
    - Initiate lifestyle changes, including diet.
    - Keep diary to identify stressors, recurrences, helpful measures.
    - Practice stress reduction measures, avoid heat, sun, or hot baths, use a lubricant during intercourse to reduce friction.

11. *Woman concerned about exposure to HIV* (see HIV section)

    a. *Risky behaviors:* exposure to contaminated body fluids, including semen and blood; discuss sexual practices and partners as well as possible IV drug use.

    b. *Testing procedure:* see Screening and Diagnosis and Counseling for HIV testing sections for description of types of tests and testing protocol, counseling required, and legal implications; nurse should witness an informed consent, tell woman how long it will take for results to be available, consider ethical issues of confidentiality and privacy, and use a nonjudgmental, empathetic approach.

    c. *Counseling protocol:* counseling should occur before and after testing, by the same person, in a private area with no interruptions; all assessments, actions, and responses should be documented.
    - Pretest: personalized risk assessment; explain meaning of test results, informed consent, plan for reducing risk and preventing infection.
    - Posttest: inform regarding results, review meaning of result obtained, reinforce self-care/prevention measures; refer for treatment if positive result is obtained.

    d. *Instructions following a negative test result:* use Sonya's risky behaviors as a basis for discussing prevention measures, including safer sex practices; discuss impact HIV could have on her health and that of her fetus when pregnant.

12. *Woman with fibrocystic breast change* (see Fibrocystic Changes section).

    a. *Assessment process to diagnose fibrocystic change:*
    - History and physical assessment including clinical breast examination
    - Ultrasonography to determine if lumps are solid or fluid filled
    - Fluid filled—fluid aspirated if necessary
    - Solid—mammography if over 50 and fine-needle aspiration (FNA)

b. *Signs and symptoms:*
  - Lumpiness both breasts; enlarge premenstrually
  - Symptoms—1 week before menses subside 1 week after it ends: dull heavy pain, fullness, tenderness
  - Cysts: soft, differentiated, mobile

c. *Nursing diagnosis:* based on assessment findings and time in menstrual cycle; can include pain, anxiety.

d. *Relief measures:* try several approaches and see which combination works the best; keep a diary.
  - Discomfort: use analgesics, support bra, heat.
  - Diet: eliminate dimethylxanthine and caffeine; limit sodium.
  - Avoiding alcohol and smoking can help.
  - Take vitamin E and mild diuretics premenstrually.

13. *Woman with lump in left breast*

a. *Diagnostic protocol:*
  - History and physical examination including clinical breast examination; document characteristics of the lump and other associated findings such as dimpling, increased venous pattern, enlarged lymph nodes.
  - Mammography; compare with previous test results if available.
  - Biopsy of lump tissue is done to confirm diagnosis.

b. *Nursing diagnoses and care management* (see Management section, Nursing Care Plan box, Home Care box, and Box 6-9):
  - Nursing diagnoses would include pain, risk for infection, impaired skin integrity, risk for deficient fluid volume.
  - Typical postoperative care along with elevation of arm; avoid using arm for BP, IV, blood draws, and medications; follow protocol for movement and use of affected arm; check for bleeding in drainage bag, on dressing, and under arm; assist with position changes, leg exercises, and coughing and deep breathing; emotional support is important for both periods.

c. *Preparing Molly for self-care at home:* see Box 6-9: Arm Exercises, Home Care box, After a Mastectomy; instructions should address pain control; signs of complications; wound, dressing, and drainage care; BSE; arm exercises and use of arm; time for follow-up appointment.

d. *Support measures:*
  - Help woman and partner deal with change in appearance; encourage open communication; meet with woman and her partner together and separately.

- Refer to community resources and support groups (e.g., Reach for Recovery).
- Discuss follow-up treatments, including adjuvant therapy, radiation therapy, reconstructive surgery, and complementary/alternative therapies.
- Discuss use of prostheses.
- Ensure that health care provider is with woman and her partner when she views wound for the first time.

CHAPTER 7: INFERTILITY, CONTRACEPTION, AND ABORTION

I. Reviewing Key Concepts and Content

1. F   2. F   3. T   4. T   5. F   6. T
7. T   8. F   9. F   10. T   11. F
12. In vitro fertilization (IVF) and embryo transfer (ET)
13. Intracytoplasmic sperm injection
14. Gamete intrafallopian transfer (GIFT)
15. Zygote intrafallopian transfer (ZIFT)
16. Therapeutic donor insemination
17. Gestational carrier (embryo host)
18. Surrogate motherhood
19. Assisted hatching
20. e   21. f   22. c   23. b   24. d   25. a
26. *Couple receiving care for infertility* (see Infertility section).

a. *Identify/describe components for normal fertility* (see Factors Associated with Infertility section and Box 7-5): normal male and female reproductive tract, hormonal support for gametogenesis, timing for intercourse, adequate sperm and ova, patent tubal system for passage of sperm and ova.

b. *Support statement that assessment for infertility must involve both partners:* see Boxes 7-1, 7-2, and 7-5 and Care Management section, which discuss findings favorable for fertility indicating male and female factors; cite statistics revealing the percentage for a female factor, a male factor, and unexplained factors and unusual problems causing infertility.

27. *Cite surgical procedures to treat infertility:* see Surgical section of Plan of Care and Implementation; remove tumors and release adhesions; hysterosalpingogram to release blockage; laparoscopy to release adhesions, destroy endometrial implants, repair tubes; reconstructive surgery of uterus; repair of varicocele and microsurgery to restore sperm ducts.

28. F   29. T   30. T   31. T   32. T   33. F
34. F   35. F   36. T   37. T   38. T   39. F
40. F   41. T   42. F   43. F   44. F   45. T
46. T   47. T   48. F   49. F   50. T

51. Coitus interruptus
52. Natural family planning
53. Fertility awareness
54. Calendar (rhythm) method
55. Basal body temperature (BBT)
56. Spinnbarkeit
57. Symptothermal
58. Spermicide
59. Condom
60. Diaphragm
61. Cervical cap
62. Contraceptive sponge
63. Norplant
64. Mifepristone (RU 486); prostaglandin
65. Intrauterine device (IUD)
66. Sterilization, occlusion, ligation, electrocoagulation, bands, clips, vasectomy, vas deferens
67. Induced abortion, elective abortion, therapeutic abortion
68. *Factors influencing contraceptive choice:* see Care Management section, Contraception; answer should include such factors as knowledge level, commitment to and confidence in the method, frequency of coitus, number of partners, willingness and comfort with touching genitalia and cervical mucus, and religious and cultural beliefs and values.
69. *Purpose for self-assessment of cervical mucus* (see Cervical Mucus, Ovulation Method section and Guidelines box, Cervical Mucus Characteristics).
    - Alert couple about reestablishment of ovulation after breastfeeding or discontinuing oral contraceptives.
    - Determine if cycles are ovulatory at any time including menopause, when planning pregnancy, or for timing infertility treatments and diagnostic procedures.
70. *Periodic abstinence or natural family planning as a method of birth control*
    a. Exact time of ovulation cannot be predicted accurately, abstain from sexual intercourse during fertile period, irregular menstrual periods (cycles).
    b. 5, 22
    c. Drop, 0.05, progesterone, rise, 0.4 to 0.8, 2 to 4 days, thermal shift
    d. Cervical mucus ovulation detection, cervical mucus, amount, consistency
    e. Basal body temperature (BBT), cervical mucus, increased libido, midcycle spotting, mittelschmerz, pelvic fullness, tenderness, vulvar fullness, cervix, slight dilation, softening, rising
    f. Luteinizing hormone (LH), 12 to 24
71. a. c   b. i   c. c   d. c   e. c
    f. i   g. i   h. i

72. *Cite four factors for seeking an abortion:* preserve life and health of the woman, genetic disorder of the fetus, rape/incest, pregnant woman's request
73. Choice b is correct; Spinnbarkeit refers to stretchiness of cervical mucus at ovulation to facilitate passage of sperm; there is an LH surge before ovulation; BBT rises in response to increased progesterone after ovulation; cervical mucus becomes thinner and more abundant with ovulation.
74. Choice b is correct; the couple should abstain from intercourse for 2 to 4 days before expected ovulation; the test is scheduled for the expected time of ovulation; report for examination within several hours.
75. Choice a is correct; oral contraception provides no protection from STIs; therefore, a condom and spermicide are still recommended to prevent transmission; choices b, c, and d reflect appropriate actions and recognition of side effects.
76. Choice a is correct; although choices b, c, and d are all temporary side effects, the most common is the irregular pattern of bleeding that occurs; women report that this bleeding is also the most distressing side effect.
77. Choice c is correct; the string should be checked after menses, before intercourse, at the time of ovulation, and if expulsion is suspected; a missing string or one that becomes longer or shorter should be checked by a health care professional.
78. Choice b is correct; spermicide should not be applied around the rim because a seal will not form to keep the cap in place; use during menses increases the risk for toxic shock syndrome; checking the cap's position is all that is required before each subsequent act of coitus.

II. Thinking Critically

1. *Couple undergoing testing for infertility*
    a. *Nursing support measures* (see Care Management, Assessment and Psychosocial sections); help couple to
        - Express feeling and openly discuss sexuality issues
        - Make decisions regarding diagnostic tests and treatment options
        - Grieve the loss of fertility and inability to have biologic children if that is the outcome
        - Refer to support groups and adoption agencies as appropriate
    b. *Procedure for semen analysis* (see Semen Analysis section); emphasize need to abstain for 2 to 3 days before test, not to use spermicide, to collect specimen in a clean container or plastic sheath, to protect it from extremes of heat and cold, and to transport to lab within 2 hours of ejaculation.

c. *Semen characteristics evaluated:* see Box 7-6 for a full list of characteristics in terms of liquefaction, volume, pH, density, and morphology.

d. *Postcoital test instructions:* see Postcoital test section; instructions should include purpose of test, when to have intercourse (expected time of ovulation), what to do afterwards, when to come for examination (within several hours of intercourse); caution that vagina must be free of infection and couple should abstain for 2 to 4 days before the test.

2. *Concerns engendered by reproductive technologies:* see Reproductive Alternatives section and Boxes 7-3 and 7-4:
   - Who should pay? insurance coverage; wealthy vs. poor couples
   - Children: Who are their biologic parents? What is their medical history?
   - Availability to married couples only
   - Ownership of ovum, sperm, embryos
   - Attempt to create the "perfect" child

3. *Woman seeking assistance with making choice regarding birth control method:*
   a. *Nursing diagnosis:* anxiety related to lack of knowledge regarding contraception.
   b. *Approach for nurse to use to assist with decision making:*
      - Assess her level of knowledge regarding how her body works; sexual practices including beliefs, practices, number of partners, frequency of coitus.
      - Fully describe different methods; determine preferences for or objections to methods described.
      - Determine level of contraceptive involvement desired: comfort with touching genitalia, myths and misconceptions, religious and cultural factors.
      - Obtain health status as determined with health history, physical examination, and laboratory testing as appropriate.

4. *Woman choosing to use combination estrogen-progestin oral contraceptive* (see Hormonal Methods, Box 7-9, Table 7-3, and Fig. 7-11).
   a. *Mode of action:* suppression of hypothalamus and anterior pituitary; altered maturation of endometrium, thickened cervical mucus; inhibition of ovulation.
   b. *Advantages:* easy to use, not connected with intercourse, improves sexual response, regular predictable menses with decreased blood loss, decrease in dysmenorrhea and PMS, some protection from GYN problems such as endometrial and ovarian cancer, functional ovarian cysts, benign breast disease, ectopic pregnancy, and some types of PID.

c. *Signs and symptoms requiring woman to stop taking the OCP and notifying her health care provider:* see Box 7-9, Signs of Potential Complications with Oral Contraceptives for an explanation of ACHES.
   d. *Instructions for the patient:*
      - Follow specific directions on package insert in terms of taking the pill and what to do if one or more are missed; take at same time of day
      - Use own pills not someone else's because OCPs vary.
      - Discuss side effects and complications.
      - Check effect of other medications being taken on the effectiveness of the OCP.
      - Importance of using STD protection and of using backup method for first cycle on OCP, when certain other medications are being taken, or if pill(s) have been missed (see Fig. 7-11).

5. *Woman using a cervical cap* (see Cervical Cap section and Home Care box, Use of Cervical Cap):
   a. *Factors making patient a poor candidate for using cap:* abnormal Pap test results, history of TSS, vaginal or cervical infection, cannot be fitted properly, insertion/removal too difficult for the woman, allergy to latex or spermicide.
   b. *Patient instructions for safe and effective use:*
      - Review when and how to insert and remove, checking placement, use of spermicide.
      - Avoid using during menses or for 6 weeks postpartum.
      - Check fit annually and after GYN surgery, birth, major weight loss or gain.

6. *Instructions following IUD insertion:*
   - See Box 7-10, Signs of Potential Complications with Intrauterine Devices, which uses the acronym of PAINS to identify signs of problems.
   - Teach how and when to check string.
   - Stress importance of appropriate genital hygiene and sexual practices.
   - Inform when IUD needs to be replaced.

7. *Couple contemplating sterilization* (see Sterilization section).
   a. *Decision making approach:* nurse acts as facilitator to help couple explore the pros and cons of sterilization itself and the options available for male and female sterilization as well as alternatives to sterilization.
   b. *Preoperative and postoperative care measures and instructions for vasectomy:*
      - Preoperative: obtain health assessment in terms of history, psychologic assessment, physical examination, and laboratory tests; preparatory instructions; witness an informed consent.

- Postoperative: discuss prevention and early detection of bleeding and infection; self-care measures in terms of hygiene, comfort, prevention and reduction of swelling with ice packs and scrotal support; activity restrictions for a couple of days, moderate activity level
  - Caution that sterility may not be immediate: an alternative method should be used until sperm count is zero for two consecutive semen analyses.
  - STI protection must be considered as appropriate.
8. *Couple using symptothermal method of natural family planning*
   a. *Components:* BBT, cervical mucus, secondary cycle phase–related symptoms
   b. *Assessing BBT and cervical mucus:*
      - BBT: see Guidelines box, BBT and Fig. 7-7 and 7-8.
      - Cervical mucus: see Guidelines box, Cervical Mucus Characteristics.
   c. *Effectiveness:* typical effectiveness rate for all fertility awareness methods is 25% during the first year of use.
9. *Woman contemplating elective abortion (see Abortion section).*
   a. *Nursing diagnosis:* decisional conflict related to unplanned pregnancy and need to complete education.
   b. *Describe approach:* use therapeutic communication techniques to establish trusting relationship; discuss alternatives available to her and the consequences of each; nurse facilitates decision making process and the patient makes the decision; make appropriate referrals to help her with the decision.
   c. *Purpose of Laminaria and procedure for vacuum aspiration:*
      - *Laminaria* is used to dilate cervix after 8 weeks of gestation; inserted 4 to 24 hours before the procedure.
      - *Aspiration:* vaginal area is cleansed; procedure takes 5 minutes; prepare her for menstrual-like cramping and sound of the machine.
   d. *Nursing diagnoses:* consider fear/anxiety, anticipatory grieving, risk for infection, pain, risk for deficient fluid volume.
   e. *Nursing measures for care and support:* assess physical condition, checking for bleeding and ability to void; keep her informed; provide support and comfort measures, rest for 1 to 3 hours before discharge; provide time for her to talk about her feelings about the experience and make referrals as needed.

   f. *Discharge instructions:* discuss hygiene measures to prevent infection; signs of complications (bleeding, infection); activity restrictions; resumption of sexual relations and use of birth control and safer sex measures; arrange for follow-up appointment and stress importance of keeping it.
10. *Woman seeking assistance following unprotected intercourse* (see Emergency Contraception section).
    - Explore possibility of pregnancy and options related to continuing pregnancy if it occurs, keeping baby, adoption.
    - Explore options for emergency contraception to prevent pregnancy: methods available, how each works, timing, side effects, how administered.
    - Emphasize importance of follow-up to check for effectiveness of method used and occurrence of infection.
    - Discuss methods of contraception and safer sex measures to prevent recurrence of this situation.

CHAPTER 8: GENETICS, CONCEPTION, AND FETAL DEVELOPMENT

I. Reviewing Key Concepts and Content

1. Conception
2. Gametes, sperm, ovum (egg)
3. Gametogenesis, spermatogenesis, oogenesis
4. Fertilization, ampulla, zona reaction, diploid (46)
5. Zygote, morula, blastocyst, trophoblast
6. Implantation, endometrium, chorionic villi, trophoblast, decidua, decidua basalis, decidua capsularis
7. Embryo
8. Fetus
9. Amniotic membranes, chorion, amnion
10. Amniotic fluid
11. Umbilical cord, arteries, vein, Wharton's jelly
12. Placenta, cotyledons, hormones, oxygen, nutrients, wastes, carbon dioxide
13. Viability
14. Surfactants, lecithin-sphingomyelin
15. Ductus arteriosus
16. Ductus venosus
17. Foramen ovale
18. Hematopoiesis
19. Quickening, 16, 20
20. Meconium
21. Dizygotic, fraternal
22. Monozygotic, identical

23. e	24. b	25. m	26. h	27. k	28. c
29. l	30. i	31. r	32. a	33. q	34. f
35. u	36. o	37. g	38. t	39. d	40. n
41. p	42. s	43. j			

44. *Functions of yolk sac, amniotic fluid and membranes, umbilical cord, placenta:* see individual sections for each of these structures in the embryo and fetus

45. T	46. F	47. T	48. T	49. F	50. T
51. T	52. F	53. F	54. T	55. F	56. T
57. T	58. F	59. F	60. T	61. F	62. F

63. *Complete table related to primary germ layers:* see Primary Germ Layers section of the Embryo and Fetus for identification of tissues and organs that develop from the ectoderm, mesoderm, endoderm.

64. *Factors that determine risk for inheritable disorders* (see Fig. 8-1, a risk factors questionnaire): ask questions that would elicit information regarding health status of family members, abnormal reproductive outcomes, history of maternal disorders, drug exposures, and illnesses, advanced maternal and paternal age, and ethnic origin.

65. *Explain each type of inheritance and give an example:*
    a. *Unifactorial inheritance:* inheritable characteristic is controlled by a single gene that can be dominant or recessive; Marfan's syndrome, Huntington's chorea, achondroplasia
    b. *Multifactorial inheritance:* congenital disorder resulting from a combination of genetic and environmental factors; cleft lip and palate, congenital heart defects, neural tube defects
    c. *X-linked inheritance:* transmission of abnormal genes on X-chromosome; can be recessive or dominant; both males and females can be affected but females are usually carriers; if expressed in females it tends to be less severe because they have a normal gene on their second chromosome

66. Choice d is correct; genotype is the entire genetic makeup whereas phenotype is the manner in which the genotype is expressed in the person's physical appearance.

67. Choice a is correct; autosomal dominant inheritance is unrelated to exposure to teratogens; each pregnancy has the same potential for expression of the disorder; there is no reduction if one child is already affected; if the gene is inherited, the disorder is always expressed.

68. Choice b is correct; there is a 25% chance females will be carriers; if males inherit the X-chromosome with the defective gene, the disorder will be expressed and they can transmit the gene to female offspring; females are affected if they receive the defective gene from both parents.

69. Choice d is correct; cystic fibrosis, as an inborn error of metabolism, follows an autosomal recessive pattern of inheritance; two defective genes (one from each parent) are required for the disorder to be expressed; she does not have the disorder and the father does not have the defective gene, therefore, none of their children will have the disorder but there will be a 50% chance they will be carriers of the defective gene.

70. Choice c is correct; feeling of movement is called quickening; the sex of a baby is determined at conception; the heart begins to pump blood by the third week, and a beat can be heard with ultrasound by the eighth week of gestation

II. Thinking Critically

1. *Questions from pregnant women to nurse midwife during prenatal care:*
   a. *Progress of development at 2 months, 5 months, and 7 months:* see Table 8-2 to formulate your answer; use of illustrations and life-size models would facilitate learning.
   b. *Survival after 35 weeks' gestation:* discuss how the respiratory system develops including the critical factor surfactant production; describe how surfactant helps the newborn breathe.
   c. *Quickening:* explain that this is the woman's perception of fetal movement that occurs at about 16 to 20 weeks of gestation; use Box 8-5 to describe how the fetus moves; it will not hurt but can be uncomfortable and interfere with sleep toward the end of pregnancy; fetus will develop its own sleep-wake cycle.
   d. *Fetal-sensory perception:* discuss sensory capability of the fetus using Sensory Awareness subsection of Fetal Maturation section; fetus can hear sounds such as parents' voices, respond to light and touch, and perceive temperature and taste.
   e. *Sex determination:* discuss function of X and Y chromosomes; sex of her fetus will become recognizable around 12 weeks of gestation.
   f. *Multiple gestation—twins:* discuss monozygotic (identical) and dizygotic (fraternal) twinning and how each occurs; emphasize that fraternal twinning tends to occur in families.

2. Couple facing a genetic disorder:
   a. *Nurse's role in determining genetic risk:* Tay-Sachs is an autosomal recessive disorder that follows a unifactorial pattern of inheritance; Mr. G. needs to be tested because he must also be a carrier to produce a child with the disorder; emphasize the nurse's role in terms of emotional support, facilitation of the decision-making process, and interpretation of diagnostic test results and how they can influence future childbearing decisions.
   b. *Inheritance possibility when both parents carry the defective recessive gene:* there is a 25% chance child will be normal, a 25% chance that child will express the disorder, and a 50% chance that child will be a carrier; this pattern is the same for every pregnancy; there is no reduction in risk from one pregnancy to another.

c. *Education and emotional support*: discuss the nature of this disorder, extent of risk, and consequences if the child inherits the disorder; options available including amniocentesis, continuing or not continuing the pregnancy if the child is affected; use of reproductive technology or adoption; be sensitive to cultural and religious beliefs; encourage expression of feelings; refer for further counseling or support groups as appropriate.

CHAPTER 9:   ASSESSMENT FOR RISK FACTORS

I.   Reviewing Key Concepts and Content

1. F	2. F	3. T	4. T	5. F	6. F
7. T	8. T	9. T	10. F	11. T	12. F
13. T	14. F	15. F	16. T	17. F	

18. *Factors placing a pregnant woman and her fetus/newborn at risk:* see Box 9-1, which describes several risk factors in each category listed.

19. *Role of nurse when caring for high risk pregnant women undergoing antepartal testing:* see Nurse's Role in Antepartal Assessment for Risk section; answer should emphasize education, support measures as well as assisting with or performing the test and follow-up care.

20. *Woman scheduled for vaginal ultrasound* (see Ultrasonography section):
    a. *Cite reason for test for this woman:* to determine location of gestational sac because PID could have resulted in narrowing of fallopian tube, thereby increasing risk for ectopic pregnancy; in addition, a determination of gestational age and estimation of date of birth would be done related to irregular cycles and unknown date of last menstrual period (LMP).
    b. *Preparation for the test:* explain purpose of test, how it will be performed, and how it will feel; assist her into a lithotomy position or supine position with hips elevated on a pillow; point out structures on monitor as test is performed.

21. *Nurse's role in abdominal ultrasound for monitoring fetal growth:* see Ultrasonography section; instruct woman to come for test with full bladder if appropriate; explain purpose of test and method of examination; assist her into a supine position with head and shoulders elevated on pillow and hip slightly tipped to right or left side; observe for supine hypotension during test and orthostatic hypotension when rising to upright position after test; indicate how the fetus is being measured and point out fetus and its movements.

22. *Risk factors for pregnancy-related problems:* see Box 9-3, which lists risk factors for each pregnancy-related problem identified.

23. High risk pregnancy

24. Fetal compromise, asphyxia, fetal anomalies, intrauterine environment

25. Daily fetal movement count, 12 hours, 3 movements within 1 hour, nonstress test, contraction stress test, biophysical profile, sleep cycle, depressant, alcohol, smoking a cigarette, decrease

26. Ultrasonography, abdominally, vaginally, transabdominally, transvaginally, vagina, pelvic, intrauterine pregnancy, ectopic, embryo, abnormalities, gestational age

27. Doppler blood flow analysis, hypertension, intrauterine growth restriction, diabetes mellitus, multiple fetuses, preterm labor

28. Biophysical profile, ultrasonography, fetal monitoring, fetal breathing movements, body or limb movement, fetal tone/posture, cardiotocogram (nonstress test), amniotic fluid volume, biophysical, central nervous system, hypoxemic

29. Magnetic resonance imaging

30. Amniocentesis, transabdominally, amniotic fluid, genetic, congenital, pulmonary, hemolytic

31. Percutaneous umbilical blood sampling (PUBS), cordocentesis, blood sampling, transfusion, umbilical vessel

32. Chorionic villus sampling, genetic makeup, 10, 12

33. Maternal serum alpha-fetoprotein, 15, 22

34. Triple marker, 16, 18, maternal serum alpha-fetoprotein, unconjugated estriol, human chorionic gonadotropin, age

35. Nonstress, fetal activity, accelerate

36. Contraction stress, late deceleration, nipple-stimulated contraction stress, oxytocin-stimulated contraction stress

37. Choice d is correct; an amniocentesis with analysis of amniotic fluid for the L/S ratio and presence of phosphatidylglycerol (Pg) is used to determine pulmonary maturity; choice b refers to a contraction stress test; choice c refers to serial measurements of fetal growth using ultrasound.

38. Choice c is correct; food/fluid is not restricted before the test to stimulate fetal movement; the test will evaluate the response of the fetal heart rate (FHR) to fetal movement—acceleration is expected; external not internal monitoring is used.

39. Choice b is correct; the triple marker test is used to screen the older pregnant woman for the possibility that her fetus has Down syndrome; serum levels of alpha fetoprotein (AFP), unconjugated estriol, and hCG are measured; maternal serum alpha-fetoprotein alone is the screening test for open neural tube defects such as spina bifida; a 1 hour, 50 g glucose test is used to screen for gestational diabetes; amniocentesis would be used to check for Rh antibodies.

40. Choice c is correct; a suspicious result is recorded when late decelerations occur with less than 50% of the contractions; a negative test result is recorded when no late decelerations occur during at least 3 uterine contractions lasting 40 to 60 seconds each, within a 10 minute period; a positive test is recorded when there are persistent late decelerations with more than 50% of the contractions; unsatisfactory is the result recorded when there is a failure to achieve adequate uterine contractions.

41. Choice a is correct; a supine position with hips elevated enhance the view of the uterus; a lithotomy position may also be used; a full bladder is not required for the vaginal ultrasound but would be needed for most abdominal ultrasounds; during the test the woman may experience some pressure but medication for pain before the test is not required; contact gel is used with the abdominal ultrasound; water-soluble lubricant may be used to ease insertion of the vaginal probe.

II. Thinking Critically

1. *Woman having biophysical profile* (see Table 9-4 for identification of variables tested; scoring):
   a. Nursing diagnosis: anxiety related to unexpected need to undergo a biophysical profile.
   b. *Nurse's response to woman's concern about the test:* describe how the test will be performed using ultrasound and external electronic fetal monitoring; explain that the purpose of the test is to view the fetus within its environment, to determine the amount of amniotic fluid, and assess the FHR response to fetal activity.
   c. *Meaning of score obtained:* a score of 8 to 10 is a normal result.

2. *Amniocentesis* (see Amniocentesis section and Nurse's Role in Antepartal Assessment for Risk section:
   a. *Preparing woman:* explain procedure, witness informed consent, assess maternal vital signs and health status and FHR before the test; ensure that ultrasound is performed to locate placenta and fetus before the test.
   b. *Supporting woman during the procedure:* explain what is happening and what she will be feeling; help her relax; encourage her to ask questions and voice concerns and feelings; assess her reactions.
   c. *Postprocedure care and instructions:* monitor maternal vital signs and status and FHR; tell her when test results should be available and whom to call; administer RhoGAM since she is Rh negative; teach her to assess herself for signs of infection, bleeding, rupture of membranes, and uterine contractions; make a follow-up phone call to check her status.

3. *Nonstress test* (see Nonstress Test subsection of Electronic Fetal Monitoring section):
   a. *Tell woman about purpose of test:* test measures response of FHR to fetal activity to determine adequacy of placental perfusion and fetal oxygenation.
   b. *Preparation of woman for test:* tell her that she can eat before and during the test; schedule test at a time of day that fetus is usually active; assist woman into a semi recumbent or seated position.
   c. *Indicate how test is conducted:* attach tocotransducer to fundus and Doppler transducer at site of point of maximum intensity (PMI); instruct woman to indicate when fetus moves; assess change, if any, in FHR following the movement.
   d. *Analyze the results:* see Table 9-6 for the criteria to determine the test result and to document it as reactive: good variability and normal baseline with accelerations following fetal movement that meet criteria for a reactive result; as nonreactive—no accelerations with movement or the accelerations that do occur do not meet the criteria and limited variability; or as unsatisfactory: quality of FHR recording is inadequate.

4. *Contraction stress test* (see Contraction Stress Test subsection of Electronic Fetal Monitoring section):
   a. *Tell woman about purpose of test:* the test is a way of determining how her fetus will react to the stress of uterine contractions as they would occur during labor; uterine contractions decrease perfusion through placenta leading to fetal hypoxia; late decelerations during this test could be interpreted as an early warning of fetal compromise.
   b. *Preparation:* assess woman's vital signs, general health status, and contraindications for the test; attach external electronic fetal monitor and assess FHR and uterine activity; assist woman into a lateral, semi recumbent, or seated position.
   c. *Indicate how the test is performed:* see Protocol for a Nipple-Stimulation Contraction Stress Test; stimulate nipple(s) according to protocol until 3 contractions of good quality occur in a 10 minute period; make sure that contractions subside after the test and assess maternal and fetal responses.
   d. *Use of oxytocin to stimulate contractions:* see Protocol for an Oxytocin-Stimulated Contraction Stress Test; administer Pitocin intravenously (similar to induction of labor but with lower dosages) according to protocol, increasing rate until uterine contractions meet

criteria indicated for a Nipple-Stimulated Contraction Stress Test; monitor woman, fetus, and contractions during the test and afterward until contractions subside.

e. *Analyze the results:* see Table 9-7 for criteria used to interpret the test results and to document it as negative—no late decelerations are noted; as positive—late decelerations with more than half of the contractions, limited variability; suspicious—late decelerations with less than half of the contractions; hyperstimulation—late decelerations with excessive uterine contractions or tone; or unsatisfactory—recording is inadequate.

CHAPTER 10: ANATOMY AND PHYSIOLOGY OF PREGNANCY

I. Reviewing Key Concepts and Content

1. Gravidity
2. Parity
3. Gravida
4. Nulligravida
5. Nullipara
6. Primigravida
7. Primipara
8. Multigravida
9. Multipara
10. Viability
11. Preterm
12. Term
13. Postdate, postterm
14. Human chorionic gonadotropin (hCG)
15. c 16. p 17. k 18. t 19. s 20. u
21. j 22. n 23. v 24. b 25. g 26. a
27. o 28. i 29. q 30. e 31. m 32. w
33. f 34. h 35. d 36. r 37. l
38. *Complete table regarding signs and symptoms of pregnancy:* see Table 10-2 and Signs of Pregnancy section to insert information into this table regarding presumptive, probable, and positive signs and symptoms of pregnancy.
39. *Obstetric history:* Nancy (1-1-0-1 or 3-1-1-0-1); Marsha (2-0-1-2 or 4-2-0-1-2); Linda (1-1-1-3 or 4-1-1-1-3)
40. T 41. T 42. F 43. T 44. F 45. T
46. T 47. F 48. F 49. T 50. T 51. F
52. T 53. F 54. T 55. T 56. F 57. T
58. T
59. *Changes in vital signs as pregnancy progresses:*
a. and b. Blood pressure and heart rate patterns: see Box 10-3; systolic and diastolic blood pressure decrease in the second trimester by 5 to 10 mm Hg and return to first trimester levels during the third trimester; pulse increases during the second trimester by 10 to 15 beats per minute; murmurs and palpitations can occur.

c. Respiratory patterns: see Box 10-4; breathing becomes more thoracic in nature and volume is deeper with a slight increase in rate; some shortness of breath may be experienced in the second trimester as the diaphragm is pushed up the enlarging uterus; continues until lightening occurs.

d. *Temperature:* baseline temperature increases by about 0.4° to 0.8°C as a result of the increase in BMR and the progesterone effect; women may complain of heat intolerance.

60. Mean arterial pressure (MAP) calculation: use the following formula (see Box 10-2):

$$\frac{\text{Systolic} + 2(\text{diastolic})}{3}$$

Answers are 91, 81, 90, 110.

61. *Specify value changes for selected laboratory tests during pregnancy:*
a. *CBC:* see Box 10-3 and Table 10-3.
b. *Clotting activity:* see Circulation and Coagulation Times section of Cardiopulmonary System and Table 10-3.
c. *Acid-base balance:* see Acid-Base Balance section and Table 10-3.
d. *Urinalysis:* see Box 10-5 and Fluid and Electrolyte section.

62. *Expected adaptations in elimination during pregnancy:*
a. *Renal:* see Renal System section; slowed passage of more alkaline urine and dilation of the ureters as a result of progesterone increases the risk for UTIs; bladder irritability, nocturia, urinary frequency and urgency (first and third trimester after lightening).
b. *Bowel:* see Esophagus, Stomach, and Intestines section; constipation and hemorrhoids; effect of increased progesterone, which decreases peristalsis and intestinal displacement by enlarging uterus

63. *Changes in endocrine function and secretions of hormones:* see Table 10-4 for a description of each hormone and how it changes with pregnancy.

64. Choice a is correct; hCG indicates a positive pregnancy test and is a probable sign; breast tenderness and morning sickness are presumptive signs; fetal heart sounds are a positive sign of pregnancy.

65. Choice d is correct; gravida (total number of pregnancies including the present one is 5); para (term birth of daughter at 39 weeks = 1; stillbirth at 32 weeks and triplets at 30 weeks = 2; spontaneous abortion at 8 weeks = 1; total number of living children = 4).

66. Choice c is correct; while little change occurs in respiratory rate, breathing becomes more thoracic in nature with the upward displacement of the diaphragm; women normally experience a greater awareness to breathe and may even complain of dyspnea at rest as pregnancy progresses; supine hypotension syndrome with a decrease in systolic pressure as much as 30 mm Hg occurs as a result of vena cava and aorta compression by the uterus when the woman is in a supine position; baseline pulse rate increases by 10 to 15 beats per minute; systolic and diastolic pressure decreases by approximately 5 to 10 mm Hg beginning in the second trimester returning to first trimester levels in the third trimester.

67. Choice d is correct; recording cycle information assists with accuracy of diagnosis; choice c reflects the most common error of performing this test too soon; she will need to repeat the test in 1 week if the result is negative; first-voided morning specimens should be used since they are the most concentrated and apt to have the largest amount of hCG; anticonvulsants, tranquilizers, diuretics, and promethazine can result in inaccurate results.

68. Choice b is correct; friability refers to cervical fragility resulting in slight bleeding when scraped or touched; Chadwick's sign refers to a deep bluish color of cervix and vagina as a result of increased circulation; Hegar's sign refers to softening and compressibility of the lower uterine segment.

II. Thinking Critically

1. *Responses to patient concerns and questions:*
   a. *Spotting after intercourse:* discuss cervical and vaginal friability and increased vascularity; makes the vagina and cervix softer and more delicate so spotting after intercourse is expected; caution that any bleeding should be reported so it can be evaluated.
   b. *Use of home pregnancy test:* emphasize the importance of following directions because each brand of test is slightly different; use first-voided morning specimen for the most concentrated urine and notify health care provider regardless of the test result.
   c. *Bladder and vaginal infections:* discuss impact of increased vaginal secretions and impact of stasis of urine that contains nutrients and has a high pH; review prevention measures at this time.
   d. *Breast changes with pregnancy:* discuss changes in breasts such as enlargement of Montgomery's glands and development of lactation structures resulting in larger breasts that are tender during the first trimester;

changes in consistency and presence of lumpiness during BSE; changes are bilateral.
   e. *Effects of pregnant woman's position:* discuss supine hypotensive syndrome and importance of the lateral position when at rest.
   f. *Nosebleeds:* discuss impact of estrogen stimulated increase in upper airway vascularity, which increases edema, congestion, and hyperemia of the tissue making nose bleeds more common.
   g. *Ankle edema:* explain that the swelling of her ankles is a result of the pressure of the enlarging uterus and the dependent position of her legs; elevating her legs and exercising them helps decrease edema; caution her to never take someone else's medications or to self-medicate herself.
   h. *Posture and low back pain:* lordosis occurs as a result of the enlargement of the uterus, which decreases abdominal muscle tone and increases mobility of the pelvic joints, tilting the pelvis forward and resulting in lower back pain, a change in posture, and a shifting forward of the change of gravity.
   i. *Braxton Hicks:* the woman is describing false labor contractions because they diminish with activity; these contractions facilitate blood flow and promote oxygen delivery to the fetus; compare these contractions with true labor contractions.
   j. *Shortness of breath (SOB):* explain that what she is experiencing is a result of increased sensitivity of her respiratory center to carbon dioxide and the elevation of her diaphragm by the enlarging uterus; assess the woman for signs of pulmonary edema to be sure the SOB is physiologic rather than pathologic.

2. *Blood pressure protocol:* consider the effects of maternal age, activity and stress level, health status, arm, and position; protocol should emphasize consistency in arm and position used, size of cuff, time provided for relaxation before measurement; repeat if finding is inconsistent with woman's baseline or is abnormal.

CHAPTER 11: NURSING CARE DURING PREGNANCY

I. Reviewing Key Concepts and Content

1. Nägele's, estimated date of birth (EDB), 3 months, 7 days, 1 year, last menstrual period (LMP), 7 days, first day of last menstrual period, 9 months, trimesters,
2. Supine hypotension, vena cava, aorta, pallor, dizziness, faintness, breathlessness, tachycardia, nausea, clammy skin, sweating

3. Fundal height, pinch
4. Fetal movement, fetal heart rate pattern, fundal height, gestational age
5. Developmental, accepting pregnancy, identifying with role of parent, reordering personal relationships, establishing relationship with fetus, preparing for childbirth
6. Biologic fact of pregnancy, "I am pregnant," growing fetus as distinct from herself, person to nurture, "I am going to have a baby," birth, parenting of the child, "I am going to be a mother"
7. Emotional lability
8. Ambivalence
9. Couvade
10. Prescriptions, proscriptions, taboos
11. Triple screen, Down syndrome, 16, 18, alpha-fetoprotein, human chorionic gonadotropin, unconjugated estriol
12. Calculate expected date of birth: use Nägele's rule: subtract 3 months and add 7 days, and 1 year to the first day of the last menstrual period
    a. February 12, 2006
    b. October 21, 2005
    c. April 11, 2006
13. *Cultural beliefs and practices:* see Cultural Influences subsection of Variations in Prenatal Care section:
    a. *Describe how cultural beliefs affect participation in prenatal care:* consider the following factors: beliefs that conflict with typical Western prenatal practices, lack of money and transportation, communication difficulties, concern regarding modesty and gender of health care provider, fear of invasive procedures, view of pregnancy as a healthy state whereas health care providers imply illness, view pregnancy problems as a normal part of pregnancy.
    b. *Prescriptions and proscriptions:* see specific subsections for emotional responses, clothing, physical activity and rest, sexual activity, diet.
14. *Complete table regarding components of initial and follow-up visits;* see subsections for the Initial Visit and Follow-up Visits in the Care Management assessment section.
15. *Components of fetal assessment:* measurement of fundal height, determination of gestational age, assessment of health status of the fetus, including FHR pattern, fetal movements, and unusual or abnormal maternal or fetal signs and symptoms; see specific subsections for each component in the Follow-up Visits section.
16. *Warning signs of potential complications during pregnancy*
    a. *List signs of complications:* see Box 11-5 Signs of Potential Complications, which lists signs according to the first, second, and third trimesters.

b. *Nursing approach when discussing signs of complications with pregnant woman and her family:*
   - Discuss the signs, possible causes, when and to whom to report.
   - Present the signs verbally and in written form.
   - Provide time to answer questions and discuss concerns; make follow-up phone calls.
   - Gather full information of signs that are reported; use information as a basis for action.
   - Document all assessments, actions, and responses.

17. T	18. F	19. T	20. T	21. T	22. F
23. F	24. F	25. F	26. T	27. T	28. F
29. T	30. F	31. F	32. T	33. T	34. T
35. F	36. T	37. T	38. T	39. T	40. F
41. T					

42. *Protocol for fundal measurement:* consider woman's position, type of measuring tape used, measurement method (Fig. 11-8), and conditions of the examination such as an empty bladder and relaxed or contracted uterus.
43. *Factors used to estimate gestational age:* menstrual history, contraceptive history, pregnancy test result, and specific findings related to the maternal-fetal unit, for example, time of appearance of the specific signs of pregnancy, uterine size/fundal height, ultrasound examination.
44. *Prevention of injury:*
    a. *Principles of body mechanics:* see Figs. 11-14 and Home Care box related to Posture and Body Mechanics.
    b. *Safety Guidelines:* see Patient Teaching box, Safety during Pregnancy and prevention measures identified in subsections of Education for Self-Care section such as physical activity, rest and relaxation, employment, clothing, and travel.
45. *Contraindications for breastfeeding:* deep-seated aversion to breastfeeding by woman or partner, need to take certain medications that can be harmful to the newborn, medical disorders such as active tuberculosis, newly diagnosed breast cancer, and HIV-positive status (in developed countries).
46. *Male styles of involvement in pregnancy:* see Family Focus box, Paternal Adaptation for a description of each involvement style listed: observer, expressive, instrumental.
47. Choice b is correct; choices a and c are probable signs and choice d is a positive sign, diagnostic of pregnancy.
48. Choice a is correct; use Nägele's rule by subtracting 3 months and adding 7 days and 1 year to the first day of the last menstrual period, which in this case is September 10, 2005.

49. Choice d is correct; supine hypotension related to compression of aorta and vena cava is being experienced; the first action is to remove the cause of the problem by turning the woman on her side; this should alleviate the symptoms being experienced, including nausea; assessment of vital signs can occur after the woman's position is changed.

50. Choice c is correct; during this quiet period a woman focuses on her fantasy child; sexual desire is decreased during the first and third trimesters and is increased in second; ambivalence is a common response when preparing for a new role; safe passage and birth preparation is a concern during the third trimester.

51. Choice a is correct; intake of at least 2 to 3 liters per day is recommended; choices b, c, and d are all accepted methods of preventing urinary tract infections along with frequent, regular urination, good genital hygiene, and avoiding wearing tight-fitting jeans for long periods.

52. Choice d is correct; continuous support is critical and involves praise, encouragement, reassurance, comfort measures, physical contact, as well as explanations; the doula does not get involved in clinical tasks; she is not a substitute for the father but rather encourages his participation as a partner with her in supporting the laboring woman.

II. Thinking Critically

1. *Health history interview:* see Initial Visit and Follow-up Visits subsections of Assessment section.
   a. *Purpose of the health history interview:*
      - Establish therapeutic relationship with the pregnant woman and her family
      - Planned time for purposeful communication to gather baseline data related to the woman's subjective appraisal of her health status and to gather objective information based on observation of the woman's affect, posture, body language, skin color, and other physical and emotional signs
      - Update information and compare to baseline information during follow-up interviews
   b. *Write for each component of initial health history interview:* be sure questions reflect principles of effective questioning; consider the need to ask follow-up questions to clarify and gather further information when a problem is identified.
   c. *Write four questions for the follow-up health history interviews:* focus on updating baseline information and asking questions related to anticipated events and changes for the woman's gestational age at the time of the visit.

2. *Care of woman at initial visit who is anxious and unsure about prenatal care:* answer should emphasize
   - Establishing a therapeutic, trusting relationship so woman will feel comfortable continuing with prenatal care
   - Teaching the woman about the importance of prenatal care for her health and that of her baby
   - Involving her boyfriend in the care process so he will encourage her participation in prenatal care
   - Following guidelines for health history interview, physical examination, and laboratory testing; ensure privacy and comfort during the examination and teach her about how her body is changing and will continue to change with pregnancy
   - Evaluating the desire for this pregnancy and the need for community agency support

3. *Couple during first trimester—concerns and questions:*
   a. *Accuracy of EDB:* reliability depends on the accuracy of date used and the regularity of her menstrual cycles; birth can normally occur 2 weeks before or after the date or from week 38 to 42.
   b. *Kegel exercises:* pelvic muscle exercises to maintain muscle tone and ability to support pelvic organs; see Kegel Exercises subsection of Education for Self-Care section and Patient Teaching box, Kegel Exercises.
   c. *Effect of pregnancy on sexuality:* see Sexual Counseling section, Guidelines box, Sexuality in Pregnancy, and Fig. 11-21; emphasize that intercourse is safe as long as pregnancy is progressing normally and it is comfortable for the woman; sexual expression should be in tune with the woman's changing needs and emotions; inform that spotting can normally occur related to the fragility of the vaginal mucosa and cervix and that changes in positions and activities may be helpful as pregnancy progresses.
   d. *Morning sickness:* see Table 11-2 (first trimester section); fully assess what she is experiencing, then discuss why it happens, how long it will likely last, and relief measures that are safe and effective (also see Coping with Nutritional-Related Discomforts of Pregnancy section of Chapter 12).

4. *Physical activity and exercise in pregnancy:* see Physical Activity subsection of the Education for Self-Care section and Home Care box, Exercise Tips for Pregnant Women; assess her usual pattern of exercise and activity and consider their safety during pregnancy; discuss precautions and guidelines for safe, effective exercise; emphasize that moderate physical activity benefits her and her baby and will prepare her for the work of labor and birth; caution her to take note of the effects of exercise in terms of temperature, heart rate, and feeling of well-being.

5. *Nursing diagnoses, expected outcomes and nursing measures for women in various situations during pregnancy:*

   a. *Risk for urinary tract infection related to lack of knowledge regarding changes of the renal system during pregnancy:*
      • Woman will drink at least 2 to 3 liters of fluids per day; will empty bladder at first urge.
      • Explain changes that occur in the renal system during pregnancy; increase fluid intake, use acid-ash forming fluids, void frequently to keep bladder empty, perform good perineal hygiene, use lateral position to enhance renal perfusion and urine formation.

   b. *Pain in lower back related to neuromuscular changes associated with pregnancy at 23 weeks of gestation:*
      • Woman will experience lessening of lower back pain following implementation of suggested relief measures.
      • Explain basis for lower back pain and relief measures, including back massage, pelvic rock, and posture changes (see Table 11-2 and Fig. 11-13); encourage woman to change her footwear for better stability and safety.

   c. *Anxiety related to lack of knowledge concerning the process of labor and birth and appropriate measures to cope with the pain and discomfort:*
      • Couple will enroll in a childbirth education program in the seventh month of pregnancy.
      • Explain the childbirth process and describe the many nonpharmacologic and pharmacologic measures to relieve pain; discuss role of coach and possibility of hiring a doula; make a referral to a childbirth education program and assist with the preparation of a birth plan; discuss childbirth options and prebirth preparations.

6. Woman in the second trimester—questions and concerns:

   a. *Purpose of fundal height:* indirect assessment of how her fetus is growing.

   b. *Determining fetal health status:* discuss FHR (let her listen) and fetal movement assessments (tell her how); begin week 27.

   c. *Clothing choices during pregnancy:* consider safety and comfort in terms of low-heeled shoe and nonrestrictive clothing.

   d. *Gas and constipation:* see Table 11-2 (second trimester section); assess problem and lifestyle factors that may be contributing to the problem; discuss why it occurs and appropriate relief measures (fluids, roughage, activity).

   e. *Itchiness:* if the woman is experiencing noninflammatory pruritus, use Table 11-2 (second trimester section) for basis of discomfort and relief measures; be sure to rule out rashes related to infection or allergic reactions.

   f. *Travel during pregnancy:* see Travel subsection of Self-Care section; tell her that she may travel if her pregnancy is progressing normally; emphasize importance of staying hydrated, wearing seat belt, doing breathing and lower extremities exercises, ambulating every hour for 15 minutes, and voiding every 2 hours.

7. *Woman experiencing supine hypotension syndrome* (see Emergency Box, Supine Hypotension):

   a. *Explanation of assessment findings:* supine hypotension.

   b. *Immediate action:* turn her on her side and maintain the position until vital signs stabilize and signs and symptoms diminish; place wedge to maintain a lateral tilt then continue the assessment; when completed, help her to rise slowly to an upright position— observe for signs of postural hypotension (decrease in blood pressure when rising from a supine to an upright position).

8. *Woman during third trimester—questions and concerns:*

   a. *Nipple condition for breastfeeding:* perform pinch test to see if nipples will evert; if they do not, the woman can be taught to use a nipple shell to help her nipples protrude; no special exercises are recommended because they could stimulate preterm labor in susceptible woman as a result of secretion of oxytocin; keep nipples and areola clean and dry.

   b. *Ankle edema:* see Table 11-2 (third trimester section); discuss basis of the edema and encourage use of lower extremities exercises and elevation of legs periodically during the day (Fig. 11-17); emphasize importance of fluid intake.

c. *Leg cramps:* see Table 11-2 (third trimester section) and Fig. 11-18; discuss basis of leg cramps then demonstrate relief measures such as pressing weight onto foot when standing or dorsiflexing the foot while lying in bed; avoid pointing the toes; ensure adequate intake of calcium.

9. *Woman concerned about preterm labor:*

a. *Nursing diagnosis:* anxiety related to perceived risk for preterm labor and birth; woman will identify signs suggestive of preterm labor and the action to take if they occur.

b. *Signs of preterm labor:* see Home Care box, How to Recognize Preterm Labor and Fig. 11-20; emphasize that signs are vague so she must be alert for even subtle changes; teach her how to palpate her abdomen to detect uterine contractions.

c. *Action if signs are detected:* empty bladder, drink 3 to 4 glasses of water, assume a side-lying position, and count contractions for another hour; if contractions continue call health care provider.

10. *Sibling reactions to mother's pregnancy:* see Sibling Adaptation section of Adaptation to Pregnancy, Family Focus box, Sibling Adaptation to Pregnancy and Birth, and Box 11-1, which provides tips for sibling preparation; emphasize importance of considering each child's developmental level; prepare children for prenatal events, time during hospitalization, and the homecoming of the new baby; refer to sibling classes and encourage sibling visitation after birth; suggest books and videos that parents could use to prepare their children for birth; provide opportunities to spend time with newborns/infants if possible.

11. *Expectant father concerned about wife's mood swings:*

a. *Nursing diagnoses:* deficient knowledge related to pregnant spouse's mood changes; Tom will explain basis for wife's mood swings and strategies that he can use to cope with these changes and support his spouse.

b. *Nurse's response:* see Maternal Adaptation section, Family Focus box, Maternal Adaptation and Table 11-2 (first trimester section); discuss the basis for the mood swings and experiences during the first trimester including ambivalence; identify measures he can use to support her.

12. *Decision making regarding birth setting:* see Birth Setting Choices section; answer should include:
    - Descriptions of each option along with the criteria for use and the advantages and disadvantages.
    - Onsite visits and interaction with health care providers responsible for care at each site should be encouraged.
    - speak to couples who gave birth in these setting to get their impressions.
    - Emphasize that the decision is theirs and that they should choose what is comfortable for them; a decision should be made on the basis of a full understanding of each option.

13. *Doulas (see Care Provider Options section):*

a. *Role of doula:* describe what a doula is, what they do; cite research that illustrates the benefits of using a doula for labor support; emphasize that the doula's role is to provide physical, emotional, and informational care and that her role does not involve the performance of clinical tasks

b. *Finding a doula:* community contacts, other health care professions, especially those involved in childbirth care or education, organizations such a DONA, persons who have used a doula; emphasize the importance of starting early so that there is time to make the right choice.

c. *Questions to ask during an interview with a prospective doula:* use Box 11-19 for question ideas; discuss these questions with the woman and put them in writing so that the woman will have them to refer to during the interview.

14. *Home birth (see Home Birth subsection of Birth Setting Choices section):*

a. *Discuss decision-making process:*
   - Fully review advantages and disadvantages of home birth so an informed decision can be made and appropriate arrangements can be devised to enhance the advantages and offset the disadvantages.
   - Speak to couples who have experienced a home birth.

b. *Preparation measures:*
   - Preparation of home including obtaining supplies and equipment, arranging for medical backup and transportation in the event of an emergency; measures to increase safety should be emphasized.
   - Choosing and preparing the persons who will be attending, including children and grandparents.

CHAPTER 12: MATERNAL AND FETAL NUTRITION

I. Reviewing Key Concepts and Content

1. Healthful diet before conception, folic acid (folate), neural tube defects, 400 mcg
2. Intrauterine growth restriction, low birth weight (LBW), preterm, small for gestational age (SGA)
3. Macrosomia, fetopelvic disproportion, operative birth, emergency cesarean birth, birth trauma, postpartum hemorrhage, fetal mortality

4. Age, activity level, current weight, number of fetuses, gestation, energy, 300 kcal
5. Pregnant adolescents, poor women, women adhering to unusual diets
6. Iron deficiency anemia, adolescents, African-American women
7. Lactose intolerance
8. Pica, clay, dirt, laundry starch, ice, baking powder, baking soda, cornstarch, food cravings, nutrients
9. Obstetric/gynecologic effects on nutrition, medical history, usual maternal diet, anthropometric (body), height, weight, body mass index (BMI)
10. Vegetables, fruits, legumes, nuts, seeds, grains, semi-vegetarians, lacto-ovo vegetarians, vegetarians, vegans
11. *Complete table related to nutrient requirement during pregnancy:* see Table 12-1 to complete this activity.
12. *Indicators of nutritional risk:* see Box 12-2 to identify the five risk indicators.
13. *Guidelines for strict vegetarians during pregnancy:* see Vegetarian Diets section of Plan of Care and Interventions.
    - These diets tend to be low in vitamins B$_{12}$ and B$_6$, iron, calcium, zinc, and perhaps calories; supplements may be needed.
    - Food needs to be combined to ensure that all essential amino acids are provided.
14. *Signs of good and inadequate nutrition:* see Table 12-4 for several signs of good and inadequate nutrition.
15. *Nursing measures appropriate for each nursing diagnosis:* see appropriate subsection in Coping with Nutritional-Related Discomforts of Pregnancy section.
    a. *Imbalanced nutrition: less than body requirements related to inadequate intake associated with nausea and vomiting:* see Nausea and Vomiting section for several relief measures.
    b. *Constipation related to decreased intestinal motility associated with effects of increased progesterone and enlarging uterus:* see Constipation section; include adequate fluid and roughage/fiber intake, exercise and activity, regular time for elimination.
    c. *Pain related to reflux of gastric contents into esophagus associated with progesterone effect on gastric motility:* see Pyrosis section; small frequent meals, drink fluids between not with meals, avoid spicy foods, remain upright after eating.
16. *Determining recommended pregnancy weight gain pattern:* see Weight Gain and Pattern of Weight Gain sections to determine weight gain patterns based on each woman's BMI; keep in mind that each woman should gain 1 to 2.5 kg in the first trimester; weight gain per week is recommended for the second and third trimester.

a. June: BMI 21 (normal); total 11.5 to 16 kg; 0.4 kg/week
b. Alice: BMI 29 (overweight); total 7 kg to 11.5 kg; 0.3 kg/week
c. Ann: BMI 16 (underweight); total 12.5 to 18 kg; 0.5 kg/week

17. T 18. F 19. T 20. T 21. F 22. F
23. T 24. T 25. T 26. F 27. F 28. T
29. F 30. T 31. F 32. F 33. T 34. F

35. *Nutrition guidelines for lactation:* adequate calcium intake, a balanced intake of nutrients (about 500 kcal above nonpregnant intake) or at least 1800 kcal/day, adequate fluid intake (should not experience thirst), and avoid tobacco, alcohol, and excessive caffeine.
36. *Factors that increase nutritional needs during pregnancy:* growth and development of uterine-placental-fetal unit, expansion of maternal blood volume and RBCs, mammary changes, increased basal metabolic rate (BMR).
37. Choice d is correct; bran, tea, coffee, milk, oxalate-containing vegetables, and egg yolks all decrease iron absorption; tomatoes and strawberries contain vitamin C, which enhances iron absorption; meats contain heme iron, which also enhances absorption; ideally, iron is best absorbed on an empty stomach and should be taken between, not with, meals.
38. Choice b is correct; BMI indicates woman is at a normal weight; total gain should be 11.5 to 16 kg representing a gain of 0.4 kg/week and 1.6 kg/month during the second and third trimesters
39. Choice c is correct; small, frequent meals are better tolerated than large meals that distend the stomach; hunger can worsen nausea; therefore, meals should not be skipped; dry, starchy foods should be eaten in the morning and at other times during the day when nausea occurs; fried, fatty, and spicy foods should be avoided; a bedtime snack is recommended.
40. Choice b is correct; legumes are a good source for folic acid along with whole grains and fortified cereals, oranges, asparagus, liver, and green leafy vegetables; choices a, c, and d are not good sources of folic acid though they do supply other important nutrients for pregnancy (see Box 12-4).
41. Choice a is correct; up to 6 oz total are suggested for meat, poultry, fish, dry beans, eggs, and nut group during pregnancy; choices b, c, and d are all appropriate for pregnancy; orange juice contains vitamin C will enhance iron absorption (see Table 12-3).

II. Thinking Critically

1. *Nutrition and weight gain concerns during pregnancy:*
   a. *Concern regarding amount of recommended weight gain during pregnancy:*
   - Identify components of maternal weight gain (see Table 12-2); use Fig. 12-2 to illustrate how the weight gain is distributed over weeks of gestation.
   - Discuss impact of maternal weight gain on fetal growth and development; association between inadequate maternal weight gain and low birth weight and infant mortality.
   - Discuss weight gain total and pattern recommended for a woman with a BMI of 18 (underweight).
   b. *Eating for two during pregnancy:*
   - Place emphasis on quality of food that meets nutritional requirements, not on the quantity of food.
   - Discuss expected weight gain total and pattern for a woman with a normal BMI of 21.4.
   - Excessive weight gain during pregnancy may be difficult to lose after pregnancy and could lead to chronic obesity; excessive fetal size and childbirth problems could also result.
   c. *Vitamin supplementation during pregnancy:* determine what and how much she takes; compare to recommendations for pregnancy; discuss potential problems with toxicity, especially with overuse of fat-soluble vitamins.
   d. *Heartburn:* recommend relief measures such as small frequent meals, fluids between not with meals, avoiding spicy, fatty, foods, and remaining upright after meals.
   e. *Weight reduction diets during pregnancy:*
   - BMI indicates overweight status; a gain of 7 to 11.5 kg during pregnancy.
   - Discuss hazards of inadequate caloric intake during pregnancy in terms of growth and development of fetus and pregnancy-related structures; impact of ketoacidosis.
   - Discuss quality foods and development of good nutritional habits to be used during the postpartum period as part of a sensible weight loss program.
   - Discuss importance of exercise and activity during pregnancy.
   f. *Reduction of water intake:* Discuss importance of fluid to meet demands of pregnancy-related changes, regulate temperature, prevent constipation and urinary tract infections (UTIs); consider possible association between dehydration and preterm labor and oligohydramnios.
   g. *Lactose intolerance:* discuss basis for problem; reduce lactose intake by using lactose-free products, nondairy sources of calcium and calcium supplements; take lactase supplements.
   h. *Weight loss lactation:* discuss weight loss patterns with lactation; emphasize that pregnancy fat stores are used during lactation with a resultant weight loss; inform her of increased need for nutrients, calories, and fluids, which are used up with lactogenesis.

2. *Taking iron supplements effectively:* see Iron subsection of Nutrient Needs section, Iron Supplementation subsection of Plan of Care and Implementation, and Table 12-1 for iron sources.
   - Discuss importance of iron.
   - Emphasize importance of vitamin C for iron absorption; discuss food sources high in iron and vitamin C.
   - Discuss ways to take iron supplements to enhance absorption and minimize side effects including GI upset and constipation.

3. *Native-American woman—nutritional needs:*
   a. *Counseling approach:*
   - Assess her current nutritional status and habits; obtain a diet history.
   - Analyze current patterns as a basis for menu planning.
   - Discuss weight gain pattern for an underweight woman.
   - Use a variety of teaching methods; keep woman actively involved.
   - Emphasize importance of good nutrition for herself and her newborn.
   b. *Menu plan:* use Table 12-5 for Native-American foods and Table 12-3 for servings of required nutrients for a 1-day menu; distribute throughout day—meals/snacks.

CHAPTER 13: PREGNANCY AT RISK: PREEXISTING CONDITIONS

I. Reviewing Key Concepts and Content

1. *Interrelationship of the clinical manifestations of diabetes mellitus:* see Pathogenesis section of Diabetes Mellitus for a full description of each of the clinical manifestations listed in terms of cause and interrelationship with one another.
2. Hyperglycemia, insulin secretion, insulin action
3. Polyuria, polydipsia, polyphagia, glycosuria
4. Pregestational
5. Gestational; second half
6. Glucose, conception, pregnancy
7. Hypoglycemia
8. Hyperglycemia, diabetic ketoacidosis (DKA)
9. Glycosylated hemoglobin, 60 mg/dl, 90 mg/dl, 100 to 120 mg/dl, 90 to 120 mg/dl, euglycemia, 60 mg/dl, 120 mg/dl

10. Blood glucose, 30 to 35, 50% to 60%, simple, complex, fiber, 12% to 20%, 20% to 30%, 10%, 12 kg

11. Breakfast, lunch, dinner, 2 hours after meals, bedtime, middle of the night, postprandial hyperglycemia, second, third, increased, hypoglycemia, hyperglycemia, insulin dosage, diet, nausea, vomiting, diarrhea, infection

12. Ketones, diabetic ketoacidosis (DKA)

13. Two-thirds, breakfast, longer acting (NPH), short-acting (regular or lispro), one-third, dinner, hypoglycemia, short-acting, dinner, longer acting, bedtime, short-acting, longer acting

14. *Maternal and fetal/neonatal risks and complications related to pregestational diabetes:* see Maternal Risks/Complications and Fetal Risks/Complications sections
    - *Maternal:* increased rate of childbirth complications, preeclampsia, hydramnios, premature rupture of membranes (PROM), postpartum hemorrhage, infection, hypoglycemia, DKA
    - *Fetal/newborn:* congenital anomalies, macrosomia with related birth injuries, intrauterine growth restriction (IUGR), respiratory distress syndrome (RDS), neonatal hypoglycemia, hypocalcemia, hypomagnesemia, hyperbilirubinemia, polycythemia

15. *Complete table related to metabolic changes in pregnancy and impact on diabetes:* see Metabolic Changes Associated with Pregnancy section of Diabetes Mellitus for a description related to changes associated with pregnancy and the postpartum period.

16. *Recommendations for screening for and diagnosing gestational diabetes:* see Screening for Gestational Diabetes Mellitus section of Care Management of Gestational Diabetes Mellitus.
    - Avoid screening low risk women.
    - Screen with 50 g, 1-hour glucose test at 24 to 28 weeks of gestation.
    - If result is >140 mg/dl (positive screen), follow with a 3-hour, 100 g glucose test.
    - Diagnosis of gestational diabetes is made if more than 2 values of the 3-hour glucose test are met or exceeded.

17. *State effect of thyroid disorders on reproduction and pregnancy:* see Thyroid Disorders section for a description of hyperthyroidism and hypothyroidism; consider effects of these disorders on reproductive development, sexuality, fertility in terms of ability to conceive and to sustain a pregnancy to viability, potential fetal/newborn complications related to maternal treatment of her thyroid disorder.

18. T 19. T 20. F 21. T 22. F 23. F
24. F 25. T 26. T 27. T 28. F 29. F
30. F 31. F 32. T 33. T 34. F 35. F
36. T 37. F 38. T 39. F 40. T 41. F

42. F 43. F 44. T 45. T 46. T 47. F
48. T 49. T 50. F 51. F 52. F 53. T
54. F 55. F 56. T 57. F 58. F 59. T
60. T 61. T 62. F 63. T 64. F

65. *Maternal and fetal complications related to maternal cardiovascular problems:* see Cardiovascular Disorders section; increased risk for miscarriage, preterm labor and birth, IUGR, maternal mortality, and stillbirth.

66. *Modifications in CPR and Heimlich maneuver when a woman is pregnant:* see Cardiopulmonary Resuscitation of the Pregnant Woman subsection including Emergency box, CPR for Pregnant Woman, and Fig. 13-5; modifications include:
    - Use standard CPR but with uterus tipped laterally.
    - Place paddles of defibrillator one rib interspace higher.
    - Monitor fetus and prepare for immediate cesarean birth.
    - Heimlich: place arms under axilla, across chest with thumbside of fist against middle of sternum, then perform backward chest thrusts.

67. Cardiac decompensation, 28, 32, childbirth, 24, 48

68. Classifications of functional capacity of patients with heart disease, asymptomatic at normal levels of activity, symptomatic with ordinary activity, symptomatic with less than ordinary activity, symptomatic at rest

69. Rheumatic heart disease, penicillin G benzathine

70. Mitral valve stenosis

71. Infective endocarditis

72. Mitral valve prolapse

73. Sickle cell hemoglobinopathy, anemia, African-American, Mediterranean

74. Thalassemia (Mediterranean or Cooley's anemia)

75. Bronchial asthma, hyperactive airways, breathe, wheezing, cough, sputum, dyspnea

76. Cystic fibrosis

77. Epilepsy

78. Systemic lupus erythematosus (SLE)

79. Cholelithiasis

80. Cholecystitis

81. *T-ACE and TWEAK tests*
    a. *Purpose for the tests:* both tests screen for alcohol use; they are specifically designed to screen for alcohol use during pregnancy.
    b. *Questions represented by each letter:* T-ACE (see Box 13-8) and TWEAK (see Box 13-9).
    c. *Interpretation and scoring for each tool:* see Substance Abuse during Pregnancy section and Boxes 13-8 and 13-9 to determine scoring; both tests use a point system with a score of 2 or greater as indicative of a risk drinker.

82. *Reasons for delaying prenatal care:* see Substance Abuse, Barriers to Treatment section for a list of several reasons women might delay care.

83. Choice d is correct; the woman is exhibiting signs of DKA; insulin is the required treatment with the dosage dependent on blood glucose level; intravenous fluids may also be required; choice a is the treatment for hypoglycemia; choices b and c, although they may increase the woman's comfort, are not priorities.

84. Choice c is correct; a 2-hour postprandial blood glucose should range between 90 to 120 mg/dl; choices a, b, and d all fall within the expected normal ranges

85. Choice b is correct; calories should be increased to 30 to 35 kcal/kg; a minimum of intake of 250 g of carbohydrates is recommended daily; protein intake should range between 12% and 20%.

86. Choice d is correct; washing hands is important but gloves are not necessary for self-injection; vial should be gently rotated not shaken; regular insulin should be drawn into the syringe first; because she is obese, a 90° angle with skin taut is recommended.

87. Choice d is correct; other signs of cardiac compensation include moist, productive, frequent cough, and crackles at bases of lungs; supine hypotension is a common finding during pregnancy related to compression of vena cava and aorta not cardiac decompensation.

88. Choice a is correct; this woman is exhibiting signs of cardiac decompensation; further information regarding her cardiac status is required to determine what further action would be needed.

89. Choice c is correct; furosemide is a diuretic; propranolol is used to manage hypertension and tachycardia; although warfarin is an anticoagulant, it can cross the placenta and affect the fetus (congenital anomalies and hemorrhage), whereas heparin, which is a large molecule, does not.

90. Choice b is correct; bed rest is not required for a woman with a Class II designation; she will need to avoid heavy exertion and stop activities that cause fatigue and dyspnea; actions in a, c, and d are all appropriate and recommended for Class II.

II. Thinking Critically

1. *Preconception counseling for a woman with diabetes mellitus:* see Preconception Counseling section.
   - Discuss purpose in terms of planning pregnancy for the optimum time when glucose control is established within normal ranges, since this will decrease incidence of congenital anomalies; diagnose any vascular problems; emphasize the importance of her health before the pregnancy, helping to ensure a positive outcome.
   - Discuss how her diabetic management will need to be altered during pregnancy; include her husband, because his health is important, as is his support during the pregnancy.

2. *Pregnant woman with pregestational diabetes experiencing hypoglycemia:* see Guidelines box, Treatment for Hypoglycemia, and Metabolic Changes associated with Pregnancy and Pregestational Diabetes Mellitus sections.
   a. *Problem:* signs and symptoms suggest hypoglycemia resulting from insufficient caloric intake with no adjustment in insulin dosage.
   b. *Action:* check blood glucose level if possible, eat or drink something that contains 10 to 15 g of simple carbohydrate, rest for 15 minutes, recheck blood glucose level, repeat if glucose level remains too low.

3. *Woman with pregestational diabetes: care management*
   a. *Additional antepartal fetal assessments:* see Fetal Surveillance section of Plan of Care and Implementation: tests can include ultrasound examination (growth, congenital anomalies such as spina bifida), maternal serum alpha-fetoprotein, fetal echocardiography (increased risk for cardiac disorders), Doppler blood flow analysis, daily fetal movement counts, nonstress test (NST), biophysical profile (BPP), contraction stress test (CST).
   b. *Stressors facing woman and family:* alteration in daily living, including usual diabetes management, need for additional antepartal testing and prenatal visits, financial implications.
   c. *Nursing diagnoses:* consider both physiologic and psychosocial concerns; consider areas of deficient knowledge, anxiety/fear, ineffective coping, risk for maternal or fetal injury, imbalanced nutrition.
   d. *Activity/exercise recommendations:* see Exercise section of Plan of Care and Implementation; recommend exercises according to her diabetic status; discuss when she should exercise and emphasize the importance of checking blood glucose level before, during, and after, taking care to adjust caloric intake and insulin administration accordingly.
   e. *Complete table related to care management during antepartum, intrapartum, and postpartum periods:* see specific sections for diet, glucose monitoring, and insulin in Plan of Care and Implementation and the Home Care boxes for information regarding interventions and health teaching; the Plan of Care for a Pregnancy Complicated by Pregestational Diabetes may also be helpful in completing the table.
   f. *Birth control recommendations:* see Postpartum section; discuss risks and benefits of methods including their impact on glucose levels

(hormone based) and infection (IUD); barrier method is preferred starting with condom and spermicide until diaphragm or cervical cap can be refitted; stress importance of delaying intercourse until healing is complete to prevent infection.

4. *Hispanic woman with gestational diabetes* (see Gestational Diabetes section).

a. *Complication of pregnancy exhibited with validating findings:* gestational diabetes; 50 g glucose test result 152 mg/dl (>140 mg/dl); 3-hour glucose test reveals three values exceeding the normal range (fasting, 1-hour result, and 2-hour result—see Fig. 13-4).

b. *Risk factors exhibited:* over 30 years of age, obese, mother with type 2 diabetes, previous birth of baby over 9 pounds.

c. *Pathophysiology of gestational diabetes;* pancreas unable to meet demands for increased insulin to compensate for the insulin resistance during the second and third trimesters; cannot maintain euglycemic state.

d. *Maternal and fetal/newborn risks:* see Maternal-Fetal Risks subsection of Gestational Diabetes section; similar risks as for pregestational diabetes except for congenital anomalies, which are the same as for the nondiabetic population,

e. *Ongoing assessment:* see Antepartum section of Plan of Care and Implementation; emphasize importance of monitoring blood glucose levels at recommended times, antepartal fetal surveillance measures, and increased frequency of prenatal visits.

f. *Nursing diagnoses:*
   - Anxiety or deficient knowledge related to ineffective glucose metabolism during pregnancy associated with gestational diabetes
   - Risk for fetal injury related to excessive intrauterine growth associated with gestational diabetes

g. *Dietary changes:* see Diet section and Home Care box, Dietary Management of Diabetic Pregnancy; woman is placed on a standard diabetic diet for pregnancy at 30 to 35 kcal/kg/day for a total of 2000 to 2500 kcal/24 hours; spaced over 3 meals and 4 snacks, including 1 at bedtime; because she is obese, kcal requirement may be decreased, depending on blood glucose levels.

h. *Implications of gestational diabetes mellitus (GDM):* see Postpartum subsection; most women return to normal glucose levels, but GDM is likely to recur in subsequent pregnancies; the risk for developing diabetes later in life is increased especially if she remains obese; the infant is more likely to be obese and have diabetes mellitus in the future;

discuss lifestyle changes including weight reduction and a regular exercise program.

5. *Woman with type 2 diabetes unable to take oral hypoglycemic agents:* inform her that these agents are still unproven in terms of their ability to maintain the fine blood glucose control required during pregnancy; help her self-inject insulin through teaching, demonstration, practice, and support; see Patient Teaching box, Administration of Insulin.

6. *Pregnant woman with mitral valve stenosis—Class II* (see Cardiovascular Disorders section).

a. *Two nursing diagnoses:* several nursing diagnoses and expected outcomes of care are listed in the Nursing Diagnoses section; use assessment findings to determine the priority for a specific pregnant woman.
   - Fear and deficient knowledge would be top priority psychosocial nursing diagnoses for this woman because it is her first pregnancy and she does not really know what to expect; expected outcome would be: woman/couple will openly express concerns and seek information as needed.
   - Physiologically activity intolerance and risk for self-care deficit would be priorities as pregnancy advances and the cardiac work-load increases; expected outcome: woman will follow recommended therapeutic regimen to reduce stress on her heart.

b. *Recommended therapeutic plan for a pregnant woman designated as Class II:* see Antepartum section of Plan of Care and Implementation focusing on specific guidelines for Class II; see Patient Teaching box, Pregnant Woman at Risk for Cardiac Decompensation.
   - *Rest/sleep/activity patterns:* avoid heavy exertion, stop if signs of decompensation occur; sleep 8 to 10 hours/night; 30-minute naps after meals; keep a record of the effect of various activities.
   - *Prevention of infection:* good hygiene and health habits to maintain resistance; identify early and treat promptly; use of prophylactic antibiotics.
   - *Nutrition:* well-balanced diet with iron and folic acid; high protein, adequate calories, sodium restriction as appropriate for her cardiac condition, need for roughage; keep weight gain at lower end of recommended range for her BMI.
   - *Bowel elimination:* prevent constipation to avoid Valsalva maneuver; activity, fluids, and roughage/fiber.

c. Factors increasing stress: see Care Management section.
   - Physiologic stress: anemia, infection, edema, constipation

- Psychosocial stress: depression, anxiety and fear, financial concerns, anger, impaired social interactions, feelings of inadequacy, cultural expectations, inadequate support system

d. *Subjective symptoms of cardiac decompensation:* see Box 13-5, Signs of Potential Complications, Cardiac Decompensation.

e. *Objective signs of cardiac decompensation:* see Box 13-5, Signs of Potential Complications, Cardiac Decompensation

f. *Care during labor:* see Intrapartum subsection.
- Initiate comprehensive assessment for decompensation.
- Decrease fear and anxiety with one-on-one care and support in a calm atmosphere; keep couple informed about what is happening and how woman and fetus are progressing.
- Provide pain relief (epidural is recommended); use of comfort measures.
- Vaginal birth is the best approach from a lateral position; avoid Valsalva maneuver; use open glottis pushing with assistance of low forceps/vacuum, oxygen via mask, antibiotic therapy.

g. *Risk for postpartum cardiac decompensation* (see Nurse Alert section): problems occur as a result of hemodynamic changes associated with birth of baby and the circulatory and hormonal changes occurring with separation and expulsion of the placenta.

h. *Nursing diagnoses for early postpartum period:*
- Risk for imbalanced fluid volume related to extravascular fluid shifts and blood loss following birth would be the top priority physiologic nursing diagnosis.
- Ineffective breastfeeding, risk for impaired mother-infant attachment, OR situational low self-esteem can be priority psychosocial nursing diagnoses related to the woman's need for activity reduction and limited ability to care for newborn on her own.

i. *Stress reduction during postpartum period:* see Postpartum subsection; encourage rest in a lateral position; assist with activities of daily living (ADLs) and progressive ambulation; provide for pain relief and comfort; emphasize measures to prevent infection and constipation; assist with newborn care.

j. *Breastfeeding:* breastfeeding is allowed but the woman will need extra support and rest due to the increased energy demands associated with lactation, and medications used need to be evaluated.

k. *Discharge plan:* emphasize the following:
- Follow-up with health care providers for assessment of postpartum recovery and cardiac status
- Contraception, future pregnancy, and sexuality issues
- Assistance with infant, self, and home care; make referrals as needed
- Importance of balancing rest and activity
- Instruction regarding the healing process, how to assess progress, and prevent complications

7. *Pregnant woman with cardiac disorder needs to take heparin* (see Plan of Care and Implementation section).

a. *Explain why heparin instead of Coumadin will be used:* discuss importance of taking an anticoagulant to prevent thrombus formation; inform that Coumadin will cross placenta and could cause congential anomalies and fetal hemorrhage; heparin does not cross the placenta.

b. *Information to ensure safe use of heparin:*
- Safe administration; teach subcutaneous injection technique to Allison and family.
- Stress importance of routine blood tests to assess clotting ability; discuss alternative sources for folic acid.
- Review side effects, including unusual bleeding and bruising and measures to prevent injury (soft toothbrush, no razors to shave legs).

8. *Pregnant woman with epilepsy:* see Epilepsy section of Neurologic Disorders; inform her that effects of pregnancy on epilepsy are unpredictable; convulsions may injure her or her fetus and lead to miscarriage, preterm labor, or separation of the placenta; medications that will be given in the lowest therapeutic dose, must be taken to prevent convulsions; folic acid supplementation is important because anticonvulsants can deplete folic acid stores.

9. *Pregnant woman who is HIV positive:* see Care Management section of HIV and AIDS;

a. Antepartum: include tests for other STIs; treat with zidovudine; provide vaccinations as recommended; encourage measures to support function of immunologic system; discuss safer sex practices; refer to substance abuse treatment if indicated.

b. Intrapartum: IV zidovudine; avoid invasive procedures; deliver within 4 hours of rupture of membranes (ROM); recommend cesarean birth before ROM.

c. Postpartum: implement infection control measures, especially if immune system is suppressed; discourage breastfeeding.

10. *Principles to follow for providing care to women who abuse alcohol or drugs:* see Care Management section of Substance Abuse section for description of principles to follow; emphasize:
- Family focus including, child care and education and support for parenting

- Empowerment building
- A community-based interdisciplinary approach with multiplicity of services, including those related to sexual and physical abuse and lack of social support
- Continuum of care
- Pregnancy as a window of opportunity related to motivation for change

CHAPTER 14: PREGNANCY AT RISK: GESTATIONAL CONDITIONS

I. Reviewing Key Concepts and Content

1. Chronic hypertension, gestational hypertension, chronic hypertension, gestational hypertension
2. Preeclampsia, 20, hypertension, proteinuria, mild, severe
3. Hypertension, 140 mm Hg, 90 mm Hg, 105 mm Hg, 2, 4 to 6
4. Proteinuria, 30 mg/dl (1+ or greater on a dipstick), 2, 6
5. Pathologic edema, 12, 2 kg
6. Severe preeclampsia, 160 mm Hg, 110 mm Hg, 2+ to 3+, oliguria, cerebral, visual, hepatic, thrombocytopenia, 150,000/mm^3, pulmonary, cardiac, eclampsia, HELLP, creatinine, growth restriction
7. Eclampsia
8. HELLP, hemolysis (H), elevated liver enzymes (EL), low platelets (LP)
9. Transient hypertension, 12
10. venospasm, placental perfusion, intrauterine growth restriction (IUGR), oliguria
11. Hyperemesis gravidarum, 5%, dehydration, electrolyte imbalance, ketosis, acetonuria, overweight, nulliparous, twin
12. *Principles for ensuring accurate blood pressure measurement:* see Box 14-1; emphasize consistency in position of woman and her arm, the arm used, proper size of cuff, and provision of a rest period before the measurement.
13. F   14. T   15. F   16. T   17. T   18. F
19. T   20. F   21. T   22. F   23. F   24. F
25. F   26. T   27. T   28. T   29. F   30. F
31. F
32. *Risk factors associated with preeclampsia:* see Box 14-3 for a list of factors, including chronic renal and hypertensive disease, family history of preeclampsia, multifetal gestation, first pregnancy, maternal age, diabetes mellitus, and Rh incompatibility, obesity.
33. *Assessment techniques to determine findings associated with preeclampsia:* see specific sections for each assessment technique in Physical Examination.
    a. *Hyperreflexia and ankle clonus:* see Table 14-3, which grades deep tendon reflex (DTR)

responses and Fig. 14-4 *A, B, C* for illustrations depicting performance of DTRs and ankle clonus.
    b. *Proteinuria:* describe dipstick and 24-hour urine collection methods to determine level of protein in urine.
    c. *Pitting edema:* see Fig. 14-3, which illustrates assessment of pitting edema and classifications.
34. e   35. c   36. b   37. a   38. d
39. *Preeclampsia and eclampsia: effect on fetal well-being*
    a. *Describe effect:* see Significance and Incidence, Morbidity and Mortality, and Pathophysiology sections, Table 14-2, and Fig. 14-2; major effects on fetus relate to insufficient uteroplacental circulation leading to IUGR, intrauterine fetal death, or perinatal mortality (especially if abruptio placentae occurs); preterm labor and birth, acute hypoxia and abruption can occur with a convulsion.
    b. *Fetal surveillance measures:* see Mild Preeclampsia and Home Care section in Plan of Care and Implementation; measures can include FHR, serial ultrasounds to evaluate fetal growth, NST, BPP, and daily fetal movement counts by the mother.
40. F   41. F   42. T   43. T   44. F   45. T
46. T   47. F   48. F   49. T   50. T   51. T
52. F   53. F   54. T   55. T   56. F   57. F
58. T   59. F   60. T
61. Miscarriage (spontaneous abortion), ectopic pregnancy
62. Placenta previa, premature separation of the placenta (abruptio placentae)
63. Miscarriage (spontaneous abortion), viability, extrauterine, 20, 500 g, miscarriage, threatened, inevitable, incomplete, complete, missed
64. Human chorionic gonadotropin (hCG), gestational sac, ultrasonography
65. Recurrent premature dilation of the cervix, length, composition, stress, lifestyle, labors, recurring loss
66. Ectopic, fertilized ovum, ampulla, tube, Cullen, hematoperitoneum
67. Hydatidiform mole, molar pregnancy, complete (classic), partial
68. Placenta previa, internal cervical os, marginal placenta previa, internal os, low-lying placenta, lower uterine segment, contract, placenta previa, cesarean birth, suction and curettage
69. Premature separation of the placenta, detachment, implantation, Couvelaire, coagulopathy, hypertension, cocaine, blunt external abdominal, smoking, nutrition
70. Velamentous insertion of the cord (vasa previa), membranes (ROM), cord, Battledore, succenturiate

71. Disseminated intravascular coagulation (DIC), bleeding, platelets, clotting factors

72. *DIC* (see Disseminated Intravascular Coagulation section of Clotting Disorders During Pregnancy).
    a. *Predisposing conditions:* abruptio placentae, severe preeclampsia, HELLP syndrome, retained dead fetus, amniotic fluid embolism, gram-negative sepsis
    b. *Pathophysiology of DIC:* pathologic diffuse clotting that consumes large amounts of clotting factors, leading to widespread external and/or internal bleeding
    c. *Clinical manifestations:* unusual and/or excessive bleeding, abnormal results on clotting tests (PT, PTT, platelet count, fibrinogen level, presence of fibrin split products, clot retraction test)
    d. *Priority nursing care measures:* careful and thorough assessment, including renal function and fetal well-being, lateral position, careful administration of blood/blood products and oxygen as ordered, education and emotional support of woman and family

73. *TORCH infections during pregnancy:* see TORCH infections section and Table 14-9.
    a. Crossing, development, influenza-like
    b. *Complete the table related to TORCH infections:* see Table 14-9 for information needed to complete the table.

74. *Pregnant women requiring abdominal surgery* (see Surgery during Pregnancy section).
    a. *Factors that complicate diagnosis and treatment for abdominal problems:* enlarged uterus and displaced internal organs interfere with palpation, alter position of the affected organ and/or change the usual clinical manifestations associated with a specific disorder
    b. *Common conditions requiring abdominal surgery:* appendicitis, intestinal obstruction, and gynecologic problems
    c. *Major fear expressed by women undergoing surgery:* fear of losing baby; women should be encouraged to express their fears, concerns, and questions
    d. Fetus, FHR, uterine contraction, lateral tilt, compression of vena cava, FHR, uterine, preterm labor, tocolysis
    e. *Discharge planning:* see Home Care section and Box 14-9; teach woman and family about what to watch for, care of incision site, activity and rest considerations, and nutrition guidelines for healing and recovery.

75. Choice c is correct; the woman should be seated or in a lateral position, she should rest for at least 5 minutes, and the cuff should cover 80% of the upper arm.

76. Choice a is correct; with severe preeclampsia, the DTRs would be >3+ with possible ankle clonus, the BP would be >160/110; platelet levels would be decreased or <150,000 mm³.

77. Choice d is correct; a respiratory rate of 12 breaths per minute or less indicates dangerous central nervous system (CNS) depression by the magnesium sulfate; the loading dose should be an IV of 4 to 6 g diluted in 100 ml of intravenous fluid; assessment should occur every 15 to 30 minutes, and the maintenance dose should be 1 to 3 g/hour.

78. Choice b is correct; magnesium sulfate is a CNS depressant given to prevent seizures.

79. Choice d is correct; the woman should weigh herself in the morning, after voiding, before breakfast using the same scale and wearing the same clothing; a clean catch, midstream urine specimen should be used to assess urine for protein using a dipstick; fluid intake should be 8 to 10 glasses a day along with roughage to prevent constipation; gentle exercise improves circulation and helps preserve muscle tone and a sense of well-being.

80. Choice a is correct; she should be kept NPO for 48 hours after cessation of vomiting; oral hygiene is important when NPO and after vomiting episodes to maintain the integrity of oral mucosa; taking fluids between, not with, meals reduces nausea, thereby increasing tolerance for oral nutrition.

81. Choice a is correct; the woman is experiencing a threatened abortion; therefore, a conservative approach is attempted first; choices b and c reflect management of an inevitable and complete or incomplete abortion; cerclage or suturing of the cervix is done for recurrent, spontaneous abortion associated with premature dilation (incompetent) cervix.

82. Choice c is correct; choices a, b, and d are appropriate nursing diagnoses, but deficient fluid is the most immediate concern, placing the woman's well-being at greatest risk.

83. Choice b is correct; methotrexate destroys rapidly growing tissue, in this case the fetus and placenta, to avoid rupture of tube and need for surgery; follow-up with blood tests is needed for 2 to 8 weeks, alcohol and vitamins containing folic acid increase the risk for side effects with this medication or exacerbating the ectopic rupture.

84. Choice c is correct; the clinical manifestations of placenta previa are described; dark red bleeding with pain is characteristic of abruptio placentae; massive bleeding from many sites is associated with DIC; bleeding is not a sign of preterm labor.

85. Choice a is correct; hemorrhage is a major potential postpartum complication because the implantation site of the placenta is in the lower uterine segment, which has a limited capacity to contract after birth; infection is another major complication but it is not the immediate focus of

care; choices b and d are also important but not to the same degree as hemorrhage, which is life threatening

II. Thinking Critically

1. Woman with mild preeclampsia: home care
   a. *Signs and symptoms:* see Table 14-2, which differentiates between mild and severe preeclampsia in terms of maternal and fetal manifestations.
   b. *Three priority nursing diagnoses:* nursing diagnoses should consider physiologic effects of preeclampsia such as ineffective tissue perfusion—placenta, risk for injury to mother or fetus; psychosocial effects anxiety, ineffective individual/family coping, powerlessness, ineffective role performance, interrupted family processes; assessment findings should guide the choice and priority of nursing diagnoses, especially with regard to those that apply to psychosocial impact.
   c. *Organization of home care:* see Mild Preeclampsia and Home Care sections and the Plan of Care; help couple mobilize their support system, make referrals to home care if needed, discuss frequency of prenatal visits and antepartal testing.
   d. *Teaching regarding assessment of status and signs of a worsening condition:* see Table 14-2 and Home Care box, Assessing and Reporting Clinical Signs of Preeclampsia; discuss signs, including those indicating a worsening condition and put them in writing so couple can refer to them at home; have woman keep a daily diary of her findings, feelings, and concerns; teach woman and family to take blood pressure (BP), weigh accurately, assess urine, do daily fetal movement counts, and whom to call if problems or concerns arise.
   e. *Instructions about nutrition and fluid intake:* see Diet section and Guidelines box, Nutrition; emphasize the importance of protein, calcium, balance of roughage and fluids, and avoiding foods that are high in salt or contain alcohol; explain rationale for dietary recommendations.
   f. *Coping with bed rest:* see Activity Restriction section, Home Care box, Coping with Bed Rest, and the Plan of Care; explain rationale for bed rest and activity restrictions; clarify what this restriction means (e.g., how long she can be out of bed in a day and what type of activity is okay); discuss importance of lateral position when in bed, relaxation and nonstressful, calming diversional activities, and gentle exercise.
   g. *Constipation:* see Home Care box, Coping with Bed Rest and Guidelines box, Nutrition;

roughage (whole grains, bran, raw fruits and vegetables), 8 glasses of fluid each day, keep fruit and fluids nearby.

2. *Woman with severe preeclampsia—hospital care*
   a. *Signs and symptoms:* see Table 14-2, which differentiates between mild and severe preeclampsia in terms of maternal and fetal manifestations.
   b. *Three priority nursing diagnoses:* ineffective tissue perfusion, risk for impaired gas exchange, and injury take priority as the physiologic nursing diagnoses, since her condition is worsening and the safety of the maternal-fetal unit is jeopardized; anxiety or fear would be the priority psychosocial nursing diagnosis.
   c. *Precautionary measures:* see Box 14-5, which lists hospital precautionary measures in terms of environmental modifications, seizure precautions, and readiness of emergency medications and equipment.
   d. *Administration of magnesium sulfate:* see Box 14-6, Nurse Alert in Magnesium Sulfate section of Severe Preeclampsia and HELLP Syndrome and Emergency box, Magnesium Sulfate Toxicity.
      • *Guidelines:* list the guidelines for preparing and administering the medication solution safely; include essential assessment measures that must be completed and documented before and during the infusion.
      • *Nursing diagnosis:* risk for ineffective breathing pattern related to the CNS depressant effects of magnesium sulfate infusion
      • *Explain expected therapeutic effect:* discuss that this medication is used for its CNS depressant effects to prevent convulsions; describe how it will be given, how she will feel, and what will be done while she is receiving the infusion.
   e. *Maternal-fetal assessments:* VS, FHR pattern, intake and output, urine for protein, DTRs and ankle clonus, signs of improvement or worsening condition, including signs of an imminent seizure.
      • *Signs of magnesium sulfate toxicity:* hyporeflexia, respiratory depression, decreased blood pressure and pulse, oliguria, diminished level of consciousness (LOC), toxic serum magnesium levels, signs of fetal distress.
      • *Immediate action:* discontinue magnesium sulfate infusion, administer calcium gluconate slowly IV push; continue to monitor maternal-fetal status.
   f. *Seizure occurs:* see Eclampsia section and Emergency box, Eclampsia.

- *Emergency measures at onset of convulsion and immediately following include:*
  —Emphasize importance of maintaining a patent airway, preventing injury, and calling for help.
  —Observe effect of seizure on mother and fetus.
  —Document the event and care measures implemented during and after seizure.
  —Provide comfort and reassurance after the convulsion; orient to what happened; never leave alone because another seizure could occur or signs of complications can begin; inform family.
  —Suction as needed, administer oxygen.
- *List potential complications that can occur:* rupture of membranes, preterm labor and birth, altered LOC, abruptio placentae, fetal distress.

g. *Postpartum period recovering from eclampsia:* see Postpartum Nursing Care section.
- Perform close and comprehensive assessment with emphasis on signs of hemorrhage (low platelets, DIC, effect of magnesium sulfate), impending seizures, and status of preeclampsia.
- Continue hospital precautionary measures.
- Continue magnesium sulfate, antihypertensive medications; Pitocin is oxytocic of choice, since methergine could elevate BP even further, especially if given parenterally.
- Provide emotional and psychosocial support for woman and her family; provide time for them to be together and with their baby, but be careful to keep environmental stimuli at a low level until the danger of seizures passes.
- Discuss how her recovery is progressing and the prognosis for the rest of the postpartum period and for future pregnancies.

3. *Woman with hyperemesis gravidarum* (see Hyperemesis Gravidarum section).
   a. *Predisposing/etiologic factors:* see Etiology subsection, which lists physiologic and psychologic factors, including the factors present in this situation: primigravida, obesity, ambivalence about pregnancy, difficult relationship with parents; lifestyle alterations; additional factors include multifetal pregnancy, molar pregnancy, body change concerns; occurs within the first 10 weeks of pregnancy.
   b. *Assessment of physiologic and psychosocial factors upon admission:*
      - *Physiologic:* full description of nausea and vomiting, presence of other GI symptoms; relief measures used; weight, including changes; vital signs; signs of fluid, electrolyte, and acid/base imbalances; urine check for ketones and specific gravity; CBC; serum electrolytes; liver enzymes; bilirubin levels; thyroid function.
      - *Psychosocial:* discuss concerns regarding self and pregnancy; assess support system.
   c. *Priority nursing diagnoses:* deficient fluid volume, risk for fetal and maternal injury, anxiety, powerlessness, ineffective individual or family coping; woman's condition and circumstances will determine the priority, with physiologic diagnoses taking precedence in the acute phase.
   d. *Care measures during hospitalization* (see Collaborative Care section and Nursing Care Plan).
      - Restore fluid and electrolyte balance with intravenous administration of fluids, electrolytes, and nutrients.
      - Restore ability to tolerate oral nutrition: gradually progress from NPO to full diet; administer medications appropriately.
      - Monitor progress to determine effectiveness of therapeutic regimen, readiness for discharge, and need for continuing treatment with home care.
      - Provide comfort measures and create a restful environment.
      - Provide psychosocial support for woman and her family; make referrals as appropriate.
      - Teach woman and family about the disorder, how it is treated, its effect on pregnancy and fetus.
   e. *Home care* (see Follow-up Care section and Nursing Care Plan).
      - Discuss follow-up care requirements, types of foods to eat and ways to eat (similar to recommendations for morning sickness).
      - Include family in plan of care, especially with regard to meal preparation and support and encouragement of the woman; make appropriate referrals.
      - Teach woman how to assess herself in terms of weight, urine for ketones, signs of developing problems that should be reported, including weight loss, return of nausea and vomiting, pain, dehydration.

4. *Woman with ruptured ectopic pregnancy* (see Ectopic Pregnancy section).
   a. *Risk factors:* see Incidence and Etiology subsection; history of sexually transmitted infections (STIs), pelvic inflammatory disease (PID), tubal sterilization and surgical reversal of tubal sterilization.
   b. *Assessment of findings:* see Clinical Manifestations section; findings begin with signs of an unruptured tubal pregnancy (missed period, adnexal fullness and tenderness, dull or colicky pain), vaginal bleeding; these signs are subtle and often missed; signs of rupture are more acute

(abnormal bleeding, acute abdominal pain and referred shoulder pain, signs of hemorrhage and shock) and may be mistaken for other acute abdominal conditions.

c. *Differential diagnosis:* see Table 14-6; appendicitis, salpingitis, ruptured ovarian cyst, miscarriage.

d. *Major care management problem:* hemorrhage; much of the blood accumulates in the abdominal cavity.

e. *Two priority nursing diagnoses:* deficient fluid volume and acute pain as well as fear/anxiety and anticipatory grieving.

f. *Nursing measures for the preoperative and postoperative period:* see Collaborative Care, Hospital Care section; assessment, general preoperative and postoperative care measures, fluid replacement, major emphasis on emotional support to facilitate grieving, discussion of impact of rupture on future pregnancies, referral for counseling as appropriate, prepare for discharge with instructions for postoperative self-care, including self-assessment for complications such as infection, measures to enhance healing, importance of follow-up appointment to assess progress of recovery.

5. *Woman with signs of spontaneous miscarriage* (see Table 14-5).

a. *Basis for signs and symptoms:* signs indicate the woman is experiencing a threatened abortion.

b. *Expected care management:* bed rest, sedation, avoidance of stress and orgasm; follow progress with hCG levels and ultrasound to assess integrity of gestational sac; watch for signs of progress to inevitable abortion; caution her to save peripads and tissue passed.

6. *Woman with signs of spontaneous miscarriage* (see Box 14-7, Table 14-5, and Guidelines/Guías box).

a. *Questions:* determine what she means by a lot of bleeding, and if she is experiencing any other signs and symptoms related to miscarriage such as pain and cramping; determine the gestational age of her pregnancy and if there is anyone to bring her to the hospital if inevitable abortion is suspected.

b. *Assessment findings indicative of an incomplete abortion:* heavy, profuse bleeding, severe cramping, passage of tissue, cervix remains dilated.

c. *Priority nursing diagnosis at this time:* deficient fluid volume related to blood loss secondary to incomplete abortion.

d. *Nursing measures:* prompt termination of pregnancy: assess before and after procedure, explain what will occur, provide emotional support, refer for counseling if needed, prepare for discharge, and arrange for follow-up to assess physical and emotional status.

e. *Discharge instructions:* see Home Care section and Patient Teaching box, Discharge Teaching for Woman after Early Miscarriage; advise regarding signs and symptoms of complications (bleeding, infection), what to expect regarding progress of healing (pain, discharge), measures to prevent complications (hygiene, nutrition, rest).

f. *Nursing measures for anticipatory grieving:* see Home Care section and Patient Teaching box, Discharge Teaching for Woman after Early Miscarriage; acknowledge her loss and provide time for her to express her feelings; inform her about how she may feel (mood swings, depression); refer her for grief counseling, support groups, clergy; make follow-up phone calls.

7. *Woman with complete hydatidiform mole* (see Hydatidiform Mole section).

a. *Typical signs and symptoms:* see Clinical Manifestations section; scant to profuse vaginal bleeding (dark brown to bright red), larger uterus for dates, anemia, hyperemesis gravidarum, abdominal cramps, early signs of preeclampsia or gestational hypertension.

b. *Post-treatment instructions:* see Home Care section; frequent physical and pelvic examinations, regular measurement of serum hCG levels following protocol for frequency for at least 1 year; emphasize importance of follow-up assessments and strict birth control to prevent pregnancy until hCG levels have been normal for a specified period of time.

c. Choriocarcinoma, hCG, uterus

8. *Comparison of a woman with marginal placenta previa to a woman with abruptio placentae, Grade II:*

a. *Comparison of findings:* see Placenta Previa and Abruptio Placentae sections and Table 14-7 to compare findings for each disorder in terms of characteristics of bleeding, uterine tone, pain and tenderness, and ultrasound findings regarding location of placenta and fetal presentation/position.

b. *Priority nursing diagnoses:* consider diagnoses related to major physical problems such as deficient fluid volume related to blood loss, ineffective tissue perfusion (placenta), and risk for fetal injury; major psychosocial nursing diagnoses could include fear/anxiety, interrupted family processes, and anticipatory grieving.

c. *Comparison of care management approaches* (see Fig. 14-11): consider home care versus hospital care for woman with placenta previa; hospital care is the safest approach for woman experiencing abruptio placentae; discuss active versus expectant management for each disorder.

d. *Postpartum considerations:* potential complications should be the basis for the special postpartum care requirements; hemorrhage (placenta previa related to limited contraction of lower portion of the uterus; abruptio placentae related to Couvelaire uterus and DIC) and infection (lower implantation site, anemia from blood loss) are the major physiologic complications that need to be addressed; emotional and psychosocial support are important related to the high risk nature of the pregnancy, especially if fetal loss was an outcome.

9. *Trauma during pregnancy* (see Trauma during Pregnancy section).
   a. *Significance of problem:* see Significance subsection; 8% incidence during pregnancy making it one of the leading nonobstetric causes of maternal mortality; risk increases as pregnancy progresses with most injuries occurring in the third trimester; most common causes are motor vehicle crashes, falls, and direct assaults to the abdomen (battering).
   b. *Effects of trauma:* increased risk for miscarriage, preterm labor, abruptio placentae, stillbirth; effects are influenced by length of gestation, type and severity of the trauma, degree of disruption of uterine and fetal physiologic features.
   c. *Impact of trauma on fetus:* fetal injury (skull fracture, intracranial hemorrhage, prematurity); death related to maternal death or abruptio placentae; hypoxia related to altered placental perfusion.
   d. Resuscitate, stabilize, fetal, fetal, maternal, airway, breathing, circulation
   e. *Outline assessment and care of a pregnant woman experiencing trauma:* see Care Management section to highlight the important components of each area cited; answer should reflect the unique characteristics of the pregnant woman and how they can influence finding, including vital sign values and the pain experience.
   f. *Components of discharge planning:* see Discharge Planning subsection; emphasize the importance of self- and fetal assessment, measures to prevent future trauma, and making needed referrals.

CHAPTER 15:   LABOR AND BIRTH PROCESSES

I.   Reviewing Key Concepts and Content

1. Passenger (fetus, placenta), passageway (birth canal), powers (contractions), position of the mother, psychologic response
2. Fontanels, sutures
3. Molding
4. Presentation, cephalic, breech, shoulder
5. Presenting part, occiput, mentum (chin), sacrum, scapula
6. Vertex presentation, occiput
7. Lie, longitudinal (vertical), transverse (horizontal, oblique)
8. Attitude (posture), flexion
9. Biparietal, suboccipitobregmatic, flexion
10. Position
11. Engagement, ischial spines, zero
12. Presenting part, ischial spines, centimeters, ischial spines, descent
13. Effacement, first, percentage
14. Dilation, centimeters, 1, 10
15. Lightening, 2, uterine contractions, true labor
16. Involuntary uterine contractions, bearing down, pushing
17. Bloody show, mucous plug, ripens
18. Mechanism of labor, cardinal movements, engagement, descent, flexion, internal rotation, extension, external rotation, restitution, expulsion
19. Valsalva, glottis, breath, bearing down, hypoxia, acidosis, perineal tears
20. Onset of regular uterine contractions, dilation, latent, active, transition
21. Dilated, birth
22. Birth of the fetus, placenta
23. Recovery, hemostasis, 2 hours
24. Position, blood pressure, uterine contractions, umbilical cord blood flow
25. *Describe five factors and how they affect the process of childbirth:* see separate sections for each of the five factors in Factors of Labor; consider the factors of passenger, passage, powers, position of mother, psychologic response.
26. *Explain how the cardinal movements of labor facilitate birth:* see Mechanism of Labor section in the Process of Labor and Fig. 15-13; describe engagement and descent, flexion, internal rotation, extension, external rotation and restitution, expulsion.
27. Label illustrations:
    Fetal skull: A. mentum (chin); B. occipitofrontal diameter; C. frontal bone (sinciput); D. suboccipitobregmatic diameter; E. parietal bone (vertex); F. occipitomental diameter; G. occiput; H. sagittal suture; I. lambdoid suture; J. posterior fontanel; K. biparietal diameter; L. coronal suture; M. frontal suture; N. anterior fontanel (bregma)

Maternal pelvis: A. symphysis pubis;
B. anteroposterior diameter of inlet; C. transverse diameter of the inlet; D. sacral promontory;
E. sacrum; F. sacroiliac joint; G. ischial spine;
H. pubic bone; I. sacrotuberous ligament; J. pubic arch; K. ischial tuberosity; L. coccyx; M. sacroiliac joint

28. *Indicate presentation, presenting part, position, lie, and attitude represented by each illustration*
    a. Cephalic (vertex), occiput, LOA, longitudinal, flexion
    b. Cephalic (vertex), occiput, LOT, longitudinal, flexion
    c. Cephalic (vertex), occiput, LOP, longitudinal, flexion
    d. Cephalic (vertex), occiput, ROA, longitudinal, flexion
    e. Cephalic (vertex), occiput, ROT, longitudinal, flexion
    f. Cephalic (vertex), occiput, ROP, longitudinal, flexion
    g. Cephalic (face), mentum, LMA, longitudinal, extension
    h. Cephalic (face), mentum, RMP, longitudinal, extension
    i. Cephalic (face), mentum, RMA, longitudinal, extension
    j. Breech, sacrum, LSA, longitudinal, flexion
    k. Breech, sacrum, LSP, longitudinal, flexion
    l. Shoulder, scapula, ScA, transverse, flexion

29. F 30. T 31. F 32. F 33. T 34. T
35. F 36. T 37. F 38. F 39. T 40. T
41. F 42. T 43. T 44. F 45. T 46. F

47. Choice b is correct; attitude is extension of head and neck as indicated by the mentum (chin) as the presenting part; the lie is longitudinal as indicated by the cephalic presentation.

48. Choice c is correct; systolic blood pressure increases with uterine contractions in the first stage while both systolic and diastolic blood pressure increase during contractions in the second stage; WBC increases; gastric motility decreases and can lead to nausea and vomiting, especially during the transition phase of the first stage of labor.

49. Choice c is correct; the first stage can last up to 20 hours for the primigravid woman; the second stage of labor lasts an average of 50 minutes or longer and up to 2 hours, especially in nulliparous labors or if an epidural was used; fourth stage lasts approximately 1 to 2 hours

50. Choice d is correct; quickening refers the woman's first perception of fetal movement at 16 to 20 weeks of gestation; urinary frequency, lightening, weight loss of 0.5 to 1.0 kg occur to signal that the onset of labor is near; backache, stronger Braxton Hicks and bloody show are also noted.

II. Thinking Critically

1. *Analysis of vaginal examinations:*
   - *Examination I:* ROP (right occiput posterior, cephalic [vertex] presentation, longitudinal lie, flexed attitude), −1 (station at 1 cm above the ischial spines), 50% effaced, 3 cm dilated
   - *Examination II:* RMA (right mentum anterior, cephalic [face] presentation, longitudinal lie, extended attitude), 0 (station at the ischial spines, engaged), 25% effaced, 2 cm dilated
   - *Examination III:* LST (left sacrum transverse, breech presentation, longitudinal lie, flexed attitude), +1 (station at 1 cm below the ischial spines), 75% effaced, 6 cm dilated
   - *Examination IV:* OA (occiput anterior, cephalic [vertex] presentation, longitudinal lie, flexed attitude), + 3 (station at 3 cm below the ischial spines near or on the perineum), 100% effaced, 10 cm (fully dilated)

2. *Woman with questions and concerns about process of labor:*
   a. *Onset of labor:* see Onset of Labor section of the Process of Labor; explain in simple terms the interaction of maternal and fetal hormones, uterine distention, placental aging, fetal fibronectin, prostaglandins.
   b. *Signs preceding labor:* see Box 15-1 for the signs that occur before the onset of labor, including lightening, urinary frequency, backache, Braxton Hicks contractions, weight loss, energy surge, bloody show, possible rupture of the membranes; health care provider would detect cervical changes such as ripening, effacement, and dilation.
   c. *Duration of labor:* see Stages of Labor section for approximate times for each stage; give woman ranges rather than absolute numbers, especially since this will be her first labor; discuss her role in facilitating the progress of labor.
   d. *Position changes during labor:*
      - Emphasize that the position of the woman is one of the 5 *P's* of labor.
      - Discuss each position and describe its effect (see Fig. 15-12).
      - Demonstrate each position and have her practice them with her partner.
      - Emphasize the beneficial effects of ambulation and changing positions on fetus, circulation, comfort, and progress.

CHAPTER 16: MANAGEMENT OF DISCOMFORT

I. Reviewing Key Concepts and Content

1. Visceral, cervical, distention, ischemia, first, lower portion
2. Somatic, second, perineal tissues, pelvic floor, peritoneum, uterocervical, lacerations
3. Referred, uterus, abdominal, lumbosacral, iliac crests, gluteal, thighs
4. Gate control, massage, stroking, music, focal points, imagery, cognitive, breathing, relaxation
5. Endorphins
6. Dick-Read method, Lamaze method, Bradley method
7. Dick-Read, fear-tension-pain, deep abdominal breathing, shallow breathing, relaxation
8. Lamaze, conditioned, relaxation, breathing
9. Bradley, harmony, breath, abdominal breathing, relaxation, darkness, solitude, quiet
10. Walk, talk, slow-paced (abdominal), half
11. Modified-paced (chest), shallow, twice
12. Deep cleansing breath
13. Patterned-paced, transition, hyperventilation, alkalosis, lightheadedness, dizziness, tingling, numbness, breathe into a paper bag held tightly around her nose and mouth, carbon dioxide, twice
14. Effleurage, counterpressure, heel, fist, gate control
15. Water therapy (hydrotherapy), active
16. Transcutaneous electrical nerve stimulation (TENS), thoracic, sacral, placebo, endogenous opiates
17. *Factors influencing nursing diagnosis of pain:* major factors include culture, previous experience, knowledge and expectations, childbirth preparation, anxiety and fear, available support, physical condition of the woman at the onset of labor, history of substance abuse or sexual abuse, environment.
18. *Theoretical basis for effectiveness of massage, stroking, music, and imagery in reducing sensation of pain:* discuss the gate control theory of pain.
19. b 20. f 21. h 22. a 23. g 24. j
25. m 26. d 27. i 28. l 29. c 30. e
31. k
32. *Complete table related to types of regional anesthetics:* see appropriate sections for each regional anesthetic listed.
33. *Systemic analgesics effect on fetus* (see Systemic Analgesics section of Pharmacologic Management of Discomfort).
   a. *Factors influencing effect of systemic analgesics on fetus:* maternal dosage, pharmacokinetics of the specific drug, route, time when administered during labor.
   b. *Fetal effects:* CNS depression as a result of the direct effect of the drug when it crosses the placenta and/or the indirect effect of maternal hypotension and hypoventilation resulting from the drug's action on maternal function; CNS depression slows the FHR and decreases variability and leads to respiratory depression and hypoxia.
34. *Complete table related to medications used during labor:* see specific sections for each medication classification in Pharmacologic Management of Discomfort.
35. *Intravenous administration of systemic analgesics as the preferred route:* onset of action is faster and more reliable and predictable when administered intravenously.
36. T 37. T 38. F 39. T 40. T 41. F
42. T 43. F 44. T 45. F 46. T 47. F
48. T 49. T 50. F
51. Choice d is correct; maternal temperature must be monitored, because an elevation can increase the FHR; woman can and should change her position while in the bath, using lateral and hand-and-knees when indicated; as long as amniotic fluid is clear or only slightly meconium tinged a whirlpool can continue; there is no limit to the time she can spend in the water—she can stay as she wishes.
52. Choice b is correct; Narcan is an opioid antagonist; Stadol is an opioid agonist-antagonist analgesic; Sublimaze is an opioid agonist analgesic.
53. Choice d is correct; onset of effect is within 30 to 60 seconds of IV injection; a 25 mg dose is appropriate for IV administration; this medication is a potent opioid agonist analgesic; therefore, respiratory depression is a concern.
54. Choice c is correct; as an opioid antagonistic, it will reverse the effects of the opioid agonist analgesic administered for pain; maternal side effects include hypotension, tachycardia, nausea, and vomiting; Narcan is administered parenterally at a dose of 0.1 to 2 mg; it may be repeated in 2 to 3 minutes up to 2 times if needed.
55. Choice a is correct; position with a curved back separates the vertebrae and facilitates administration of the anesthetic; alternating lateral positions after administration will prevent supine hypotension; ambulation could be unsafe and difficult, related to weakness and numbness of the legs; because the dura is not punctured, there is no leakage of cerebrospinal fluid that could cause a spinal headache.

II. Thinking Critically

1. *Explaining basis of childbirth pain to expectant fathers:* see Neurologic Origins of Pain section of Discomfort During Labor; describe why pain occurs and its very real basis; discuss how women experience the pain and factors that influence the experience; identify measures they can use to help their partners reduce and cope with the pain.

2. *Working with couple with unrealistic, inaccurate views regarding pain and pain relief during labor* (see Care Management section).
   - Inform couple regarding the basis of pain and its potentially adverse effects on the maternal-fetal unit and the progress of labor.
   - Discuss a variety of nonpharmacologic and pharmacologic measures that are safe and effective to use during labor and can have beneficial effects on the maternal-fetal unit and can enhance the progress of labor.
   - Emphasize that the mother and fetus will be thoroughly assessed before, during, and after use of any measure to ensure safety.

3. *Benefits of water therapy:*
   - Describe the beneficial effects of water therapy and how it can facilitate the labor process by promoting relaxation and relieving discomfort and tension and shortening the duration of labor, thereby decreasing the possibility of cesarean birth; use research findings to substantiate these claims.
   - Describe the successful experiences of other agencies that have implemented water therapy; state how it has affected the number of births.
   - Use favorable reports of women who have used water therapy; consider how this could affect other women preparing for childbirth.

4. *Occurrence of hypotension after administration of epidural block during labor* (see Emergency box, Maternal Hypotension with Decreased Placental Perfusion).
   a. *What is being experienced by this woman:* maternal hypotension related to effect of epidural anesthesia, which can cause a rapid vasodilation, thereby decreasing placental perfusion; results in an alteration in fetal oxygen level, reflected in nonreassuring changes in FHR pattern.
   b. *Nursing diagnosis:* ineffective tissue perfusion to placenta related to maternal hypotension associated with epidural block anesthesia.
   c. *Immediate nursing actions:* turn on her side or put a wedge under her hip to displace the uterus and enhance cardiac output; maintain circulating volume by continuing or increasing rate of IV infusion; administer oxygen via mask; elevate legs from hip; assess effects of actions taken on maternal-fetal unit; notify primary health care provider for further instruction, including the possible administration of a vasopressor such as ephedrine.

5. *Woman receiving an epidural block:* (see Epidural Block section of Pharmacologic Management of Discomfort and Plan of Care and Implementation section).
   a. *Assessment before induction of block:* determine status of maternal-fetal unit, progress of labor in terms of phase, contraindications to use.
   b. *Preparation measures:* answer should reflect actions related to explanation of procedures used, informed consent, hydration, bladder condition.
   c. *Positions for induction:* (see Fig. 16-12) lateral (modified Sims with back curved forward) or sitting with back curved forward to separate vertebrae; assist her with assuming and maintaining the position without movement during the induction.
   d. *Nursing management during the epidural block:* assess the response on the maternal-fetal unit and progress of labor; maintain hydration; assist with bladder emptying and positioning of legs safely; change position frequently from side to side; maintain site to prevent infection.

CHAPTER 17: FETAL ASSESSMENT DURING LABOR

I. Reviewing Key Concepts and Content

1. Reassuring, nonreassuring, compromise, hypoxemia, hypoxia
2. Auscultation, fetoscope, ultrasound device
3. Electronic fetal monitoring, ultrasound transducer, tocotransducer, spiral electrode, intrauterine pressure catheter (IUPC)
4. Oligohydramnios, variable deceleration, amnioinfusion, normal saline, Ringer's lactate
5. Tocolytic, tocolysis, blood flow, placenta, uterine contractions
6. *Factors that affect fetal oxygen supply and expected characteristics of FHR and uterine activity* (see Fetal Response section of Basis for Monitoring).
   a. *Factors that can reduce fetal oxygen supply:* reduction in blood flow through maternal vessels, reduction in oxygen content of maternal blood, alterations in fetal circulation, and reduction in placental perfusion
   b. *Characteristics of reassuring FHR patterns:* baseline rate of 110 to 160 beats/min, no periodic changes, moderate baseline variability, accelerations with fetal movement

c. *Characteristics of normal uterine activity:* frequency every 2 to 5 minutes, duration less than 90 seconds, moderate to strong intensity less than 80 mm Hg, rest period of at least 30 seconds with an average intrauterine pressure (IUP) of 20 mm Hg or less

7. *Characteristics of nonreassuring FHR pattern:* see Fetal Compromise section; characteristics are fully identified in terms of changes in baseline rate, variability, and the occurrence of periodic and episodic changes.

8. i	9. j	10. h	11. g	12. k	13. f
14. c	15. b	16. d	17. e	18. a	19. l

20. 20
21. 30 minutes, 15 minutes
22. 15 minutes, 5 minutes
23. *Intermittent auscultation to assess fetal status during labor*
    a. *State advantages and disadvantages:*
       • Advantages: high touch/low tech approach, natural method facilitating activity, comfortable, noninvasive
       • Disadvantages: inconvenient and time consuming, increased anxiety if nurse has difficulty locating PMI, less information about FHR pattern is obtained, less accurate
    b. *Guidelines to follow:* see Intermittent Auscultation section of Monitoring Techniques; cite the 6 specific guidelines that should be used.
24. *Legal responsibilities related to fetal monitoring during childbirth:* see Legal Tip, Fetal Monitoring Standards in Plan of Care and Implementation section; evaluate FHR pattern at frequency that reflects professional standards, agency policy, and condition of maternal-fetal unit; correctly interpret FHR pattern as reassuring or nonreassuring; take appropriate action; evaluate response to actions taken; notify primary health care provider in a timely fashion; know the chain of command if a dispute about interpretation occurs; document assessment findings, actions, and responses.

25. T	26. F	27. T	28. F	29. T	30. T
31. T	32. F	33. F	34. T	35. T	36. T
37. F	38. T				

39. *Nonreassuring pattern noted upon evaluation of a monitor tracing:* see Box 17-3 and tables for each individual nonreassuring pattern to determine appropriate actions that most often involve repositioning the mother, administering oxygen, altering rate of IV, discontinuing Pitocin, assessing for possible causes, notifying primary health care provider, assisting with other methods of assessment, preparing for emergency treatment such as operative vaginal birth or cesarean birth.

40. *Nursing care measures for woman being monitored externally:* see Boxes 17-3 and 17-4 and Patient and Family Teaching section for information related to teaching and explanations, assessing tracings and maternal responses, and caring for woman in terms of comfort, changing position, and transducer placement site care.

41. Choice d is correct; the resting pressure should be 20 mm Hg or less; choices a, b, and c are all findings within the expected ranges

42. Choice b is correct; Leopold's maneuvers are used to locate the PMI for correct placement of the ultrasound transducer; the tocotransducer is always placed over the fundus; reposition the ultrasound transducer every 2 hours and as needed and the tocotransducer every 2 hours and as needed; it is not the nurse's role to apply a spiral electrode.

43. Choice a is correct; the baseline rate should be 110 to 160 beats/min; accelerations should occur with fetal movement; no late deceleration pattern of any magnitude is reassuring, especially if it is repetitive.

44. Choice c is correct; the FHR increases as the maternal core body temperature rises; therefore, tachycardia would be the pattern exhibited; it is often a clue of intrauterine infection since maternal fever is often the first sign.

45. Choice b is correct; the pattern described is an early deceleration pattern, which is considered to be benign, reassuring, and requiring no action other than documentation of the finding; it is associated with fetal head compression; changing a woman's position and notifying the physician would be appropriate if nonreassuring signs such as late or variable decelerations were occurring; prolapse of cord is associated with variable decelerations as a result of cord compression.

II. Thinking Critically

1. *Woman concerned about use of external monitoring to assess her fetus and labor:* see Box 17-3 for care measures related to fetal monitoring and Box 17-4 for teaching points.
   • Discuss how fetus responds to labor and how the monitor will assess these responses.
   • Explain the advantages of monitoring.
   • Show her a monitor strip and explain what it reveals; tell her how to use the strip to help her with breathing techniques
2. *Woman whose labor is being induced and monitored externally* (see Table 17-5 and Fig. 17-7, *B*).

a. *Pattern described and causative factors:* late deceleration patterns as a result of uteroplacental insufficiency associated with intense uterine contractions, supine position, and placental aging related to postterm gestation.

b. *Nursing interventions:* discontinue Pitocin to stop stimulation of contractions; change to lateral position to enhance uteroplacental perfusion; administer oxygen via mask to increase oxygen availability to fetus; assess response to actions and notify primary health care provider regarding assessment findings, actions taken, and responses; document.

3. *Analyze monitor tracings:*

a. *Reassuring FHR pattern with normal uterine activity:* see Fetal Response section in Basis for Monitoring; compare the criteria of a reassuring FHR pattern and normal uterine activity with monitor tracing; see Fig. 17-4 as a guide for evaluation of a monitor tracing.

b. *Late deceleration pattern with minimal variability:* see Fig. 17-5 and 17-7, *B* and Tables 17-2 and 17-5.

c. *Bradycardia with minimal variability:* average FHR is 90 beats/min; see Fig. 17-5 and Tables 17-2 and 17-3.

d. *Early deceleration:* recognize this as reassuring pattern; see Fig. 17-7, *A* and Table 17-4.

e. *Tachycardia:* average FHR is 210 beats/min; see Table 17-3.

f. *Variable deceleration pattern:* see Fig. 17-7, *C* and Table 17-5.

CHAPTER 18: NURSING CARE DURING LABOR AND BIRTH

I. Reviewing Key Concepts and Content

1. TL   2. FL   3. FL   4. TL   5. TL   6. FL
7. TL   8. FL   9. TL   10. TL   11. TL
12. Regular uterine contractions, effacement, dilation, mucous plug
13. 0, 3, 6, 8, 4, 7, 3, 6, 20, 40, 8, 10
14. Infant is born, cervical dilation, effacement, baby's birth, perspiration on upper lip, vomiting, increased bloody show, shaking of extremities, restlessness, involuntary bearing down efforts, latent, descent, transition, 2 hours
15. Birth of the baby, placenta is expelled, separation, firmly contracting fundus, discoid, globular ovoid, gush of dark blood, lengthening of umbilical cord, vaginal fullness, fetal membranes
16. f   17. g   18. j   19. h   20. b   21. m
22. a   23. e   24. k   25. n   26. d   27. c
28. i   29. l

30. Uterine contractions
31. Increment
32. Acme
33. Decrement
34. Frequency
35. Intensity
36. Duration
37. Resting tone
38. Interval
39. Bearing-down effort
40. Characteristics of uterine contractions:

a. *Label illustration:* A. beginning (onset of a contraction); B. duration; C. frequency; D. relaxation (interval between contractions); E. intensity; 1. increment; 2. acme; 3. decrement.

b. *Method of assessment:* place hand on fundus and determine changes in tone for several contractions and rest periods; press finger into fundus at acme (peak) of contraction to determine intensity.

41. *Admission of woman in labor* (see Assessment section of Care Management, First Stage of Labor).

a. *Information from prenatal record:* see Prenatal Data section; include such information as age, weight gain, health status and medical problems during pregnancy, past and present obstetric history (gravida, para), including outcomes and problems encountered, laboratory and diagnostic test results, estimated date of birth (EDB), baseline data from pregnancy, including vital signs and fetal heart rate (FHR).

b. *Information regarding status of labor:* factors distinguishing false from true labor, uterine contractions (onset, characteristics), show, status of membranes, fetal movement, discomfort (location, characteristics), any other signs of the onset of labor experienced.

c. *Information regarding current health status:* health problems, respiratory status, allergies, character and time of last oral intake, emotional status.

42. F   43. F   44. T   45. F   46. T   47. F
48. T   49. T   50. T   51. T   52. F   53. F
54. F   55. F   56. T   57. F   58. F   59. F
60. T

61. *Complete table regarding labor stressors and support measures:* see Stress in Labor, Supportive Care during Labor and Birth, Support of Father or Partner during Labor and Birth, Culture and Father Participation sections; see Tables 18-1, 18-5, and 18-7, Box 18-8, Care Paths, and Nursing Care Plans; answer should reflect physical and emotional stressors as well as the changing nature of stressors as labor progresses; support measures

identified should reflect the changing nature of the stressors; a couple's birth plan often identifies the type of support measures they are most likely to respond to in a positive manner.

62. *Signs of potential complications:* see Box 18-6: Signs of Potential Complications, Labor for a list of signs to consider throughout labor.

63. *Complete table regarding labor positions and their advantages:* see Box 18-7 and Ambulation and Positioning section of Plan of Care and Implementation, First Stage of Labor

64. *Critical maternal-fetal factors to assess during labor:* see appropriate sections that discuss general systems assessment, Leopold's maneuvers, assessment of FHR and pattern, assessment of uterine contractions, and vaginal examination; see Tables 18-2, 18-3 and 18-6, Boxes 18-5 and 18-6, and Care Paths.
    - *Maternal factors:* vital signs, uterine activity, cervical changes, show/bleeding/amniotic fluid, behavior, appearance, mood, energy level, bearing down effort, use of childbirth preparation methods
    - *Fetal factors:* FHR pattern, activity level, progress in cardinal movements of labor, passage of meconium

65. *Laboratory and diagnostic tests during labor:* see Laboratory and Diagnostic Tests section of Assessment, First Stage of Labor; CBC, blood type and Rh factor, analysis of urine, dipstick for protein, glucose, acetone, Nitrazine and ferning tests for amniotic fluid; additional tests may be done depending on state laws and maternal condition such as HIV or drug screening, vaginal cultures.

66. *Complete table for events/behaviors and support measures for second stage of labor:* see Tables 18-6 and 18-7 and Care Path to complete table.

67. *Factors influencing duration of second stage of labor:* use of regional anesthesia such as epidural block, quality of bearing-down efforts and positions used, parity, size, presentation, and position of fetus, maternal pelvic adequacy, maternal physical status, including energy level, support measures provided.

68. *Second stage positions:* see Maternal Position section; see Figs. 18-19 and 18-20; describe squatting, side-lying, semirecumbent, standing, hands-and-knees.

69. Choice a is correct; although choices b, c, and d are all important questions, the first question should gather information regarding whether or not the woman is in labor.

70. Choice c is correct; pH of amniotic fluid is 6.5 or higher, ferning is noted when examining fluid with a microscope, and the fluid is relatively odorless; a strong odor is strongly suggestive of infection.

71. Choice c is correct; O or occiput indicates a vertex presentation with the neck fully flexed and the occiput in the transverse section (T) of the woman's pelvis; the station is 2 cm below the ischial spines (+2); the woman is entering the active phase of labor; the lie is longitudinal because the head (cephalic/vertex) is presenting.

72. Choice b is correct; maternal BP, pulse, and respirations should be assessed every 30 minutes; temperature should be assessed every 2 hours once the membranes rupture; vaginal examinations are performed as indicated by labor events and not on a regular basis.

73. Choice b is correct; research has indicated that enemas are not needed during labor; according to research findings a, c, and d have all been found to be beneficial and safe during pregnancy.

II. Thinking Critically

1. *Woman thinking she is in labor calls nurse* (see Patient Teaching Box, How to Distinguish True Labor from False Labor and Box 18-1).
    a. *Nursing approach:* determine the status of her labor, asking her to describe what she is experiencing and comparing her description to the characteristics of true and false labor.
    b. *Write questions:* questions should be clear, concise, open-ended, and directed toward distinguishing her labor status and determining the basis for action.
    c. *Instructions for home care of woman in latent labor:* discuss comfort measures, distracting activities, measures to reduce anxiety, and measures to enhance the labor process; inform regarding assessment measures to determine progress and identify signs of problems, when and whom to call, and when to come to the hospital; nurse can make follow-up calls to determine how the woman is progressing.

2. Women in first stage of labor at various phases:
    a. *Identify phase of labor:* see Table 18-2 to determine phase; Denise (active); Teresa (transition); Danielle (latent).
    b. *Describe behavior and appearance:* see Tables 18-2 and 18-5 for descriptions; consider the phase of the woman's labor when formulating your answer.
    c. *Specify physical care and emotional support required:* see Tables 18-1, 18-4, and 18-5 and Care Path for care measures required by each woman according to her phase of labor.

3. *Procedure for locating point of maximum intensity (PMI) before auscultation of FHR or application of ultrasound transducer:* realize that presentation and position affect location of PMI (see Box 18-5 and Figs. 18-6, 18-7, and 18-8) and that Leopold's maneuvers will facilitate location of this point; the

PMI will change as the fetus progresses through the birth canal.

4. *Woman experiencing difficulty with vaginal examinations during labor* (see Vaginal Examination section of Physical Examination).

   a. *Nurse's response to concern:* explain purpose of the examination and the information that will be obtained during each examination in terms of the progress of labor and the status of the fetus; compare findings obtained from a vaginal examination with information on the monitor tracing.

   b. *Measures to enhance comfort and safety:* deep breathing and gentleness during the examination; limit frequency and explain why each examination is needed, what you are doing, and the results you are obtaining; acknowledge her feelings and ensure her privacy; use infection control measures such as perineal care before, sterile gloves and lubricant to perform; never perform when active bleeding is present.

5. *Actions and rationale when membranes rupture:* immediate assessment of the FHR and pattern (prolapse of the cord could have occurred, compressing the cord and leading to variable deceleration patterns); vaginal examination (status of cervix, check for cord prolapse); assess fluid, document findings and notify primary health care provider; strict infection control measures after rupture because risk for infection increases.

6. *Sara, a 17-year-old primigravida in the latent phase of labor:*
   • *Nursing diagnosis:* anxiety related to lack of knowledge and experience regarding the process of childbirth.
   • *Expected outcome:* couple will cooperate with measures to enhance progress of labor as their anxiety level decreases.
   • *Nursing measures:* provide full, simple explanations about each aspect of labor and care measures required as they occur; demonstrate and assist with simple breathing and relaxation techniques; make use of phases of labor to tailor health teaching (doing more during latent phase and less as labor progresses); model coaching and comfort measures father can perform.

7. *Cultural and religious beliefs and practices during labor:*
   a. *Questions to determine cultural and religious preferences:* see Callister (1995) topics for questions in Cultural Factors section of Assessment, First Stage of Labor.
   b. *Importance of determining cultural preferences:* see Cultural Awareness box; consider preferences so couple can act in ways that are comfortable to enhance the progress of labor

and their view of health care providers; such an approach demonstrates respect, concern, and caring.

8. *Couple surprised by changes in approaches to facilitate the labor process:*
   • Discuss advantages of new approaches: internal locus of control (listening to her own body); maternal positions that enhance circulation to the placenta and apply the principle of gravity to facilitate and even shorten labor; new bearing-down efforts are safer (better oxygenation for fetus) and more effective (less tiring while applying effective force to facilitate descent).
   • Use illustrations, model, and video to help couple learn techniques.
   • Demonstrate positions; help them to try.

9. *Home birth* (see Mechanism of Birth Vertex Presentation and Immediate Assessment and Care of Newborn sections and Box 18-9).
   a. *Measures to reassure and comfort:* use eye contact; assume a relaxed, calm, and confident manner; explain what is happening and what you are going to be doing to help her give birth; inform her and her husband about what they will need to do.
   b. *Crowning* (guideline 6): break membranes, tell her to pant or blow to reduce force, use Ritgen's maneuver to control delivery of the head without trauma to fetus or to maternal soft tissues
   c. *Actions after appearance of head* (guideline 7): check for cord around neck, support head during external rotation and restitution, and ease shoulders out one at a time with anterior first then posterior.
   d. *Prevention of neonatal heat loss* (guidelines 11 and 12): dry baby, wrap up with mother, cover head.
   e. *Infection control* (Box 18-4): use Standard Precautions during childbirth adapting to the home setting; use handwashing, clean materials, wear gloves if available.
   f. *Prevention of bleeding* (guideline 17): breastfeed, assess fundus and massage prn, expel clots if present once fundus is firm, assess bladder and encourage voiding, allow placenta to separate naturally.
   g. *Documentation* (guideline 20, items a-i): include date, time, assessment of mother and newborn, family present, events, blood loss, Apgar.

10. *Criteria of effective pushing:* see Maternal Position and Bearing-Down Efforts sections of Second Stage of Labor; cleansing breaths to begin and end each contraction; open glottis pushing with no breath holds longer than 5 to 7 seconds; frequent catch breaths; strong expiratory grunt; upright or lateral position.

11. *Second stage of labor with reluctance to bear down and give birth* (see Bearing-Down Efforts section).
    a. *Reasons for reluctance:* many are listed in the subsection and can include not feeling ready to become a mother, waiting for someone to come, embarrassment about pushing and what happens during bearing-down effort, including passage of feces, fear for self and baby, giving up, previous negative experience with birth.
    b. *Nursing interventions:* recognize and acknowledge her feelings, identify her reason for not continuing, address her concerns and help her to continue.
12. *Is an episiotomy needed?* see Perineal Trauma related to Childbirth section; compare episiotomies with spontaneous lacerations in terms of tissue affected, long-term sequelae, healing process, discomfort; compare reasons given for performing an episiotomy with what research findings demonstrate to be true.
13. *Siblings at childbirth:* include research findings regarding effect of sibling participation on family and on the sibling; consider the developmental readiness of the child and use developmental principles to prepare him or her for the experience; offer family and sibling classes to prepare them for participation in the birth process; evaluate parental comfort with this option; arrange for a support person to remain with the child during the entire childbirth process.
14. *Primipara exhibiting disinterest in newborn during the fourth stage of labor* (see Interactions with Newborn following Birth and Family, Newborn Relationships sections).
    a. *Factors accounting for the behavior:* exhaustion, discomfort, cultural beliefs, disappointment, difficult labor and birth, taking-in stage of recovery.
    b. *Nursing measures:* continue to assess response to newborn, provide time for close contact with newborn when she is more comfortable and rested, help her meet her needs during the taking-in stage in terms of comfort, rest, and desire to review what happened during the process of labor and birth.

CHAPTER 19: LABOR AND BIRTH AT RISK

1. Reviewing Key Concepts and Content

1. Preterm birth
2. Preterm labor
3. Length of gestation (≤37 weeks of gestation), weight at the time of birth (2500 g or less)
4. Preterm birth, intrauterine growth restriction (IUGR), nourished, uteroplacental, hypertension
5. Biochemical markers, fetal fibronectins, salivary estriol

6. Fetal fibronectins, cervical canal, 24, 34, high, lower, vaginal
7. Salivary estriol, increase, high, lower
8. Endocervical length, ultrasound, cervical length, 35, 24 to 28, 40
9. Premature rupture of membranes (PROM)
10. Preterm premature rupture of membranes (PPROM), infection, chorioamnionitis, prolapse, oligohydramnios
11. Dystocia, five factors affecting labor
12. Dysfunctional, dilation, effacement, primary, descent, secondary
13. Hypertonic uterine dysfunction, painful, frequent, dilation, effacement, latent, therapeutic rest
14. Hypotonic uterine dysfunction, weak, inefficient, stop
15. Pelvic dystocia
16. Soft tissue dystocia, placenta previa, leiomyoma (uterine fibroids), ovarian tumors, bladder, rectum
17. Fetal dystocia, cephalopelvic disproportion (CPD), fetopelvic disproportion (FPD), occipitoposterior, breech
18. Multifetal pregnancy
19. Dilation, descent, prolonged latent phase, protracted active phase, secondary arrest, protracted descent, arrest of descent, failure of descent, precipitous labor, hypertonic uterine contractions, tetanic-like
20. External cephalic version (ECV)
21. Trial of labor
22. Induction of labor
23. Bishop score, dilation (cm), effacement (%), station (cm), cervical consistency, cervical position, prostaglandins, ripen
24. Amniotomy, induce, augment
25. Augmentation of labor, oxytocin, amniotomy, nipple
26. Forceps-assisted
27. Vacuum-assisted birth, vacuum extraction
28. Cesarean birth
29. Postterm, postdate
30. Shoulder dystocia, fetopelvic disproportion related to excessive fetal size (macrosomia), pelvic abnormalities
31. Prolapse of umbilical cord, long cord, malpresentation (breech), transverse lie, unengaged presenting part, modified Sims, Trendelenburg, knee-chest, presenting part
32. Amniotic fluid embolism (AFE), meconium
33. T 34. T 35. T 36. F 37. F 38. T
39. F 40. T 41. T 42. F 43. T 44. T
45. T 46. F 47. T 48. F 49. T 50. T
51. F 52. T 53. T 54. F 55. T 56. F
57. *Identify factors associated with risk categories for preterm labor and birth:* use Boxes 19-1 and 19-2 to complete this activity.

58. *Bed rest more harmful than helpful:* see Bed Rest section of Plan of Care and Implementation and Box 19-4.
    - Discuss the adverse effects of bed rest in terms of maternal physical and psychosocial effects and the effects on the woman's support system.
    - Cite the fact that there is no research evidence to support the effectiveness of bed rest in preventing preterm birth or decreasing preterm birth rates.

59. c   60. b   61. d   62. f   63. a   64. e
65. g   66. e   67. f   68. c   69. d   70. a
71. g   72. b

73. *Five factors that cause dystocia:* see Dystocia section and specific sections for each factor.
    - Powers: dysfunctional labor (ineffective uterine contractions or bearing-down efforts)
    - Passage: altered pelvic diameters/shape
    - Passenger: malpresentation or malposition, anomalies, size, number
    - Psychologic status of mother: past experiences, preparation, culture, support system, stress and anxiety level
    - Position of mother: ability and willingness to assume positions that facilitate uteroplacental perfusion and fetal descent

74. *Therapeutic rest:* see Hypertonic Uterine Dysfunction section.
    - Purpose: help woman experiencing hypertonic uterine dysfunction to rest/sleep so active labor can begin usually after a 4- to 6-hour rest period
    - What: use of shower or warm bath for relaxation, comfort measures, administration of analgesics to inhibit contractions, reduce pain, and encourage rest/sleep and relaxation

75. *Complete table related to dysfunctional labor:* see Dysfunctional Labor section, Table 19-1, and Nursing Care Plan, Dysfunctional Labor for information related to each dysfunctional labor pattern in terms of causes, maternal-fetal effects, changes in labor progress, and care management.

76. *Signs of amniotic fluid embolism:* see Emergency box, Amniotic Fluid Embolism for a list of signs.

77. *Recommended care management for amniotic fluid embolism:* see Emergency box, Amniotic Fluid Embolism; consider interventions related to oxygenation, maintaining cardiac output, replacing fluid losses, observing for and correcting coagulation failure (DIC), preparing for emergency birth, and providing emotional support.

78. *Indications and contraindications for oxytocin induction of labor:* see Oxytocin section of Plan of Care and Interventions, Dystocia; several indicators and contraindications are listed.

79. Choice d is correct; women less than 17 or more than 34 in age represent a higher risk for preterm labor and birth, along with parity of 0 or >4, history of preterm birth, multiple abortions, or short interpregnancy interval; infections of the genitourinary tract, including urinary tract infections (UTIs) and reproductive tract such as bacterial vaginosis.

80. Choice a is correct; the woman should count contractions for 1 more hour and drink 2 to 3 glasses of water or juice after emptying bladder; conservative measures are tried before coming to the clinic for evaluation; she can resume light activity if contractions subside but should call for further instructions if they do not.

81. Choice b is correct; weight loss, not gain, occurs; sleep disturbances lead to fatigue and emotional changes; lack of weight-bearing activity leads to bone demineralization.

82. Choice a is correct; increase in heart rate is associated with beta agonists such as ritodrine or terbutaline; magnesium sulfate is a central nervous system (CNS) depressant; woman should alternate lateral positions to decrease pressure on cervix, which could stimulate uterine contractions; calcium gluconate would be used if toxicity occurs.

83. Choice c is correct; it is inserted into the posterior vaginal fornix; the woman should remain in bed for 2 hours; caution should be used if the woman has asthma; therefore, ensure that physician is aware; the insert is removed for severe side effects such as tachysystole or hyperstimulation of the uterus; Cervidil often stimulates contractions and may even induce the onset of labor, eliminating or reducing the need for Pitocin.

84. Choice d is correct; a Bishop score of 9 indicates that the cervix is already sufficiently ripe for successful induction; 10 units of Pitocin is usually mixed in 1000 ml of an electrolyte solution such as Ringer's lactate; the Pitocin solution is piggybacked at the proximal port (port nearest the insertion site).

85. Choice a is correct; frequency of uterine contractions should not be less than every 2 minutes to allow for an adequate rest period between contractions; choices b, c, and d are all expected findings within the normal range.

86. Choice b is correct; at 6 cm the woman is in active labor with progress that is less than 1.5 cm/hr; secondary arrest indicates no progress for ≥2 hours; precipitous labor refers to rapid dilation of 10 cm in 1 hour for a multiparous woman.

87. Choice c is correct; the presentation of this fetus is breech; the soft buttocks are a less efficient dilating wedge than the fetal head; therefore, labor may be slower; the ultrasound transducer should be placed to the left of the umbilicus at a level at or above it; passage of meconium is an expected finding as a result of pressure on the abdomen

during descent; knee-chest position is most often used for occipitoposterior positions.

II. Thinking Critically

1. *Preterm labor and birth prevention program:* see Predicting Preterm Labor and Birth and Prevention and Early Recognition and Diagnosis sections.
   - Why: preterm birth is a major factor contributing to perinatal morbidity and mortality; early detection is critical for successful tocolysis and antenatal glucocorticoid therapy.
   - Many risk factors for preterm labor have been identified (Boxes 19-1, 19-2), but risk scoring systems miss 50% of women who go into preterm labor.
   - All women should be taught signs of preterm labor and measures to prevent based on risk factors identified that can be manipulated by changes in lifestyle behaviors (see Box 19-3).
2. *Woman with a history of preterm labor and birth*
   a. *Identify signs of preterm labor:* see Box 19-3 as a guide for teaching Sara about preterm labor; see if Sara can retrospectively remember experiencing these vague signs with her first pregnancy.
   b. *Implementation of plan to prevent preterm labor:*
      - Evaluate Sara's lifestyle for risky behaviors and health history for risk factors for preterm labor.
      - Discuss how certain factors identified could be changed to reduce her risk, especially related to lifestyle (see Lifestyle Modifications section).
      - Consider modification of sexual activity, stress level, activity (work, home), and hygiene (prevent genitourinary [GU] tract infections).
   c. *Woman begins to experience uterine contraction* (see Guidelines/Guías box): empty bladder, drink 2 to 3 glasses of water/juice, lie down on left side and count contractions by palpating abdomen for 1 hour; call if contractions continue and progress; resume light activity if they do not.
   d. *Criteria for use of tocolysis:* assess Sara to make sure that she is indeed in labor and that she does not exhibit contraindications to tocolysis (see Suppression of Uterine Activity section and Box 19-5).
   e. *Nursing measures during ritodrine infusion to suppress preterm labor:* see Box 19-6, Suppression of Uterine Activity, Tocolysis section, including Nurse Alert, and Medication Guide, Tocolytic Therapy for Preterm Labor.
      - Assess for labor progress and maternal-fetal responses to ritodrine.
      - Monitor and regulate infusion following protocol for increments in dosage of ritodrine.
      - Measure intake and output.
      - Provide support and encouragement.
      - Maintain bed rest in lateral position.
   f. *Administration of betamethasone:* see Promotion of Fetal Lung Maturity section.
      1. *Purpose:* stimulation of fetal surfactant production.
      2. *Protocol:* see Medication Guide, Antenatal Glucocorticoid Therapy; assess Sara for signs of infection, explain action and indications for use, administer IM deep into gluteal muscle, 12 mg, twice, 12 hours apart, observe for adverse effects.
3. *Woman experiencing preterm labor discharged to home care* (see Suppression of Uterine Activity and Home Care subsections of Preterm Labor Care Management section and Plan of Care for Preterm Labor).
   a. *Nursing diagnoses:* risk for maternal/fetal injury related to effects of terbutaline therapy and bed rest requirement for the suppression of preterm labor; interrupted family processes related to demands of labor suppression regimen.
   b. *Instructions for maintaining terbutaline pump:* discuss use of pump, including signs of problems and site care; site change and adjustment of settings may be done by woman or by home care nurse; identify side effects of terbutaline and whom to call if they should appear; teach her how to assess her vital signs, especially how to count her pulse and assess for changes in her respiratory status
   c. *Side effects of terbutaline:* see Medication Guide, Tocolytic Therapy for Preterm Labor, which lists signs that should be taught to the patient
   d. *Instructions regarding palpating uterine activity:* see Guidelines/Guías box; discuss how often to monitor (once or twice a day while lying on side); teach her how to palpate abdomen for uterine contractions: palpate over fundus where uterine contractions are most intense to determine characteristics and then palpate over entire uterus to determine generalized tone; tell her what activity could indicate preterm labor and who to call.
   e. *Coping with bed rest:* see Home Care section, Home Care box, Suggested Activities for Women on Bed Rest, Family Focus box, Activities for Children of Women on Bed Rest, and Fig. 19-2; identify the members of her support system and include them in discussions of how bed rest will be managed

and how they can help; make referrals to home care agencies if needed.

4. *Woman with occipitoposterior position and difficulty bearing down* (see Dystocia, Secondary Powers and Fetal Causes, Malposition sections, Table 19-1, and Box 19-7).

a. *Identifying factors that have a negative effect on bearing-down efforts:* amount of analgesia/anesthesia used, exhaustion, maternal position, lack of knowledge about how to push effectively, lack of sleep, inadequate food and fluid intake.

b. *Measures to facilitate bearing-down efforts:* coach her in BDE, help her into an appropriate position, apply counterpressure to sacrum, demonstrate open-glottis pushing and coach her efforts with every contraction, help her to begin pushing when Ferguson reflex is perceived.

c. *Recommended positions:* hand and knees or lateral when the fetus is in an occipitoposterior position can be very effective in facilitating internal rotation and reducing back pain (see Box 19-7 for additional techniques).

5. *Emergency cesarean birth* (see Cesarean Birth section and Table 19-4, Care Path).

a. *Preoperative measures* (see Preoperative section): implement typical preoperative care measures as for any major surgery in a calm and professional manner, explaining the purpose of each measure that must be performed; use a family-centered approach; discuss what will happen; witness an informed consent; assess fetal-maternal unit, insert Foley catheter, start or maintain IV infusion, provide emotional support.

b. *Immediate postoperative measures:* see Immediate Postoperative Care section and Table 19-4, Care Path; assess for signs of hemorrhage, pain level, respiratory effort, renal function, circulatory status to extremities, signs of postanesthesia recovery, emotional status, and attachment/reaction to newborn.

c. *Ongoing postoperative care measures:* see Postpartum Care section, Table 19-4, Care Path, Patient Teaching box, Pain Relief after Cesarean Birth, and Home Care box, Signs of Postpartum Complications after Discharge; measures include assessment of recovery, pain relief, coughing and deep breathing, leg exercises and assistance with ambulation, nutrition and fluid intake (oral, IV); provide opportunities for interaction and care of newborn, assisting her as needed; provide emotional support to help her deal with her disappointment and feelings of failure; help her and her family prepare for discharge making referrals as needed.

d. *Nursing diagnosis:* situational low self-esteem related to inability to reach goal of a vaginal birth secondary to occurrence of fetal distress.

- Discuss and review why Anne needed a cesarean birth, how she performed during labor, and that she had no control over the fetal distress.
- Discuss vaginal birth after cesarcan (VBAC) and likelihood of it being an option since the reason for her primary cesarean (fetal distress) may not occur again; discuss trial of labor next time to determine her ability to proceed to vaginal birth.
- Use follow-up phone calls to assess progress in accepting cesarean birth.

6. *Fetal position/presentation—RSA:* see Malpresentation subsection of Dystocia section; right sacrum anterior (RSA) indicates a breech presentation; consider that descent may be slower, meconium is often expelled, increasing danger of meconium aspiration, and risk for cord prolapse is increased; depending on progress of labor and maternal characteristics, cesarean or vaginal birth may occur or external cephalic version (ECV) may be attempted (see Evidence-Based box).

7. *Induction of labor* (see Induction of Labor section and Box 19-9).

a. *Bishop score:* see Table 19-3 for factors assessed to determine degree of cervical ripening in preparation for labor process; it is used to determine if a cervical ripening method will need to be used to increase the chances of a successful labor induction.

b. *Score of 5 for a nulliparous woman:* her score should be greater than 9 to ensure a successful induction; cervical ripening will be needed before induction.

c. *Administration of Cervidil:* see Cervical Ripening Methods subsection and Medication Guide.

- Insert into posterior fornix of vagina.
- Side effects include headache, nausea and vomiting, fever, diarrhea, hypotension, hyperstimulation of uterine contractions with or without fetal distress.
- After administration the woman should remain in bed in a lateral position for approximately 2 hours; she may then be allowed to ambulate and be discharged if stable, returning in morning for induction.
- Monitor vital signs, uterine activity, and fetal heart rate (FHR) pattern.

d. *Amniotomy:* see Box 19-8 Procedure: Assisting with Amniotomy; explain what will happen, how it will feel, and why it is being done; assess maternal-fetal unit before and after the procedure; document findings; support woman during procedure telling her what is happening; document procedure and outcomes/reactions appropriately.

   e. *Induction protocol:*

     1. A   2. A   3. A   4. A   5. NA
     6. NA   7. NA   8. A   9. NA 10. A
     11. NA

   f. *Major side effects of Pitocin induction:* hyperstimulation of the uterus, uterine rupture, nonreassuring FHR patterns, water intoxication.

   g. *Actions if hyperstimulation occurs:* see Emergency box, Uterine Hyperstimulation with oxytocin, which lists signs related to uterine contractions and nonreassuring FHR patterns as well as immediate interventions such as discontinuing the induction, maintaining the primary infusion of fluid, turning the woman on her side, administering oxygen via mask, monitoring response of maternal-fetal unit to actions, notifying primary health care provider, and preparing for possible administration of terbutaline to suppress contractions

8. Postterm pregnancy (see Postterm Pregnancy, Labor, and Birth section).

   a. *Maternal-fetal risks related to postterm pregnancy:* see Maternal-Fetal Risks section; maternal risk relates to excessive size of fetus and hardness of fetal skull, which increases risk for dystocia; fetal risk relates to postmaturity syndrome as the placenta ages and a stressful prolonged labor and birth process, including increased risk for birth injury and neonatal hypoglycemia; macrosomia can result in shoulder dystocia and maternal/fetal birth injury.

   b. *Clinical manifestations:* maternal weight loss, decrease in uterine size, meconium in amniotic fluid, advanced fetal bone maturation including the skull.

   c. *Nursing diagnosis:* risk for fetal injury related to placental aging and difficult birth associated with prolonged pregnancy.

   d. *Care measures to ensure safety of maternal-fetal unit:* see Care Management section.
- Continue prenatal care with more frequent visits
- Antepartal assessments, including daily fetal movement counts, NST, amniotic fluid volume assessments, BPP, CST, Doppler blood flow measurements, cervical checks for ripening
- Emotional support
- Prepare for cervical ripening, induction of labor, monitoring for late and variable deceleration patterns, amnioinfusion, forceps- or vacuum-assisted or cesarean birth

   e. *Instructions for self-care at home:* see Home Care Box, Postterm Pregnancy

- Make sure Lora knows how to assess fetal movements and signs of labor.
- Emphasize importance of keeping all appointments for prenatal care and antepartal assessments.
- Identify who to call with concerns, questions, and reports of changing status such as onset of labor or change in fetal movement pattern.

CHAPTER 20: MATERNAL PHYSIOLOGIC CHANGES

I. Reviewing Key Concepts and Content

1. T   2. F   3. F   4. T   5. T   6. T
7. T   8. F   9. F   10. F 11. T 12. F
13. T 14. F

15. *Assessing the bladder for distention* (see Urethra and Bladder section of Urinary System).

   a. *Risk for bladder distention:* birth-induced trauma to urethra and bladder; edematous urethra; increased bladder capacity and diuresis; diminished sensation of bladder fullness related to use of conduction anesthesia; pelvic soreness, lacerations, and episiotomy

   b. *Implications of bladder distention:*
- Bladder pushes uterus up and to side, inhibiting uterine contraction, which leads to excessive bleeding.
- Distention can lead to stasis of urine, increasing risk for urinary tract infection (UTI).

16. *Factors interfering with bowel elimination:* see Bowel Evacuation section of Gastrointestinal; decreased muscle tone, effect of progesterone on peristalsis, prelabor diarrhea, limited oral intake and dehydration from labor, anticipated discomfort related to hemorrhoids and perineal trauma leads to resisting the urge to defecate.

17. *Hypovolemic shock is less likely:* see Blood Volume section of Cardiovascular System; pregnancy-induced hypervolemia allows most women to tolerate a considerable blood loss; size of maternal vascular bed decreases with expulsion of placenta, loss of stimulus for vasodilation, and extravascular water stores of pregnancy is mobilized back into vascular system for excretion.

18. *Risk for thrombophlebitis:* see Coagulation Factors section of Blood Components; increase in clotting factors and fibrinogen levels during pregnancy continues into the postpartum period; hypercoagulable state combined with vessel damage during childbirth and decreased activity level of the postpartum period increases risk for thrombus formation.

19. *Compare and contrast lochial and nonlochial bleeding:* see Table 20-1 for the information to complete your answer.
20. Diaphoresis
21. Afterpains
22. Prolactin, oxytocin
23. Episiotomy
24. Atony
25. Hemorrhoid
26. Involution
27. Puerperium
28. Diastasis recti abdominis
29. Lochia serosa
30. Lochia rubra
31. Lochia alba
32. Engorgement
33. Colostrum
34. Diuresis
35. Choice d is correct; fundus should be at midline; deviation from midline could indicate a full bladder; bright to dark red uterine discharge refers to lochia rubra; edema and erythema are common shortly after repair of a wound; decreased abdominal muscle tone and enlarged uterus results in abdominal protrusion; separation of the abdominal muscle walls, diastasis rectus abdominis, is common during pregnancy and the postpartum period.
36. Choice b is correct; the woman is describing the normal finding of postpartum diaphoresis, which is the body's attempt to excrete fluid retained during pregnancy; documentation is important but not the first nursing action; infection assessment and physician notification are not needed at this time.
37. Choice d is correct; afterpains are most likely to occur in the following circumstances: multiparity, overdistention of the uterus (macrosomia, multifetal pregnancy), breastfeeding (endogenous oxytocin secretion), and administration of an oxytocic.

II. Thinking Critically

1. *Postpartum women express questions and concerns:*
   a. *Afterpains:* breastfeeding with newborn sucking causes the posterior pituitary to secrete oxytocin, stimulating the let-down reflex; uterine contraction is also stimulated, leading to afterpains, which will occur for the first few days postpartum.
   b. *Length of time fundus can be palpated:* see Involution Process section of Uterus; progress of uterine descent in the abdomen is described; within 2 weeks of childbirth, the uterus is again located within the pelvis.
   c. *Stages and duration of lochia:* see Lochia section of Uterus; discuss characteristics of rubra, serosa, and alba lochia in terms of color, consistency, amount, odor, and duration.
   d. *Protruding abdomen:* see Abdomen section; enlarged uterus along with stretched abdominal muscles with diminished tone creates a still-pregnant appearance for the first few weeks after birth; by 6 weeks the abdominal wall will return to approximately its prepregnant state: skin will regain most of its elasticity and striae will fade but remain; discuss exercise and a sensible weight-loss program to facilitate the return of tone and diminish protrusion.
   e. *Diaphoresis and diuresis:* see Postpartum Diuresis section of Urinary System; discuss normalcy of these processes designed to rid the body of fluid retained during pregnancy.
   f. *Breastfeeding as a reliable contraceptive method:* see Pituitary Hormones and Ovarian Function section; emphasize that breastfeeding is not a reliable method because return of ovulation is unpredictable and may precede menstruation; discuss appropriate contraceptive methods for a breastfeeding woman, taking care to avoid hormonal based methods until lactation is well established.
   g. *Lactation suppression in bottle-feeding woman:* see Nonbreastfeeding Mothers section of Breast; congestion of veins and lymphatics along with some filling of milk begins to occur when estrogen and progesterone levels fall with expulsion of the placenta; because milk is not removed, the cycle will shut down and the milk will be absorbed into the circulatory system; she will need to support her breasts with a snug bra/binder and avoid applying warmth on her breasts and expressing any of the milk or stimulating her nipples; ice pack application and analgesics can be used for discomfort.
   h. *Sexuality during the postpartum period of breastfeeding women:* see Vagina and Perineum section of Reproductive System and Associated Structures; discuss role of prolactin in suppressing estrogen secretion, thereby inhibiting vaginal lubrication and resulting in vaginal dryness and dyspareunia, which will persist until ovulation resumes; use of water-soluble lubricant or the spermicide used with a condom for birth control can reduce discomfort.

CHAPTER 21: NURSING CARE DURING THE FOURTH TRIMESTER

I. Reviewing Key Concepts and Content

1. Fourth stage of labor
2. Mother-baby care, single-room maternity care
3. Early postpartum discharge, shortened hospital stay, one-day maternity stay
4. Oxytocic
5. Uterine atony, excessive bleeding/hemorrhage
6. Sitz bath
7. Afterpains (after-birth pains)
8. Splanchnic engorgement, orthostatic hypotension
9. Homans' sign, warmth, redness, tenderness
10. Kegel
11. Engorgement
12. Rubella
13. RhoGAM (Rh immune globulin), intramuscularly, 72
14. *Reasons for breastfeeding in fourth stage of labor:* see Breastfeeding Promotion section; breastfeeding at this time takes advantage of the infant's alert state during the first period of reactivity; aids in contraction of the uterus to prevent hemorrhage; good opportunity to instruct mother and assess breasts; facilitates the bonding/attachment process because infant is ready to feed and success is likely; stimulates infant peristalsis, facilitating excretion of bilirubin in the meconium.
15. *Measures to assist with voiding:* see Prevention of Bladder Distention section in Plan of Care and Implementation; help her assume an upright position on bedpan or in bathroom, listen to running water, put hands in warm water, pour water over vulva with peri bottle, stand in a shower, or sit in a sitz bath, provide analgesics; put oil of peppermint in bedpan.
16. *Measures to prevent thrombophlebitis:* see Ambulation section of Plan of Care and Implementation; exercise legs with active range of motion (ROM) of knees, ankles, feet, and toes; early ambulation; wear support hose (if varicosities are present); keep well hydrated.
17. *Postanesthesia recovery:* see Postanesthesia Recovery section of Assessment, Fourth Stage of Labor.
    a. General anesthesia: LOC/alertness, orientation, vital signs, oxygen saturation of at least 95%, deep breaths, color, keep her on her side until fully oriented and gag reflex returns to prevent aspiration.
    b. Epidural or spinal anesthesia: return of movement and sensation in lower extremities, decrease in numbness, tingling/prickly sensation in legs, ability to feel bladder and to void.

18. *Measures for bottle-feeding mother to suppress lactation and relieve discomfort of engorgement:* see Breastfeeding Promotion and Lactation Suppression section of Plan of Care and Implementation; wear supportive bra or a breast binder 24 hours a day for at least the first 72 hours postpartum, avoid stimulating breasts (no warm water during shower, no infant sucking, no pumping or removal of milk), apply ice packs intermittently to relieve soreness and use cabbage leaves, mild analgesics.
19. *Two interventions to prevent postpartum hemorrhage in early postpartum period:* see Prevention of Excessive Bleeding section.
    • Maintain uterine tone: massage fundus if boggy, expel clots when fundus is firm, administer oxytocic medications, breastfeed or stimulate nipples.
    • Prevent bladder distention.
20. T 21. F 22. T 23. T 24. F 25. F
26. T 27. F 28. F 29. T 30. F 31. T
32. T 33. F
34. *Performing a postpartum assessment* (see Box 21-1).
    a. *Position for fundal palpation:* supine, head and shoulder on pillow, arms at sides, knees slightly flexed
    b. *Fundal characteristics to assess:* consistency (firm or boggy), height (above, at, below umbilicus), location (midline or deviated to the right or left)
    c. *Position for assessment of perineum:* lateral or modified Sims position with upper leg flexed on hip
    d. *Episiotomy characteristics to assess:* REEDA (redness, edema, ecchymosis, drainage, approximation); presence of hematoma; adequacy of hygiene, including cleanliness, presence of odor, method used to cleanse perineum and to apply topical preparations
    e. *Characteristics of lochia to assess:* stage, amount, odor, clots
35. *Recovery room nurse report:* see Transfer from Recovery Area section and Table 21-1 for a discussion of essential information that should be reported regarding the woman, the baby, and the significant events and findings from her prenatal and childbirth periods.
36. *Infection control measures* (see Prevention of Infection section of Plan of Care and Implementation section).
    a. *Measures to prevent transmission of infection from person to person:* clean environment, handwashing, use of standard precautions, proper care and use of equipment
    b. *Infection prevention measures to teach the woman:* avoid walking barefoot, handwashing, hygiene measures (general, breast, perineal), prevention of bladder infection, measures to

enhance resistance to infection including nutrition and rest

37. *Signs of potential complications during postpartum period:* see Box 21-4, Signs of Potential Complications, Physiologic Problems and Box 21-7, Signs of Potential Complications, Psychosocial.

38. Choice d is correct; these tremors are not related to infection or hypothermia; theories include sudden release of pressure on pelvic nerves after birth, response to a fetus-to-mother transfusion during placental separation, a reaction to increased maternal adrenaline production or epidural anesthesia; they are self-limiting, lasting only a short period of time; warm blankets and reassurance that these tremors are self-limiting would be the most effective relief measures.

39. Choice c is correct; the woman should be assisted into a supine position with head and shoulders on a pillow, arms at sides, and knees flexed; this will facilitate relaxation of abdominal muscles and allow deep palpation.

40. Choice a is correct; Methergine as an oxytocic contracts the uterus, thereby preventing excessive blood loss; lochia will therefore reflect expected characteristics.

41. Choice b is correct; a direct and indirect Coombs' must be negative, indicating that antibodies have not been formed, before RhoGAM can be given; it must be given within 72 hours of birth; the newborn needs to be Rh+; it is often given in the third trimester and then again after birth.

42. Choice d is correct; this is a medical aseptic procedure; therefore, clean not sterile equipment is used; the water should be warm at 38° to 40.6° C; it is often used 2 to 3 times a day for 20 minutes each time.

II. Thinking Critically

1. *Pain relief for a postpartum breastfeeding mother:* see Comfort section of Plan of Care and Implementation; assess characteristics of pain (severity, location, relief measures already tried and effectiveness); use a combination of pharmacologic and nonpharmacologic measures as indicated by the nature of the pain being experienced; if breastfeeding, administer a systemic analgesic just before or just after a feeding session; make sure medication is not contraindicated for breastfeeding women.

2. *Woman exhibiting signs of hemorrhage and shock* (see Prevention of Bleeding section of Plan of Care and Implementation and Emergency box, Hypovolemic Shock).
   a. *Criteria to determine if flow is excessive:* note length of time pad was worn and the degree to which it was saturated with blood; check the bed to determine if lochia has pooled under buttocks; pad saturation in 15 minutes or less indicates a profuse flow.
   b. *Priority action:* assess fundus and massage if boggy; once firm, express clots, check bladder for distention and assist to empty, and administer oxytocics if ordered; notify the primary health care provider to discuss assessment findings, actions taken, and responses.
   c. *Additional interventions:* see list of measures identified in Emergency box, Hypovolemic Shock.

3. *Administering rubella vaccine to a postpartum woman:* see Health Promotion of Future Pregnancies and Children section; recheck titer results and order; determine if woman or any household members are immunocompromised; check allergies (duck eggs); inform her of side effects and emphasize that she must not become pregnant for at least 2 to 3 months after the immunization.

4. *Administering RhoGAM to a postpartum woman:* see Health Promotion of Future Pregnancies and Children section and Medication Guide; check woman's and newborn's Rh status and Coombs' test results; obtain RhoGAM and check all identification data; administer intramuscularly; woman must be Rh and indirect Coombs' negative; newborn must be Rh positive and direct Coombs' negative; ensure that it is administered within 72 hours after birth; provide woman with documentation that she received RhoGAM.

5. *Sexual changes after pregnancy and childbirth:* see Sexual Activity and Contraception section of Discharge Teaching section and the Home Care box, Resumption of Sexual Intercourse; identify changes that may occur; discuss physical and emotional readiness of the woman; stress importance of open communication; discuss how to prevent discomfort in terms of position and lubrication; emphasize the importance of birth control because return of ovulation cannot be predicted with accuracy.

6. *Postpartum women—nursing diagnoses, expected outcomes, and nursing management:*
   a. *Nursing diagnosis:* risk for infection of episiotomy related to ineffective perineal hygiene measures.
      Expected outcome: episiotomy will heal without infection.
      Nursing management: see Prevention of Infection section of Plan of Care and Implementation and Box 21-5 for full identification of measures to enhance healing and prevent infection.
   b. *Nursing diagnosis:* constipation related to inactivity and lack of knowledge.
      Expected outcome: woman will have soft formed bowel movement.

Nursing management: see Promotion of Normal Bladder and Bowel Patterns section; determine usual elimination patterns and measures used to enhance elimination; encourage activity, roughage, fluids; obtain order for mild combination stool softener-laxative.

c. *Nursing diagnosis:* acute pain related to episiotomy and hemorrhoids.
Expected outcome: woman will experience a reduction in pain following implementation of suggested relief measures.
Nursing management: see Promotion of Comfort section, Nursing Care Plan, and Box 21-5; emphasize nonpharmacologic relief measures such as perineal care, sitz bath, topicals, side-lying position, Kegel exercises, measures to enhance bowel and bladder elimination; use pharmacologic measures if local measures are ineffective or pain is severe.

7. *Fundus above umbilicus and to the right of midline:*
   a. *Most likely basis for finding:* bladder distention; confirm by palpating the bladder and asking the woman to describe the last time she voided.
   b. *Nursing action:* assist woman to empty bladder; measure amount voided and assess characteristics of the urine; palpate bladder and fundus again to determine response; catheterization may be required if she is unable to empty her bladder fully because a distended bladder can lead to uterine atony with excessive bleeding and UTIs.

8. *Resumption of physical activity after giving birth:* see Postanesthesia section and Ambulation section of Plan of Care and Implementation section.
   • Assess postanesthesia recovery and physical stability, including return of strength, mobility, and sensation in lower extremities.
   • Assist and supervise first few times out of bed because orthostatic hypotension can cause her to be dizzy and fall.
   • Show her where the call light is and what to do if she is alone and begins to feel dizzy or lightheaded.

9. *Resumption of full oral intake after giving birth:* see Promotion of Nutrition section of Plan of Care and Implementation; assess woman for physiologic stability (vital signs [VS], fundus, lochia, perineum) before resuming full diet; determine type of anesthesia used for birth—if general anesthesia was used make sure woman is fully alert and gag reflex has returned.

10. *Woman preparing for early discharge:*
    a. *Nurse's legal responsibility:* assess woman, newborn, and family to confirm that criteria for discharge are fully met; notify primary health care provider if criteria are not met;

document all assessment findings, actions, and responses.
    b. *Criteria for discharge—maternal, newborn, general:* see Box 21-3.
    c. *Outline essential content that must be taught before discharge:* see Discharge Teaching section; include information regarding self- and newborn care, signs of complications, prescribed medications; arrange for first postpartum checkup and for a follow-up telephone call or home visit usually within 1 to 2 days after discharge.

11. *Cultural beliefs and practices* (see Impact of Cultural Diversity section of Care Management of Psychosocial Needs).
    a. *Importance of using a culturally sensitive approach:* recognition of cultural beliefs and practices is essential to meet her individual needs; such an approach demonstrates respect, caring, and concern.
    b. *Korean-American woman—heat and cold balance:* ask woman the substances and practices that she identifies to be hot and cold, then intervene appropriately; see Box 21-8.
    c. *Muslim woman in postpartum period:* see Box 21-8; emphasize diet modification and modesty.

CHAPTER 22: TRANSITION TO PARENTHOOD

I. Reviewing Key Concepts and Content

1. *Complete table related to maternal adjustment:* see Table 22-2 and specific sections for each phase in the Maternal Adjustment section.
2. *Discussion of paternal adjustment:* see Paternal Adjustment section and Table 22-3; phases of transition and nursing measures that provide for support, teaching, demonstration, and practice and time for interaction with the newborn should be emphasized in the discussion.
3. *Attachment of newborn to parents and parents to newborn* (see Parental Attachment, Bonding, and Acquaintance section).
   a. *Define attachment and bonding:*
      • Attachment: parents come to love and accept child and child comes to love and accept parents
      • Bonding: sensitive period after birth when parents have close contact with their infant
   b. *Conditions that facilitate attachment:* see Table 22-1; emotionally healthy parents, competent in communication and caregiving; parent and newborn fit in terms of state, temperament, and gender; parental proximity to infant; adequate social support system.

c. *Acquaintance process:* parents use eye contact, touch, talking, and exploring to get to know their newborn; claiming or identification in terms of likeness, differences, and uniqueness is part of this process.

d. *Assessment of process of attachment:* see Assessment of Attachment Behaviors section and Patient Teaching box, Assessing Attachment Behavior, for specific behaviors indicating the quality of the attachment that is developing; it is critical that nurses provide opportunities for parent and infant contact and to be present during these contacts to observe the interaction that is taking place.

4. *Parental tasks:* see Parental Tasks and Responsibilities section of Parental Role after Childbirth for a description of each of the tasks of reconciling actual child with fantasy child, becoming adept in infant care, and establishing a place for the newborn within the family group.

5. *Parent infant contact:* see specific sections for each form of contact in Parent-Infant Contact.

a. Early contact: important to provide time for parents to see, touch, and hold their newborn as soon as possible after birth; stress that attachment is an ongoing process; interference with this early contact because of maternal and/or newborn problems should not have a long-term effect as long at it is balanced by opportunities for close contact as soon as possible after birth as appropriate for maternal and/or newborn condition.

b. Extended contact: family-centered care, mother-baby care, and use of LDRP/LDR rooms to facilitate this type of contact

6. Attachment, bonding
7. Acquaintance, eye contact, touching, talking, exploring
8. *En face,* face to face, positioning mom and baby together after birth, dimming lights so baby can open eyes, delay eye prophylaxis
9. Claiming, likeness, differences, uniqueness
10. Entrainment, waving, lifting, kicking, dancing in tune
11. Biorhythmicity, loving care, alert, responsive, social interactions, learning
12. Reciprocity, synchrony
13. Engrossment, touch, eye-to-eye contact, features both unique and similar to himself
14. *Factors influencing parental responses to the birth of their child:* see section for each factor in the Factors Influencing Parental Responses section.
15. Choice d is correct; choice a reflects the first phase of identifying likenesses; choice b reflects the second phase of identifying differences; choice c reflects a negative reaction of claiming the infant in terms of pain and discomfort; choice d reflects the third or final stage of identifying uniqueness.

16. Choice b is correct; early close contact is recommended to initiate and enhance the attachment process.
17. Choice a is correct; engrossment refers to a father's absorption, preoccupation, and interest in his infant; choice b represents the claiming process phase I identifying likeness; choice c represents reciprocity; choice d represents *en face* or face-to-face position with mutual gazing.
18. Choice b is correct; taking-in is the first 1 to 2 days of recovery following birth; other behaviors exhibited include reliance on others to help her meet needs, being excited, and talkative.
19. Choice c is correct; approximately 50% to 80% of women experience postpartum blues; new parents should be reassured that their skills as parents develop gradually and they should seek help to develop these skills; postpartum blues that are self-limiting and short lived do not require psychotropic medications; support and care of the postpartum woman and her newborn by her partner and family is the most effective prevention and coping strategy; feelings of fatigue from childbirth and meeting demands of newborn can accentuate feelings of depression

II. Thinking Critically

1. *Teaching parents communication skills with their newborns* (see Communication between Parent and Infant section).

a. *Communication techniques:* discuss touch, eye contact, voice, and odor; demonstrate techniques, have parents try, and point out newborn response in terms of quieting, alerting, making eye contact, gazing; help parents interpret cues.

b. *Newborn's communication:* point out infant responses; discuss processes of entrainment, biorhythmicity, reciprocity, synchrony, and repertoire of behaviors.

2. *Woman following emergency cesarean birth: disappointment with lack of immediate bonding time with newborn:*

• Discuss concepts of early and extended contact.
• Emphasize that the parent-infant attachment process is ongoing—her emotional bond with her baby will not be weaker.
• Help her meet her own physical and emotional needs so that she develops readiness to meet her newborn's needs.
• Help her get to know her baby, interact with and care for him; point out newborn characteristics, including how the baby is responding to her efforts.
• Show her how to communicate with her newborn and how her newborn communicates with her.

- Arrange for follow-up after discharge to assess how attachment is progressing.
3. *Sibling adjustment to newborn:* see Sibling Adaptation section and Family Focus box, which identifies strategies parents can use to help their other children adapt; caution her that adjustment takes time and is strongly related to the developmental level and experiences of the sibling(s).
4. *Parents unsure and anxious about caring for their newborn* (see Table 22-1).
   a. *Nursing diagnosis:* risk for impaired parent-infant attachment related to lack of knowledge and feeling of incompetence regarding infant care.
   b. *Nursing measures to facilitate attachment can include the following:*
      - Perform newborn assessment with parents present, pointing out newborn characteristics and encouraging parents to participate and ask questions.
      - Demonstrate newborn care measures and provide time for parents to practice and obtain feedback.
      - Provide extended contact time with newborn, such as longer visiting hours and rooming-in, until discharge
      - Make referral for follow-up with telephone contacts and home visits; refer to parenting classes and support groups, lactation consultant and La Leche.
      - Recommend books, magazines, and videos/DVDs and interactive Internet sites that discuss newborns and their care
5. *Parental disappointment with newborn's gender and appearance:* see Parental Tasks and Responsibilities section; foster attachment, acquaintance, and claiming; help parents get acquainted with the infant and to reconcile the real child with the fantasy child; discuss the basis of molding, caput succedaneum, and forceps marks and how they will be resolved; be alert for problems with attachment and care so follow-up can be arranged.
6. *Grandparent adjustment:* see Grandparent Adaptation section; observe interaction between grandparents and parents taking note of signs of effective interaction and conflict; involve grandparents in teaching sessions as appropriate for this family; spend time with grandparents to help them be supportive without "taking over" or being critical; help the new parents recognize the unique role grandparents can play as parenting role models, nuturers, and providers of respite care.
7. *Woman experiencing postpartum blues:*
   - *Nursing diagnosis:* ineffective maternal coping related to hormonal changes and increased responsibilities following birth.

- *Expected outcome:* woman will report feeling more contented with her role as mother following the use of recommended coping strategies.
- *Nursing management:* see Postpartum Blues section of Maternal Adjustment section, Patient Teaching box, Coping with Postpartum Blues, and Fig. 22-6; use the "Am I Blue" assessment tool to determine the level of blues she is experiencing; involve both Jane and her husband in the teaching session and in the development of a plan for coping with the blues; this must occur early to prevent development of postpartum depression.
8. *Questions asked by expectant parents during a class about newborn care:*
   a. *What to do about crying infant:* see Development of Day-Night Routines and Interpretation of Crying and Quieting Techniques sections of Plan of Care and Implementation and Boxes 22-2 and Guidelines/Guías box.
   b. *Value of infant massage:* see Box 22-4 and Infant Stimulation section.
   c. *Newborn learning:* see Developmental Milestones and Infant Stimulation sections of Plan of Care and Implementation and Box 22-3.

CHAPTER 23: POSTPARTUM COMPLICATIONS

I. Reviewing Key Concepts and Content

1. Postpartum hemorrhage (PPH), uterine atony, early (acute, primary) PPH, late (secondary) PPH
2. Uterine atony
3. Hematoma, vulvar hematomas, vaginal hematomas
4. Inversion, hemorrhage, shock, pain, fundal, vigorous fundal, excessive traction, uterine atony, leiomyomas, placenta tissue
5. Subinvolution
6. Hemorrhagic (hypovolemic) shock
7. Coagulopathy, DIC
8. Thrombosis, inflammation (thrombophlebitis), obstruction, superficial venous thrombosis, deep vein thrombosis (DVT), pulmonary embolism
9. Postpartum, puerperal infection, fever, 2 successive days of the first 10 postpartum days excluding the first 24 hours, uterus, wounds, breasts, urinary tract, respiratory tract
10. Infection of the lining of the uterus, endometritis, placental
11. Mastitis, first time mothers who are breastfeeding, unilateral, flow of milk
12. Uterine prolapse

13. Cystocele
14. Rectocele
15. Urinary incontinence
16. Fistula, vesicovaginal fistula, urethrovaginal fistula, rectovaginal fistula
17. Postpartum depression without psychotic features, 10%, 15%, irritability, significant others, baby, rejection, jealousy
18. Postpartum psychosis, days, 2 to 3, 8, fatigue, insomnia, tearfulness, emotional lability, infant, kill the infant
19. F   20. T   21. T   22. F   23. F   24. T
25. F   26. F   27. T   28. F   29. F   30. T
31. F   32. F   33. T   34. T   35. F
36. *Twofold focus of management of hemorrhagic shock:* restore circulating blood volume to enhance perfusion of vital organs and treat the cause of the hemorrhage.
37. *Four priority nursing interventions for PPH:* see Nursing Interventions section of Hemorrhagic Shock; cite interventions related to improving and monitoring tissue perfusion, treating the cause of the hemorrhage, enhancing healing, supporting the woman and her family, fostering maternal-infant attachment as appropriate, and planning for discharge.
38. *Standard of care for bleeding emergencies:* provision should be made for the nurse to implement actions independently—policies, procedures, standing orders or protocols, and clinical guidelines should be established by the agency and agreed upon by health care providers including nurses; the nurse should never leave the patient alone.
39. *Measures to prevent genital tract infections:* see Care Management section of Postpartum Infections for a list of prevention measures including good prenatal nutrition to control anemia and intrapartal hemorrhage, perineal hygiene, adherence to aseptic techniques.
40. *Identification and discussion of the phases of the grief response for a woman at 24 weeks with suspected fetal death:*
   a. Acute distress
   b. Intense grief
   c. Intense grief (disorganization)
   d. Reorganization
41. *Actualizing the loss:* see Actualizing the Loss and Options for Parents sections; helping parents and family express their loss and create tangible memories of the baby can help parents actualize (make it a reality) the loss; help them participate in the options that are most appealing and comfortable for them; many different ideas are presented in these sections, including holding, bathing, and dressing the infant; spending time alone with the infant and with other family members; taking pictures and creating special memories; importance of follow-up after discharge should be emphasized to assess progress through the grief process and to offer support

42. Choice b is correct; although BP should be taken before and after administration of Methergine the woman's hypertensive status would be a contraindicating factor for its use; therefore, the order should be questioned
43. Choice d is correct; Hemabate is a powerful prostaglandin that is the third-line medication given to treat excessive uterine blood loss or hemorrhage related to uterine atony; it has no action related to pain, infection, or clotting.
44. Choice a is correct; puerperal infections are infections of the genital tract after birth; pulse will increase not decrease in response to fever; lochia characteristics will change, but this will not be the first sign exhibited; WBC count would already be elevated related to pregnancy and birth.
45. Choice c is correct; heparin and warfarin (Coumadin) are safe for use by breastfeeding women; heparin, which is administered intravenously or subcutaneously, is the anticoagulant of choice during the acute stage of DVT; woman should be fitted for elastic stockings after the acute stage is past when edema subsides.
46. Choice a is correct; although the other questions are appropriate, the potential for harming herself or her baby is the most serious and very real concern.
47. Choice a is correct; telling her to be happy that one twin survived may be interpreted that she should not grieve the loss of the daughter who died—the loss must be acknowledged and the tasks for mourners accomplished; choices b, c, and d are all appropriate responses by the nurse with choices b and c helpful in actualizing the loss.
48. Choice d is correct; choices a and b represent the intense grief phase, and choice c represents the reorganization phase.
49. Choice b is correct; see Box 23-9; note that choices a, c, and d are in the category of what not to say, whereas choice b represents a response that acknowledges the difficulty of the loss and offers an opportunity for expression of feelings.

II. Thinking Critically

1. *Postpartum woman at risk for postpartum hemorrhage*
   a. *Risk factors for early postpartum hemorrhage:* parity (5-1-0-7), vaginal full-term twin birth 1 hour ago; hypotonic uterine dysfunction treated with oxytocin (Pitocin); use of forceps for birth; increased manipulation with birth of twins.

b. *Nursing diagnosis:* risk for deficient fluid volume related to moderate to heavy blood loss associated with vaginal birth of twins.

c. *Nurse's response to excessive blood loss:* most common cause of the excessive blood loss 1 hour after birth would be uterine atony, especially because woman exhibits several risk factors.
- Assess fundus for consistency, height, and location; massage if boggy.
- Express clots, if present, once uterus is firm.
- Check bladder for distention (distended bladder will reduce uterine contraction); check perineum for swelling and ask woman about experiencing perineal pressure (hematoma formation is possible related to use of forceps for birth).

d. *Guidelines for administering Pitocin IV:* use Table 23-1 for administration guidelines in terms of dose/route, contraindications, side effects, nursing considerations.

e. *Signs of developing hemorrhagic shock:* see Emergency box, Hemorrhagic Shock, which identifies priority assessments a nurse should perform and the findings that would indicate progress from hemorrhage to hypovolemic shock; assessment includes VS, skin, urinary output, level of consciousness, mental status, and CVP; assessment should be frequent and findings compared to one another to note change.

f. *Nursing measures to support the woman and family:*
- Explain progress, including meaning of findings and need for treatment measures being used, including their purpose and effectiveness.
- Use a calm, professional, organized approach that incorporates periods of uninterrupted rest.
- Initiate comfort measures.
- Provide opportunities for interaction with newborn and updates on newborn's status.

2. *Puerperal infection:*

a. *Risk factors:* see Box 23-3; consider preconception, antepartum, and intrapartum factors.

b. *Typical signs of endometritis:* see Endometritis section; signs include fever, tachycardia, chills, anorexia, nausea, fatigue and lethargy, pelvic pain and uterine tenderness, foul-smelling, profuse lochia.

c. *Nursing diagnoses:* acute pain related to effects of infection on uterine tissue; interrupted family processes OR anxiety OR ineffective individual or family coping related to unexpected postpartum complication (use assessment findings to determine priority psychosocial nursing diagnoses).

d. *Nursing measures:* see Care Management section.
- Assess progress of healing.
- Administer antibiotics as prescribed; teach woman about correct use.
- Ensure adequate hydration, nutrition, rest to enhance healing.
- Provide comfort measures and medications for pain relief.
- Provide emotional support for woman and her family.
- Arrange for newborn interaction and care.
- Use support measures and teaching to prepare woman for discharge.

3. *Woman with mastitis (see Mastitis section):*

a. *Assessment findings associated with mastitis:* unilateral findings well after milk comes in; inflammatory edema and breast engorgement with obstructed flow of milk in region; chills, fever, malaise, localized tenderness, pain, swelling, and redness; axillary adenopathy

b. *Nursing diagnoses:* acute pain related to inflammation of right breast; ineffective breastfeeding OR anxiety related to interruption of breastfeeding while taking antibiotics or related to concerns regarding transmission of infection to newborn

c. *Treatment measures:* antibiotics, breast support, local heat and cold applications, adequate hydration and nutrition, analgesics; maintain lactation with continued breastfeeding if permitted or with breast pumping

d. *Measures to prevent recurrence of mastitis:* good breastfeeding technique (latch-on, and removal, alternating positions and starting breast), frequent feedings (avoid missing feedings or abrupt weaning), breast care, and early detection and treatment of cracks, cleanliness practices

4. *Woman with DVT (see Thromboembolic Disease section):*

a. *Risk factors:* see Incidence and Etiology subsection; in addition to hypercoagulability of pregnancy continuing into the postpartum period, other risk factors for this woman would be cesarean birth, obesity, age over 35 years, multiparity, smoking habit, and varicosities in both legs.

b. *Signs and symptoms indicative of DVT:* see Clinical Manifestations section; unilateral leg pain and calf tenderness, swelling, redness and warmth, positive Homans' sign; woman may also be asymptomatic with a DVT, depending on degree of involvement.

c. *Nursing diagnosis:* anxiety related to unexpected development of a postpartum complication.

d. *Expected care management:* see Medical Management and Nursing Interventions sections.
  - Assess for unusual bleeding, signs of pulmonary embolism, circulatory status of lower extremities.
  - Administer anticoagulant (usually heparin) as ordered.
  - Institute bed rest with elevation of affected leg; assist to change position; caution not to rub site.
  - Initiate pain management using analgesics without aspirin; local application of warm, moist heat.
  - Explain disorder and purpose and effectiveness of treatment measures used.
  - Assist with care of self and newborn.

e. *Discharge instructions:*
  - How to assess leg and for signs of unusual bleeding
  - Proper use of elastic/support stockings
  - How to take anticoagulant safely and importance of follow-up to assess progress
  - Practices to prevent bleeding while taking an anticoagulant and importance of avoiding pregnancy because warfarin is teratogenic
  - Importance of avoiding aspirin and acetaminophen and food/vitamin supplements that are sources of vitamin K because they can interact with warfarin (Coumadin)

5. *Woman diagnosed with cystocele and rectocele* (see Cystocele and Rectocele and Care Management sections of Sequelae of Childbirth Trauma).

a. *Signs and symptoms most likely exhibited:* bearing down/pelvic pressure, urinary and bowel elimination changes, bulging into the vagina noted during a vaginal examination.

b. *Two priority nursing diagnoses with expected outcomes:*
  - Constipation or diarrhea related to displacement of rectum into posterior rectal wall; woman will experience regular, soft, formed bowel elimination.
  - Impaired urinary elimination related to displacement of bladder into anterior vaginal wall; woman will fully empty bladder every 2 to 3 hours.
  - Ineffective sexuality patterns related to vaginal changes associated with cystocele and rectocele; woman will openly discuss measures to enhance sexual function.

c. *Management of cystocele and rectocele:* see Plan of Care and Implementation subsection; answer should include use of Kegel exercises, diet (fiber and fluids), stool softener, mild laxative, genital hygiene including sitz baths, and proper use of commercial products; emotional support.

d. *Using a pessary:*
  - *Nursing diagnosis:* risk for infection related to insertion of foreign object into vagina.
  - *Instructions for use:* tailor instructions for the type of pessary that is being used; include how to insert and remove, how to care for and cleanse the pessary, genital hygiene measures, and signs indicative of infection.

6. *Woman with postpartum depression:*
a. *Signs and symptoms indicative of postpartum depression* include fatigue, increased yearning for sleep, irritability, concerned about being a good mother but has a low level of self-esteem and self-confidence regarding her effectiveness, expressed jealousy of her husband's seemingly greater enjoyment when spending time with baby than with her, and angry outbursts directed against husband.

b. *Predisposing factors* include prenatal anxiety, meager social support and stressful life events (recent relocation, husband busy with new job), bottle-feeding, mother unemployed and inexperienced with newborn care, 35 years of age.

c. *Questions:* see Box 23-4 for question topics; be sure to directly ask Mary about contemplating harm to self or baby.

d. *Nursing diagnoses:* several nursing diagnoses are listed in Nursing Diagnosis section; at this point, fatigue, situational low self-esteem, ineffective individual coping, and risk for impaired parenting seem to be paramount.

e. *Measures to cope with postpartum depression:* include husband in discussions and planning, consider relationship with partner and suggest changes and resources they could seek out from their church and childrearing couples in their community; emphasize safety measures for mother or newborn; provide referral for psychiatric care with the use of antidepressant medications if postpartum depression is determined to be moderate to severe; frequent follow-up to check progress is critical; activities to prevent postpartum depression would apply here.

7. *Family experiencing miscarriage at 13 weeks of gestation:*
a. *Approach to individualize support measures:* see Assessment section.
  - Begin with assessment to determine best approach to take for this couple.
  - Determine nature of the parental attachment with the pregnancy and the meaning of the pregnancy and birth to the parents—their perception of the loss—recognizing that responses of father and mother may differ.
  - Understand circumstances surrounding the loss—listen to their story.
  - Observe the immediate response of each parent to the loss—do they match?

- Identify persons comprising their social network and how can they support them; do the parents want their support?
b. *Cite questions and observations to gather information required to create an individualized plan of care:* use each of the areas identified in section "a" of this critical thinking situation to formulate questions and organize observations.
c. *Nursing diagnoses:* see Nursing Diagnoses section; consider assessment findings to determine nursing diagnoses and their priority for a specific family.
  - Nursing diagnoses associated with emotional effects of grief: situational low self-esteem, spiritual distress, anxiety, ineffective individual coping
  - Nursing diagnoses associated with impact on family including other child and grandparents: interrupted family processes, ineffective family coping
  - Nursing diagnoses related to the physical effects of the grief process: fatigue, disturbed sleep pattern, imbalanced nutrition
d. *Therapeutic communication techniques to help couple express feelings and emotions:* see Communicating and Caring Techniques section and Box 23-9; examples of therapeutic communication techniques include encourage expression of feelings by leaning forward, nodding, reflection, saying "tell me more"; observe nonverbal cues; use touch as appropriate; listen patiently and use silence while couple tell their story.
e. *Analysis of nurse responses:* N, T, N, N, T, T, N, N, T, T.
8. *Physical needs of postpartum woman following stillbirth:* see Physical Comfort section.
  - Provide option of staying on maternity unit or transferring to another; discuss the advantages and disadvantages of each option.
  - Provide option for room assignment (away from nursery).
  - Assist with breast care and other physical care requirements that would remind her she had a baby (i.e., milk comes in, afterpains, gas pains mimic fetal movements, flow).
  - Emphasize the importance of comfort measures to help with sleep.
  - Encourage adequate nutrition, fluids, rest to enhance strength and healing.
9. *Birth of baby with anencephaly:*
a. *Making the decision to see the baby:* see Options for Parents section.
  - Tell them about the option to see the baby.
  - Give them time to think about the option so they can choose what is best for them.

- Come back and ask them their decision; if they are unsure or say no, ask again before discharge.
b. *Measures to help the couple when they see their baby:*
  - Prepare baby, making it look as normal as possible: bathe, use powder, comb hair, place under warmer, put on identification bracelet, dress, wrap in a pretty blanket (get help from a funeral director if needed).
  - Treat baby as one would a live baby when bringing baby to parents: use name, talk about baby's features emphasizing those that are normal, resemblances.
  - Provide time alone with baby and adjust length of time with the baby to meet their needs; observe for cues that tell you they need more time or that they are done.
  - Determine what else they would need to make a memory—foot print, photograph, lock of hair etc.

CHAPTER 24: PHYSIOLOGIC ADAPTATIONS OF THE NEWBORN

I. Reviewing Key Concepts and Content

1. P 2. N 3. N 4. P 5. N 6. N
7. N 8. N 9. P 10. N 11. N 12. N
13. P 14. N 15. N 16. N 17. P 18. N
19. N 20. N 21. P 22. N 23. P
24. *Factors initiating breathing after birth:* the reflex to breathe is triggered by such factors as pressure changes, chilling, noise, light, and other sensations associated with birth; chemoreceptor activation of respiratory center by lowered oxygen level, high carbon dioxide level, and lower pH.
25. Thermoregulation, hypothermia, thermogenesis, brown fat, metabolic activity
26. Produce heat, blood vessels, body surface to body weight (mass) ratio, flexed, body surface
27. Convection, 24° C, wrap
28. Radiation, nursery cribs, examination tables, windows, air draft
29. Evaporation, dry, drying
30. Conduction, warmed crib
31. *Guidelines for weighing and measuring newborn:* see Table 24-2 and Baseline Measurements of Physical Growth section of Physical Examination; wear gloves if performed before first bath.
a. *Weight:* balance scale, cover scale with clean scale paper, place undressed infant on scale, keep hand hovering over infant, never turn away; weigh at the same time of day when hospitalized.
b. *Head circumference:* measure the widest part of head just above ears and eyebrows; repeat if molding is present at birth.

c. *Chest circumference:* measure across nipple line.

d. *Abdominal circumference:* measure just above the level of umbilicus.

e. *Length:* measure from crown to rump, then rump to heels.

32. k   33. f   34. b   35. j   36. d   37. i
38. h   39. l   40. a   41. e   42. g   43. c
44. Sleep-wake
45. Deep, light
46. Drowsy, quiet alert, active alert, crying, quiet alert
47. 16 to 18, increasing
48. Habituation
49. Orientation
50. Temperament, behavioral style, easy, slow to warm up, difficult
51. *Factors influencing newborn's behavior:* see section for each factor listed in Behavioral Characteristics section; each factor is described in terms of its influence on newborn behavior.
52. *Complete table related to phases of newborn transition period to extrauterine life:* see Transition Period section at beginning of chapter for identification of each phase and description of timing/duration and typical newborn behaviors for each phase.
53. F   54. F   55. T   56. T   57. F   58. T
59. T   60. T   61. F   62. T   63. T   64. T
65. T   66. F
67. Telangiectatic nevi
68. Molding
69. Caput succedaneum
70. Cephalhematoma
71. Mongolian spots
72. Acrocyanosis
73. Vernix caseosa
74. Milia
75. Jaundice
76. Meconium
77. Erythema toxicum
78. Strabismus
79. Harlequin sign
80. Hydrocele
81. Thrush
82. Fontanel
83. Lanugo
84. Choice d is correct; the newborn at 5 hours old is in the second period of reactivity, during which tachycardia, tachypnea, increased muscle tone, skin color changes, mucus production, and passage of meconium are normal findings; although a newborn can have periods of apnea, they should be less than 20 seconds; the average heart rate of a newborn when awake is 120 to 160 beats/min.
85. Choice a is correct; the rash described is erythema toxicum; it is an inflammatory response that has no clinical significance and requires no treatment because it will disappear spontaneously.

86. Choice b is correct; physiologic jaundice does not appear until 24 hours after birth; further investigation would be needed if it appears during the first 24 hours, because this is consistent with pathologic jaundice; a, c, and d are findings within the normal range for a newborn 12 hours old
87. Choice d is correct; choices b and c are common newborn reflexes used to assess integrity of neuromuscular system; syndactyly refers to webbing of the fingers
88. Choice c is correct; telangiectatic nevi are also known as stork bite marks and can also appear on the eyelids; milia are plugged sebaceous glands and appear like white pimples; nevus vasculosus or a strawberry mark is a raised, sharply demarcated, bright or dark red swelling; nevus flammeus is a port-wine, flat red to purple lesions that do not blanch with pressure.

II. Thinking Critically

1. *Newborn—risk for cold stress* (see Cold Stress section of Thermogenic System and Fig. 24-1).
   a. *Dangers of cold stress:* metabolic and physiologic demands are placed on the newborn → increased oxygen need and consumption → oxygen and energy are diverted from brain cell and cardiac function and growth → decreased oxygen leads to vasoconstriction, respiratory distress, and reopening of the ductus arteriosus → acidosis occurs, increasing the level of bilirubin → hypoglycemia can occur as a result of increased glucose utilization.
   b. *Nursing diagnosis:* risk for imbalanced body temperature—hypothermia related to immature thermoregulation associated with newborn status; *Expected outcome:* newborn's temperature will stabilize between 36.5° to 37.2° C within 8 to 10 hours of birth.
   c. *Measures to stabilize newborn temperature and prevent cold stress:* implement measures that reflect application of heat loss mechanisms of convection, radiation, evaporation, and conduction:
      • Dry infant and cover with warmed blankets or wrap with mother.
      • Cover head and feet; double wrap.
      • Use radiant warmer to stabilize temperature, assess newborn, and perform procedures.
      • Adjust environment in terms of temperature and drafts (nursery and mother's room).
      • Place bassinet away from drafts and outside windows.
      • Maintain adequate nutrition (caloric intake).
2. *Parental concern regarding head variations:* see Integumentary System and Skeletal System sections; discuss each finding in terms of cause,

significance for the newborn's health status and adjustment, and how/when it will be resolved; refer to Figs. 24-3, *A* and 24-9 to facilitate parental understanding.

3. *Parental concern about weight loss:* see Baseline Measurements of Physical Growth section and Table 24-2; determine percentage of weight loss, making sure it does not exceed 10%; explain that their newborn's weight loss of 6% is within the expected range for weight loss after birth; discuss the cause of the loss and feeding measures, and inform them that the birth weight should be regained within 2 weeks.

4. Parental interest in newborn's sensory capabilities (see Sensory Behaviors section of Behavioral Characteristics).
   a. *What nurse should tell parents:* discuss and demonstrate newborn's capability regarding vision, hearing, touch, taste, and smell.
   b. *Stimuli parents can provide to facilitate newborn development:* face-to-face/eye to eye contact, objects (bright or black-and-white changing, complex patterns), sound (talking to infant, music, heartbeat simulator), touch (infant massage, cuddling).

5. *Parental concern regarding "bruises" on newborn's back and buttocks:* discuss the characteristics and cause of Mongolian spots (see Mongolian Spots subsection of Integumentary System section and Fig. 24-4).

CHAPTER 25: NURSING CARE OF THE NEWBORN

I. Reviewing Key Concepts and Content

1. F	2. T	3. F	4. F	5. F	6. T
7. F	8. F	9. T	10. F	11. T	12. T
13. T	14. F	15. T	16. F	17. F	18. F
19. T	20. F	21. F	22. T	23. F	24. T

25. Tetracycline, erythromycin, lower conjunctiva, inner canthus, outer canthus
26. Vitamin K, 0.5 to 1 mg, 25, ⅝ to ⅞
27. Edema, erythema (redness), drainage, sterile water, alcohol, triple blue dye, erythromycin solution, 24 hours after birth, dry
28. Blanch, nose, forehead, sternum, yellow
29. Kernicterus
30. Pathologic jaundice, hyperbilirubinemia, hearing loss, cognitive, kernicterus
31. Neonatal Postoperative Pain Scale, crying, requires oxygen for saturation >95%, increased vital signs, expression, sleepless
32. Eutectic mixture of local anesthetic
33. 48, physical, neuromuscular
34. *Creation of a protective environment in terms of infection control and safety:* see Protective Environment section of Plan of Care and Implementation.
    a. *Environment:* adequate lighting, ventilation, warmth, and humidity; elimination of fire hazards; ensure safety of electrical equipment.
    b. *Infection control:* use Standard Precautions with an emphasis on handwashing, provide adequate spacing of bassinets (3 feet), separate areas for cleaning and storing equipment and supplies, keep persons with infections away or use appropriate precautions, monitor regulation of visitors.
    c. *Safety:* ensure security precautions and identification measures—instruction for parents; photo IDs for personnel, including nurses; locked unit entry doors, alarm bands on newborns—are followed.

35. *Predisposing factors for newborn birth trauma:* see Physical Injuries section in Assessment of Common Problems to identify several maternal and fetal factors and factors related to intrapartum events and childbirth techniques.

36. *Complete table related to hypoglycemia and hypocalcemia:* see Hypoglycemia and Hypocalcemia sections in Assessment of Common Problems for a description of each deficit in terms of signs, risk factors, and management.

37. *Health teaching in preparation for discharge:* see Home Care boxes, Sponge Bathing and Newborn Home Care following Early Discharge, and specific sections for teaching topics identified in Discharge Planning and Teaching.

38. *Maintaining a patent airway and supporting respirations:*
    a. *Four conditions essential for maintaining an adequate oxygen supply:* clear, patent airway; adequate respiratory effort; functioning cardiopulmonary system; adequate thermoregulation.
    b. *Signs of respiratory distress:* see Box 25-3, Newborn Breathing, Signs of Distress; signs include nasal flaring, retractions, and increased use of intercostal muscles, chin tug, grunting with expiration, seesaw respirations, rate of less than 30 breaths/min or more than 60 breaths/min, apnea periods lasting less than 20 seconds, adventitious breath sounds; note that some of these signs may normally be present during the first period of reactivity following birth.
    c. *Three methods of relieving airway obstruction:* see Relieving Airway Obstruction section; reposition infant, use a bulb syringe or mechanical suction; take note of effectiveness of the methods used.

39. Choice d is correct; thinning of lanugo with bald spots is consistent with full-term status; pulse and weight are not part of the Ballard scale; the popliteal angle for a full-term newborn would be 100 degrees or less (see Fig. 25-1).

40. Choice c is correct; the hemoglobin should be 14 to 24 g/dl; hematocrit should be 45% to 64%; glucose should be 45 to 65 mg/dl; bilirubin should be <2 mg/dl (see Box 25-5).

41. Choice b is correct; signs of hypoglycemia include cyanosis along with apnea, jitteriness/twitching, irregular respirations, high-pitched cry, difficulty feeding, hunger, lethargy, eye rolling, and seizures.

42. Choice a is correct; the control panel should be set between 36° C to 37° C; the probe should be placed in one of the upper quadrants of the abdomen below the intercostal margin, never over a rib; axillary, not rectal, temperatures should be taken every hour.

43. Choice b is correct; the infant should be NPO for 2 to 3 hours to prevent vomiting and aspiration; the site should be checked every hour for 4 to 6 hours; diaper wipes should not be used on the site because they contain alcohol, which would delay healing and cause discomfort; the yellow exudate is a protective film that forms in 24 hours, and it should not be removed.

II. Thinking Critically

1. *Apgar scoring:*
   a. *Baby boy Smith:* heart rate: 160 (2); respiratory effort: good, crying (2); muscle tone: flexion, active movement (2); reflex irritability: cry with stimulus (2); color: acrocyanosis (1); score is 9; interpretation: score of 7 to 10 indicates that the infant is not having difficulty adjusting to extrauterine life
   b. *Baby girl Doe:* heart rate: 102 (2); respiratory effort: slow, irregular, weak cry (1); muscle tone: some flexion (1); reflex irritability: grimace with stimulus (1); color: pale (0); score is 5; interpretation: score of 4 to 6 indicates moderate difficulty adjusting to extrauterine life.

2. *Assessment of newborn girl:*
   a. *Protocol for assessment during first 2 hours:* see Table 25-1 (Apgar score) and Box 25-1 (Initial Physical Assessment by Body System), Initial Assessment section, and the Care Path, Healthy Term Newborn to prepare your outline.
   b. *Nurse's responsibility for newborn identification at birth:* see Initial Assessment section and Care Path; complete the identification process before mother and newborn are separated; attach matching ID bands to both (father also in some cases immediately after birth; take newborn's footprint and mother's finger-print(s) and place on appropriate form.
   c. *Priority nursing diagnoses for immediate postbirth period:* consider nursing diagnoses related to breathing (ineffective airway clearance, impaired gas exchange), ineffective thermoregulation (hypothermia)

   d. *Priority nursing care measures*—discuss each of the following areas:
   - Stabilization of respiration and airway patency
   - Maintenance of body temperature
   - Immediate interventions in terms of identification, prophylactic medications, promotion of bonding/attachment

3. *Performing a physical examination of newborn before discharge:*
   a. *Actions to ensure safety and accuracy:* well-lighted, warm, and draft-free environment; undress as needed; place on firm surface with constant supervision; progress in a systematic manner from cleanest to dirtiest area
   b. *Major areas assessed:* (see Tables 24-1 and 24-2); areas to include general appearance and posture; vital signs and weight; integument; head and neck; abdomen and back; genitalia and anus; elimination patterns; extremities; neurologic system, including reflexes; behavioral characteristics.
   c. *Rationale for presence of parents:* chance to observe parent-infant interactions and to identify and meet learning needs; foster active involvement in assessment and care of their newborn; encourage discussion of concerns and asking of questions; chance to explain and demonstrate newborn characteristics and capabilities.

4. *Newborn with mucus in airway* (see Stabilization and Resuscitation section).
   a. *Nursing diagnosis:* impaired gas exchange related to upper airway obstruction with mucus.
   b. *Steps using bulb syringe:* suction mouth first then nose; compress bulb before insertion; insert tip along side of mouth not over tongue, which could stimulate the gag reflex and sucking; release compression slowly; continue till breathing sounds clear; teach parents how to use bulb syringe.
   c. *Guidelines for use of mechanical suction:* suction for 5 seconds or less per insertion; use <80 mm Hg setting; lubricate catheter with sterile water; insert along base of tongue or horizontally through nose into nares; repeat until breathing/cry sounds clear.

5. *Care of circumcision and umbilical cord sites:*
   a. *Nursing diagnosis:* risk for infection related to removal of foreskin and healing umbilical cord site.
   b. *Expected outcome:* cord and circumcision site will heal without infection.
   c. *Teaching about care:* see Patient Teaching box, Care of Circumcised Newborn at Home, and Home Care box, Sponge Bathing; emphasize importance of assessing sites for infection and progress of healing; discuss measures to keep

areas clean and dry and to enhance comfort; teach parents how to assess circumcision site for bleeding and what to do if it occurs, and emphasize importance of assessing urination and what to do if the newborn has difficulty voiding; demonstrate skills and assist parents to redemonstrate.

6. *Newborn with hyperbilirubinemia* (see Therapy for Hyperbilirubinemia section, Physiologic Problems section, and Family Focus box).
   a. *Responding to parental concerns:* tell parents in simple terms that their newborn is exhibiting physiologic jaundice, explaining why it occurs, what impact it will have on their newborn's health, and how it will be resolved; emphasize that their newborn's form of jaundice is a common and naturally occurring physiologic process as the newborn adjusts to extrauterine life.
   b. *Blanch test:* apply pressure with finger over a bony area (nose, forehead, sternum) for several seconds to empty capillaries at the spot; if jaundice is present, the blanched area will appear yellow before the capillaries fill.
   c. *Expected findings of physiologic hyperbilirubinemia:* jaundice (cephalocaudal, proximodistal progression), watery greenish stools, sleepiness, alteration in bilirubin levels that follows a specific pattern and degree of elevation (see Chapter 24).
   d. *Precautions and care measures during phototherapy:* increase fluids and feed at least every 3 hours; cover eyes, removing periodically to assess condition and allow for interaction with parents; monitor temperature for increases or decreases; cleanse stools promptly; do not put lotions on skin; place undressed under lights and change position every 2 hours to expose as much skin to the lights as possible; remove from under lights for feeding, cuddling, and interaction with parents.

7. *Maternal concerns regarding immunizations:* emphasize that breastfeeding only provides temporary immunity to some infections and that immunizations must be given as recommended in terms of timing and number in order to achieve adequate immunity to what could be life-threatening infections; provide her with written materials to read and a person to call to ask questions and discuss concerns; make referrals in order to address her financial concern.

8. *Newborn scheduled for circumcision—pain concerns* (see Pain in Neonate section, Atraumatic Care box, and Table 25-4).
   a. *Common behavioral responses to pain:* body movements (withdrawal of upper and lower limbs), vocalization (cry), cry face, fussy, irritable, listless.
   b. *Using CRIES Neonatal Postoperative Pain Scale:* see Table 25-4 and Metabolic Responses section to develop this answer.
   c. *Nursing diagnosis:* acute pain related to effects of removal of foreskin.
   d. *Nonpharmacologic and pharmacologic relief measures:*
      • *Nonpharmacologic:* lamb's wool on circumcision board, keep warm, play music, apply a sucrose preparation on pacifier, swaddle afterward, nonnutritive sucking, take to mother to be fed and comforted, distract (older infant), apply Vaseline/ointment to site; change diaper frequently; position on side or back (see Patient Teaching box, Care of the Circumcised Newborn at Home).
      • *Pharmacologic:* local anesthesia, topical preparations including EMLA, dorsal penile nerve block or ring block, oral acetaminophen.

CHAPTER 26: NEWBORN NUTRITION AND FEEDING

I. Reviewing Key Concepts and Content

1. *Calculation of daily energy and fluid requirements* (calories depend on age in months; fluid requirements of all infants is 100 to 140 ml/kg/day):
   a. Jim (first 3 months—110 kcal/kg/day):
      • 110 kcal × 4 kg = 440 kcal/day
      • 400 to 550 ml/day
   b. Sue (3 to 6 months—100 kcal/kg/day):
      • 100 kcal × 6 kg = 600 kcal/day
      • 600 to 840 ml/day
   c. Sam (6 to 9 months—95 kcal/kg/day):
      • 95 kcal × 7.5 kg = 712.5 kcal/day
      • 750 to 1050 ml/day

2. Lactation structures:
   a. *Label:* A. alveolus; B. ductule; C. duct; D. lactiferous duct; E. lactiferous sinus; F. nipple pore; G. ampulla; H. areola
   b. *Fill in the blanks:*
      1. Lobes (milk glands)
      2. Alveoli
      3. Ductule
      4. Lactiferous duct
      5. Lactiferous sinuses, ampullae
      6. Myoepithelial
      7. Areola

3. *Teaching group of women about breastfeeding:* see Benefits of Breastfeeding section; emphasize the importance and benefits of breastfeeding for infants, mothers, and family/society.

4. *Four breastfeeding positions:* see Positioning section of Plan of Care and Implementation and

Fig. 26-4; describe the positions of football hold, cradle (traditional), modified cradle (across the lap), and side-lying.

5. *Feeding readiness cues* (see Frequency of Feeding section).
   a. *Cues:* hand-to-mouth or hand-to-hand movements, sucking motions, strong rooting reflex, mouthing, tongue movements; crying is a late sign.
   b. *Rationale for feeding according to these cues:* if cues are missed, baby may cry vigorously, become distraught, shut down, or withdraw into a deep sleep; these behaviors will make feeding more difficult or impossible; feeding when the infant exhibits readiness enhances the chance of success.

6. *Differences between foremilk and hindmilk:* see Uniqueness of Human Milk section.
   • Foremilk: bluish white, part skim and part whole milk providing primarily lactose, protein, water-soluble vitamins
   • Hindmilk: cream is "let down" into the feeding; denser in calories from fat to ensure optimal growth and contentment between feedings

7. *Label illustrations of lactation reflexes:*
   • Milk production reflex: A. sucking stimulus; B. hypothalamus; C. anterior pituitary gland (prolactin); D. milk production
   • Let-down reflex: A. sucking stimulus; B. hypothalamus; C. posterior pituitary gland (oxytocin); D. let-down reflex

8. *Stages of lactogenesis:* see Uniqueness of Human Milk section.
   a. Stage I: begins in pregnancy when breasts are prepared for milk production and colostrum is formed in the breasts.
   b. Stage II: Colostrum changes to mature milk; "milk coming in" on the third to fifth day after birth; onset of copious milk secretion.
   c. Stage III: milk changes over about 10 days when the mature milk is established.

9. Proper latch-on (see Latch-On section of Plan of Care and Implementation, Breastfeeding).
   a. *Steps to ensure proper latch-on:* apply colostrum/milk to areola/nipple (lubricate and entice), support the breast (see Fig. 26-5), hold baby close and tickle baby's lower lip with the breast nipple to stimulate the rooting reflex— mouth opening and extrusion of tongue occurs; pull baby onto nipple and areola; brings infant to the breast.
   b. *Signs of proper latch-on:* see Fig 26-6; nose, cheeks, and chin touch the breast, firm, tugging sensation on the nipple but no pinching or pain; baby's cheeks are rounded and jaw glides smoothly with sucking; swallow is audible.

c. *Removal of baby from breast:* see Fig. 26-7; break suction by inserting finger in the side of baby's mouth between gums and leaving the finger in until nipple is completely out of the baby's mouth.

10. F	11. F	12. T	13. F	14. T	15. F
16. T	17. T	18. F	19. T	20. F	21. T
22. T	23. T	24. F	25. F		

26. *Calming a fussy baby:* see Special Considerations section of Supplements, Bottles, and Pacifiers; mother can try holding close, perhaps with skin-to-skin contact, swaddling, gently moving, and talking soothingly; reducing environmental stimuli, and allowing the baby to suck on a clean finger; change feeding position; assess maternal food intake.

27. *Complete table related to assessment of infant and mother regarding breastfeeding;* see Infant and Mother Assessment section for information to complete the table.

28. Mastitis
29. Massage
30. Lactogenesis/lactation
31. Nipple confusion
32. Lactation consultant
33. Engorgement
34. Feeding readiness cues
35. Weaning
36. Everted, inverted, shell
37. Colostrum
38. Prolactin, oxytocin
39. Shut-down
40. Monilia, thrush
41. Football, cradle (traditional)
42. Let-down, milk ejection
43. Rooting
44. Latch-on
45. Choice b is correct; birth weight is regained in 10 to 14 days; 6 to 8 wet diapers are expected at this time; should be fed every 2 to 3 hours for at total of 8 to 10 times per day.
46. Choice a is correct; swaddling is recommended; choices b, c, and d are all appropriate actions to calm a fussy baby.
47. Choice d is correct; no soap should be used because it could dry the areola and increase the risk for irritation; vitamin E should not be used because it is a fat-soluble vitamin that the infant could ingest when breastfeeding; lanolin or colostrum/milk are the preferred substances to be applied to the area; plastic liners can trap moisture and lead to sore nipples.
48. Choice b is correct; a hormonal contraceptive could decrease the milk supply if given before lactation is well established during the first 6 weeks after birth; after 6 weeks a progestin-only contraceptive could be used because it is the least likely hormonal contraceptive to affect lactation;

even complete breastfeeding is not considered to be a reliable method because ovulation can occur unexpectedly even before the first menstrual period.

49. Choice c is correct; nipple should allow only the passage of a slow drip; tap water can be used unless the water supply is unsafe or if otherwise instructed; formula should never be heated in the microwave because it could be overheated or unevenly heated

II. Thinking Critically

1. a. –   b. +   c. –   d. –   e. +   f. –
   g. +   h. +   i. –   j. –   k. +   l. –

2. *Bottle-feeding mother wishes to give her newborn skim milk to prevent cardiac problems:* see Fat section of Nutrient Needs section; emphasize the importance of fat in the newborn's diet for energy and supplying essential fatty acids for growth and tissue maintenance, cell membranes, and hormone production; at least 15% of calories must come from fat; skim and low-fat milk lack essential fatty acids.

3. *Infant feeding method decision making during prenatal period* (see Choosing an Infant Feeding Method section).
   a. *Nursing diagnosis:* decisional conflict regarding feeding method for their newborn related to lack of knowledge and experience with newborn feeding methods.
      Expected outcome: couple will choose the feeding method for their newborn that is most comfortable for them.
   b. *Rationale for couple making the decision together:* both should learn about the pros and cons of feeding methods with an emphasis on the benefits of breastfeeding and how the partner can help with the method.
   c. *Making decision prenatally:* the prenatal period is a less stressful time, allowing for full consideration of options, how feeding methods would be incorporated into life activities (such as work outside the home), and learning about breastfeeding by attending a prenatal breastfeeding class and reading.
   d. *How the nurse can facilitate decision-making process:* provide information about feeding methods in a nonjudgmental manner while still emphasizing the importance of breastfeeding as the preferred method, dispel myths, address personal concerns of the couple, and make needed referrals to WIC, lactation consultant, breastfeeding classes, and the La Leche League.

4. *Breastfeeding mother's questions and concerns* (see Milk Production section of Overview of Lactation section for *a* and *b* below).

a. *Breast size:* discuss development of lactation structures during pregnancy; emphasize the importance of this development and not the breast size for successful lactation.

b. *Let-down reflex:* explain what it is and why it happens (including physical and emotional triggers); emphasize its importance in providing the infant with hindmilk.

c. *Signs that breastfeeding is going well:* see Assessment of Infant and Mother sections of Care Management of Breastfeeding, which identify maternal and newborn indicators of effective breastfeeding during the first week following birth; put the indicators in writing and go over each one; provide contact person if mother is concerned.

d. *Nipple soreness:* see Special Considerations section of Care of the Mother; discuss and demonstrate measures to prevent and to treat sore nipples, including, most importantly, good breastfeeding techniques such as latch-on, removal, and alternating starting breast and positions; discuss breast care measures such as air-drying nipples, avoiding soap, and applying colostrum/milk or purified lanolin after feeding.

e. *Engorgement:* see Special Considerations section of Care of the Mother; begin by describing engorgement, what it is and why it occurs and when; prevention of excessive engorgement includes frequency of feeding every 2 to 3 hours on each breast (use pumping to soften second breast if needed); relief measures include warm packs and massage before feeding, ice afterward, cabbage leaves, supportive bra; emphasize the temporary, self-limiting nature of engorgement.

f. *Afterpains and increased flow:* explain that oxytocin is released as a result of infant sucking; this triggers the let-down reflex and stimulates the uterus to contract, causing afterpains for the first 3 to 5 after birth; oxytocin also reduces excessive bleeding, though the contractions can cause flow already in the uterus to be expelled, giving the impression of an increased flow.

g. *Breastfeeding as a birth control method:* see Effect of Menstruation and Breastfeeding and Contraception sections of Care of Mother; emphasize that breastfeeding is not an effective contraceptive method; although ovulation may be delayed, its return cannot be predicted with accuracy and may occur before the first menstrual period; discuss contraceptive methods that are safe to use with breastfeeding and resuming sexual intercourse during the postpartum period.

h. *Weaning:* see Weaning section of Plan of Care and Implementation section; emphasize that weaning needs to be a gradual process, eliminating one feeding at a time, beginning with the one the baby is most likely to sleep through; discuss the use of bottles and cups; use of formula, cow's milk, and/or solids depends on the age of infant at the time of weaning.

5. *Infrequent feeding of sleeping baby* (see Frequency and Duration of Feeding and Special Considerations sections of Plan of Care and Interventions, Breastfeeding).

a. *Nursing diagnosis:* imbalanced nutrition less than body requirements related to infrequent feeding of newborn.
   Expected outcome: mother will awaken infant every 2 to 3 hours during the day and every 4 hours at night to feed the infant, achieving approximately 8 to 12 feedings per day.

b. *Nursing approach:* discuss feeding readiness cues to facilitate proper timing of feedings; discuss techniques to wake sleeping baby and signs indicating adequate intake.

6. *Bottle-feeding mother* (see Formula Feeding section and Home Care box, Formula Preparation and Feeding).

a. *Nurse's response to mother's concern:* discuss how the mother can facilitate close contact and socialization with the infant during feeding: sitting comfortably, touching, singing, and talking quietly to newborn to make feeding a pleasant time for both; reassure that properly prepared formulas will fully meet her newborn's need for nutrients and fluid.

b. *Guidelines for bottle-feeding:* discuss how to choose a formula type; amount and frequency of feedings; how to prepare formula (follow directions for dilution exactly), warming formula correctly, discarding leftover formula, and bottle and nipple cleansing; principles of the feeding process, including semi-upright position, not propping bottles, fluid filling the nipple to limit air consumption, cues of feeding readiness and satiety, and burping.

CHAPTER 27: INFANTS WITH GESTATIONAL AGE-RELATED PROBLEMS

I. Reviewing Key Concepts and Content

1. Low-birth-weight (LBW), very-low-birth weight (VLBW), extremely low-birth-weight (ELBW)
2. Premature, preterm
3. Full term
4. Postmature, postterm
5. Large for gestational age (LGA)
6. Appropriate for gestational age (AGA)
7. Small for date (SFD), small for gestational age (SGA)
8. Intrauterine growth restriction (IUGR), symmetric IUGR, asymmetric IUGR
9. Live birth
10. Fetal death
11. Neonatal death, early neonatal death, late neonatal death
12. Perinatal mortality
13. F 14. T 15. T 16. F 17. T 18. T
19. F 20. F 21. T 22. F 23. F 24. F
25. T 26. T 27. T 28. F 29. T 30. T
31. T 32. F

33. *Purpose of exogenous surfactant administration:* see Surfactant section of Oxygen Therapy; preterm infants born before 32 weeks of gestation do not have adequate amounts of pulmonary surfactant to survive extrauterine life; exogenous surfactant will facilitate alveoli expansion and stability, easing respirations, and enhancing gas exchange until the newborn can produce sufficient quantities on its own; it is administered via an endotracheal tube directly into the lungs.

34. *Kangaroo care:* see Kangaroo Care section in Developmental Care and Fig. 27-9; uses skin-to-skin holding to help preterm newborns interact with parents; benefits newborn and parents by increasing feeling of being in control and for allowing better temperature and oxygen stability with fewer episodes of crying, apnea, and periodic breathing; the newborn is in the quiet, alert state longer, thereby enhancing attachment and development.

35. *Complete the table related to physiologic problems of the preterm newborn:* physiologic functions and potential problems are discussed in specific sections of Assessment.

36. b 37. e 38. c 39. a 40. d

41. *Respiratory distress syndrome*
   a. Surfactant, atelectasis, residual capacity, ventilation-perfusion, ventilation
   b. Tachypnea, grunting, nasal flaring, retractions, hypercapnia, acidosis, hypotension, shock, birth, 6, crackles, air exchange, pallor, accessory muscles, apnea
   c. 72, surfactant
   d. Ventilation, oxygenation, surfactant, thermoneutral

42. *Pregestational diabetes:*
   a. 2 to 4 times, blood glucose, ketoacidosis, hyperglycemia, glucose, insulin, growth, macrosomia, acidotic, ketoacidosis, carbon dioxide, oxygen, macrosomia, hypoglycemia, polyhydramnios, preterm birth, lung immaturity, glucose, 100, 120

b. *Common congenital anomalies experienced by infants of diabetic mothers:* see Congenital Anomalies section of Infants of Diabetic Mothers for identification of anomalies in each category.

43. *Macrosomic infant* (see Macrosomia section of Neonatal Complications).
   a. *Characteristics:* round face, chubby body, plethoric/flushed complexion, enlarged organs, increased fat deposits, placenta and cord are larger
   b. Hypoglycemia, hypocalcemia, hyperviscosity, hyperbilirubinemia
   c. *Warning signs of potential complications:* see section for each category: birth trauma and perinatal hypoxia, RDS, hypoglycemia, hypocalcemia and hypomagnesemia, cardiomyopathy and hyperbilirubinemia, and polycythemia.

44. Choice d is correct; retractions reflect increased effort and work to breathe; choices a, b, and c are all expected findings consistent with efficient respiratory effort in the preterm newborn.

45. Choice b is correct; although choices a, c, and d are appropriate and important, respiration with adequate gas exchange takes precedence, especially because adequate surfactant is not produced before 32 weeks of gestation

46. Choice a is correct; sterile water is used to lubricate the tube; air, not sterile water, is used to check placement before feeding; because newborns are nose breathers, the mouth is the preferred route for insertion unless the infant is unable to tolerate.

47. Choice c is correct; fracture from trauma is more common in the upper body (e.g., humerus, clavicle); hypocalcemia is common; the newborn of a pregestational diabetic mother is more likely to experience congenital anomalies such as heart defects.

II. Thinking Critically

1. Oxygen therapy for the newborn experiencing respiratory distress (see Respiratory Function section of Assessment, Oxygen Therapy section of Plan of Care and Implementation section, and Table 27-2).
   a. *Criteria to determine need for oxygen* include increased effort to breathe, respiratory distress with apnea, tachycardia or bradycardia, central cyanosis, PaO_2 less than 60 mm Hg, oxygen saturation less than 92%.
   b. *Guidelines for safe and effective administration of oxygen:* observe for signs of complications every 1 to 2 hours with continuous pulse oximeter and arterial blood gas measurement as warranted, vital signs, controlled oxygen concentration, volume, temperature and humidity; oxygen should be warm and humidified.
   c. *Complete table related to oxygen administration methods:* see specific section for each method listed.

2. *Weaning from oxygen process* (see Weaning from Respiratory Assistance section).
   a. *Signs of readiness:* signs of respiratory distress are no longer exhibited, arterial blood gases and oxygen saturation are maintained within normal limits, newborn displays spontaneous adequate respiratory effort without difficulty and exhibits good color and improved muscle tone during increased activity.
   b. *Guidelines:* approach carefully from one method to another with close observation for signs of good or poor tolerance of the change; reassure and keep parents informed throughout the process of weaning, pointing out signs that their newborn is breathing effectively and is well oxygenated.

3. *Meeting nutritional needs of a preterm infant* (see Nutritional Care and Gavage Feeding sections).
   a. *Assessment to determine effectiveness of feeding method:* observe for ability to suck and swallow and the coordination of each; signs of respiratory distress during the feeding; length of time for the feeding and the amount ingested; presence of regurgitation, vomiting, or abdominal distention after feeding; daily weight gains and losses and elimination patterns.
   b. *Guidelines to follow when inserting a gavage tube:* see Box 27-4 Procedure, Inserting a Gavage Feeding Tube and Fig. 27-4; emphasize tubing choice and measurement of length, insertion without trauma and securing to maintain placement, checking placement.
   c. *Nursing diagnosis:* imbalanced nutrition: less than body requirements related to weak suck associated with premature status.
   d. *Principles to follow before, during, and after a gavage feeding:*
      • Initiate measures to prevent aspiration with proper tube insertion, removal, and position check techniques.
      • Instill breast milk or formula at a rate of 1 ml/hr.
      • Cuddle, swaddle infant during feedings; involve parents; use nonnutritive sucking.
      • Document assessment findings and specifics of the procedure.
   e. *Advancing to oral feeding:* Proceed cautiously, checking for gastrointestinal, nutritional, fluid, and electrolyte signs of tolerance or

intolerance for advancement; decrease gavage feedings as ability to suck improves.

4. *NICU environment* (see Environmental Concerns section of Plan of Care and Implementation).
   a. *Common stressors*
      - *Infant stressors:* continuous exposure to light and noise; administration of sedatives and pain medications; invasive procedures and medications required for treatment
      - *Family stressors:* size and compromised and often fluctuating health status of their newborn; difficulty interacting with newborn and making eye contact; increased learning needs regarding status of newborn and care needs; concern regarding potential disabilities
   b. *Cues related to overstimulation or relaxed state:* see Infant Communication section for a description of several cues for each state.
   c. *Measures to provide a balance of stimuli for the newborn:* see Infant Stimulation section for many ideas, including waterbeds, kangaroo care, bundling, coordinated plan of care to provide for period of interrupted rest and sleep, use pain medications and sedatives as needed, provide diurnal light patterns, decrease noise level, use stroking, talking, mobiles, decals, music, and windup toys for stimulation.
   d. *Guidelines for infant positioning:* see Positioning section; change position frequently, observing effect of position change on breathing and oxygenation and preventing aspiration; consider boundaries, body alignment, sense of security and comfort when positioning; teach parents.
   e. *Nursing measures to support parents of an infant cared for in the NICU:* see Parental Support section for descriptions of many measures, including being with parents at first visit, helping them see their infant rather than focusing on the equipment; explain characteristics of a preterm infant and the purpose for procedures and equipment; encourage expression of feelings, concerns, and questions; assess their response to the newborn; make referrals to support group and arrange for home care.

5. *Postterm pregnancy* (see Postmature Infant section).
   a. *Rationale for increased mortality:* increased oxygen demands are not met and likelihood for impaired gas exchange occurs, leading to hypoxia and passage of meconium into amniotic fluid; risk for aspiration of meconium into lungs.
   b. *Typical assessment findings:* thin, emaciated appearance (dysmature) due to loss of subcutaneous fat and muscle mass; peeling of skin; meconium staining on fingernails; long hair and nails; absence of vernix.
   c. *Two major complications:* meconium aspiration syndrome and persistent pulmonary hypertension of the newborn (PPHN); see separate section that describes each complication.

6. *Birth of a small-for-gestational-age newborn* (see Small for Gestational Age and Intrauterine Growth Restriction sections).
   a. *Major complications:* perinatal asphyxia with possible passage of meconium and aspiration, hypoglycemia, heat loss (cold stress).
   b. *Physiologic basis for each identified complication:* see separate section for each complication.

7. *Transport to tertiary center* (see Transport to a Regional Center section).
   a. *Advantages of transport before birth:*
      - Associated neonatal morbidity and mortality are decreased.
      - Infant-parent attachment is supported because separation is avoided.
   b. *Stabilization of needs before transport:* VS, oxygenation and ventilation, thermoregulation, acid/base balance, fluid/electrolyte status, glucose levels, and developmental interventions.
   c. *Support measures for family:* see Box 27-5; provide information about center (location, visiting hours, phone number, caregivers' names, rules), one parent accompany infant, see infant before transport, get status updates.

CHAPTER 28: THE NEWBORN AT RISK: ACQUIRED AND CONGENITAL PROBLEMS

I. Reviewing Key Concepts and Content

1. T	2. T	3. T	4. F	5. T	6. F
7. T	8. F	9. T	10. T	11. F	12. T
13. T	14. T	15. F	16. T	17. T	18. T
19. F	20. F	21. T	22. F	23. T	24. F
25. T	26. F	27. T	28. F	29. T	30. F
31. F	32. F	33. T	34. F	35. T	36. F
37. F	38. T	39. T			

40. *Birth injuries* (see Birth Trauma section).
   a. *Risk factors for trauma:* macrosomia, hydrocephalus, unusual presentations, very long and difficult labor necessitating the use of forceps or vacuum, precipitous labor, preterm or postterm birth, multiple gestation.
   b. *Signs of fractured clavicle:* see Skeletal Injuries section; signs include limited use of arm, absence of Moro reflex on affected side, crepitus over the bone.
   c. *Treatment:* there is no accepted standard treatment; may be limited to gently handling and supporting shoulder when changing

clothes and moving and proper alignment; support parents with the handling and care of their baby because they may be very anxious

41. *Infections represented by TORCH:* see Box 28-1 for infections represented by each letter.

42. *Sepsis* (see Neonatal Infections section, Sepsis).
    a. *Risk factors:* see Assessment subsection and Table 28-2, which identify risk factors related to mother, intrapartum process, and neonate.
    b. *Signs of neonatal sepsis:* see Table 28-3 for signs of sepsis according to body systems.
    c. *Effective nursing measures:* see Prevention and Care Management sections for several measures.

43. *Physiologic basis for ABO incompatibility:* see ABO section of Hemolytic Disorders; fetal blood is A, B, or AB and mother's blood type is O; naturally occurring antibodies can cross the placenta, resulting in hemolysis of the fetus/newborn's red blood cells; women with blood type O already have anti-A and anti-B antibodies in their blood.

44. *Specific types of postnatal tests for diagnosis of congenital anomalies:* see specific sections of Genetic Diagnosis.
    a. Newborn screening: such as PKU, galactosemia, hypothyroidism, hemoglobinopathy
    b. Cytogenetic studies: chromosomal examination is used to confirm suggestive but not diagnostic clinical appearance
    c. Dermatoglyphics: study of the pattern of ridges in the skin of the hands and feet (e.g., simian crease suggestive of Down syndrome)

45. *Congenital heart defects* (see Cardiovascular System Anomalies section).
    a. *Maternal factors associated with higher risk:* include rubella, alcohol intake, diabetes, systemic lupus erythematosus, PKU, poor nutrition, ingestion of certain medications (i.e., antiepileptics).
    b. *Signs that could indicate congenital heart defects (CHD):* weak, muffled, or loud and breathless cry, cyanosis unrelieved by oxygen, cyanosis that increases when newborn is supine or cries, pallor, mottling on exertion, respiratory signs and symptoms, activity effects, bradycardia or tachycardia, irregular heart rate or murmurs; signs of congestive heart failure

46. Inborn errors of metabolism
47. Microcephaly
48. Hypospadias, epispadias, exstrophy of the bladder
49. Hydrocephalus
50. Congential heart defects
51. Talipes equinovarus
52. Choanal atresia
53. Meningocele
54. Omphalocele, gastroschisis
55. Esophageal atresia; tracheoesophageal fistula
56. Anencephaly
57. Diaphragmatic hernia
58. Myelomeningocele
59. Choice b is correct; findings are consistent with a bone fracture, in this case, the clavicle.
60. Choice b is correct; risk of transmission of HIV is greater than the benefits of breastfeeding; isolation is not required nor are gloves for routine care measures; the nurse should be using standard precautions as would be used with all patients; zidovudine treatment begins after birth.
61. Choice d is correct; RhoGAM should be administered to the mother within 72 hours of birth; pathologic jaundice is unlikely because Coombs' test results indicate that antibodies have not been formed to destroy the newborn's RBCs; RhoGam is given to prevent formation of antibodies; it would not be given if antibodies have already been formed, as indicated by positive Coombs' test results.
62. Choice c is correct; hypotension can occur; 75% to 85% of blood is exchanged; hypocalcemia can occur related to preservatives found in donor blood.
63. Choice a is correct; lateral or prone position prevents pressure on the sac, which could cause damage; parents can hold newborn if they are supervised regarding how to hold without touching sac; sterile, moist nonadherent dressings are used to protect the cord; skin around the defect (sac) should be cleansed and dried carefully to prevent skin breakdown.

II. Thinking Critically

1. Newborn whose mother is hepatitis B positive (see Hepatitis B section of TORCH Infections section).
   a. *Protocol for newborn care:* hepatitis B immunoglobulin (HBIG) 0.5 ml intramuscularly as soon as possible after birth (within 12 hours of life); administer hepatitis B vaccine concurrently at a different site, repeating at 1 month and at 6 months of age
   b. *Safety of breastfeeding:* it is safe to breastfeed after the infant has been cleansed and the vaccine has been administered.

2. *Newborn whose mother has active herpes at the time of birth* (see Herpes Simplex Virus section of TORCH Infections).
   a. *Four modes of transmission:* transplacental; ascending infection by way of birth canal; direct contamination during passage through an infected birth canal (mode for this baby); and direct transmission to the newborn by an infected person.
   b. *Clinical signs of active infection in the newborn:* initial symptoms usually appear in the first week or sometimes the second week; localized

CNS disease, localized infection of the skin, mouth, or eyes, disseminated infection (involvement of virtually all organ systems, especially liver, adrenal glands, and lungs).

c. *Recommended nursing measures related to:*
   • Management after birth, before discharge: use standard precautions appropriately; wear gloves when handling the newborn; inspect for lesions and obtain cultures from mouth, eyes, and lesions as indicated; delay circumcision; discharge with mother if cultures are negative; breastfeeding is allowed if there are no lesions on the breasts; arrange for follow-up health care.
   • Vidarabine or acyclovir therapy: general supportive care and treatment with acyclovir; vidarabine ointment can be used for 5 days to prevent keratoconjunctivitis.

3. *Newborn whose mother is HIV positive:* see HIV/AIDS section of TORCH infections.
   a. *Potential for newborn infection:* there is a 13% to 39% risk for transmission unless AZT was used during pregnancy, intrapartally, and with the newborn, in which case the risk is reduced to 5% to 8%.
   b. *Modes of transmission* are prenatal (transplacental); perinatal (exposure to maternal blood and secretions during childbirth process), and postpartum (maternal secretions including breast milk).
   c. *Opportunistic/secondary infections:* can include *pneumocystis carinii* pneumonia and candidiasis.
   d. *Care measures:*
      • Use Standard Precautions; protect infant from further exposure to maternal body fluids; gloves for routine care and isolation are not required.
      • Cleanse skin thoroughly after birth and before invasive procedures such as injections.
      • Discuss administration guidelines for immunizations.
      • Prepare to begin HAART/AZT treatment of newborn.
      • Make arrangements for counseling, referrals, and follow-up for care and testing as indicated.
      • Teach about infant and maternal care measures.
   e. *Breastfeeding safety:* because breast milk can contain the virus, the newborn should not be breastfed; teach mother how to bottle-feed and demonstrate how she can have close contact with her newborn during feeding; teach her other measures she can use to protect her baby from infection.

4. *Infant with thrush* (see Fungal Infection section).
   a. *Signs:* white, adherent patches on mucosa, gums, and tongue that bleed when touched;

infant does not usually experience discomfort but may, in a few cases, experience difficulty swallowing with poor oral intake.
   b. *Modes of transmission:* maternal vaginal infection during birth, person-to-person contact, contaminated hands, bottles, nipples, or other articles.
   c. *Management:* infection control measures along with cleanliness and good hygiene to prevent infection; cleanse mouth and instill nystatin into both sides of the mouth or swab over mucosa, gums, or tongue; apply 1 hour before or after a feeding; check diaper area as another common site for a fungal infection; assess mother's breasts and treat with topical nystatin as indicated.

5. *Newborn with fetal alcohol syndrome—FAS* (see Alcohol section of Substance Abuse).
   a. *Typical characteristics:* see Tables 28-5 and 28-6 and Fig. 28-9 for a description of the newborn diagnosed with FAS.
   b. *Long-term effects:* impaired visualmotor perception and performance; lowered IQ scores; delayed language development; reduced capacity to process and store factual data; motor, mental, and social delays.
   c. *Nursing measures:* involve parents in care of newborn and teach them about expected effects of FAS; encourage attachment, including the infant's need for cuddling and human contact; help parents create a warm and caring home environment that enhances development; make appropriate referrals to community services for the newborn as well as treatment program for the mother to help her with her alcohol abuse problem (father may also need assistance).

6. *Effect of maternal substance abuse on the newborn* (see Substance Abuse section).
   a. *Signs of withdrawal from heroin and methadone:* see Heroin and Methadone sections.
   b. *Effect of cocaine exposure:* see Table 28-5 and Cocaine section for identification of neonatal effects in terms of physical and behavioral assessment findings.

7. *Newborn of mother suspected of abusing drugs during pregnancy:*
   a. *Signs of neonatal abstinence syndrome:* see Table 28-7 for a list of signs in terms of gastrointestinal, CNS, metabolic, vasomotor, and respiratory functions and Fig. 28-10 for a scoring system.
   b. *Nursing diagnoses:* deficient fluid volume related to inadequate fluid intake and increased fluid loss associated with heroin withdrawal; disorganized infant behavior OR disturbed sleep pattern related to withdrawal from heroin; risk for infection related to

maternal risk behaviors associated with drug abuse.

   c. *Care management* see Teaching box, Care of Infant Experiencing Withdrawal and Nursing Care Plan; encourage parent participation in care of newborn providing education and social support as needed; maintain nutrition, fluid, and electrolyte balance with careful management of feeding; infection control and respiratory care; swaddling and pharmacologic treatment; discharge planning and referral; parents may also need treatment and support for addiction

8. *Pregnant woman who is Rh negative* (see Hemolytic Disorders, Rh Incompatibility section).

   a. *Physiologic basis:* if an Rh-negative mother's blood comes in contact with the blood of her Rh-positive fetus, she will form antibodies against Rh-positive blood, which can then be transferred via the placenta to the fetus; if a fetus is Rh positive, the presence of these antibodies in its bloodstream will result in destruction of its RBCs (hemolysis).

   b. *Meaning of a positive indirect Coombs' test:* indicates that the woman has formed antibodies, probably as a result of her miscarriage and not receiving RhoGAM to prevent antibody formation.

   c. *Candidate to receive RhoGAM:* woman is not a candidate because RhoGAM cannot be given once antibodies or sensitization has occurred.

   d. *RhoGAM purpose and use:* prevents sensitization; Rh-negative mothers who are indirect Coombs' negative should receive RhoGAM after an abortion, after specific invasive tests such as CVS and amniocentesis, during the third trimester, and within 72 hours after the birth of an Rh-positive, direct Coombs'-negative newborn.

   e. *Newborn complications:*
- Erythroblastosis fetalis: fetus compensates for anemia caused by hemolysis by producing large numbers of immature erythrocytes to replace the RBCs destroyed
- Hydrops fetalis: marked anemia with cardiac decompensation, cardiomegaly, hepato-splenomegaly, hypoxia, generalized edema and effusion of fluid into body spaces

   f. *Prevention of perinatal mortality:* intrauterine transfusions and early birth if the Rh antibody titer rises to dangerous levels and bilirubin is increasing.

9. *Care management of newborn born with myelomeningocele:* see Spina Bifida section of CNS Anomalies.
- Initiate preoperative and postoperative measures including how to position newborn to protect the site, assessment of neurologic function, prevent trauma and infection of the site and the skin surrounding the sac/defect, facilitate bladder emptying.
- Provide parental support through facilitating attachment process and encouraging parent-newborn interaction; provide information and emotional care, prepare for surgical care usually in the first 24 hours, make referrals for long-term care for parents and child to help them adjust to and cope with the effects of the congenital anomaly.

10. Newborn with cleft lip and palate (see Cleft Lip and Palate section of Gastrointestinal System Anomalies).

   a. *Nursing diagnoses:* imbalanced nutrition: less than body requirements, ineffective airway clearance, impaired parent infant attachment; all of these are related to defective and incomplete development of the lip and palate.

   b. *Nursing measures:*
- Maintain airway patency while ensuring adequate hydration and nutrition using devices that prevent passage of milk into airway
- Support and facilitate parental attachment to infant and skill with feeding; prepare parents for discharge.
- Explain the condition, how it occurs, what it entails, and how and when it will be repaired.
- Refer to support group.

CHAPTER 29: CONTEMPORARY PEDIATRIC NURSING

I. Learning Key Terms

1. e	2. c	3. k	4. f	5. b	6. q
7. s	8. d	9. a	10. x	11. g	12. t
13. h	14. u	15. v	16. i	17. n	18. j
19. p	20. m	21. l	22. r	23. o	24. w
25. o	26. h	27. a	28. k	29. f	30. l
31. i	32. c	33. p	34. e	35. b	36. m
37. j	38. q	39. n	40. g	41. d	

II. Reviewing Key Concepts and Content

42. b	43. d	44. c	45. b

46. *Possible answers:* homelessness; poverty; low birth weight; chronic illnesses; foreign-born adopted; day care centers

47. a	48. a	49. c	50. a	51. e	52. g
53. h	54. c	55. b	56. i	57. d	58. j
59. a	60. f	61. e	62. i	63. b	64. g
65. f	66. d	67. c	68. h	69. a	

70. *Possible answers:* health promotion; expanded roles in ambulatory care; home care; nursing independence and advanced skills; use of unlicensed assistive personnel (UAP)

71. Unlicensed assistive personnel (UAP) are "individuals who are trained to function in an assistive role to the registered professional nurse in the provision of (student-nurse) care activities as delegated by and under the supervision of the registered professional nurse" (American Nurses Association, 1994).

III. Thinking Critically

1. *Responses might include ideas such as the following:*
   - Education about prevention of heart disease in the public school and a broad-based program to change the food in the public schools to be heart-healthy
   - Dental health care clinics in the public school system
   - Program to immunize children at the time of admission to the public schools, rather than just requiring proof of immunization
   - Transportation programs and mobile clinics to increase access to care
2. *Responses might include ideas such as the following:*
   a. Family advocacy/caring: In home health, a nurse helps the family of a child with severe head injury prepare for the decision about long-term care of their child by identifying community resources, teaching the technical skills that will be needed for the care, and expressing compassion for them as they decide whether to care for the child at home or seek placement outside the home.
   b. Disease prevention/health promotion: During a clinic visit, the nurse takes time to teach a young mother about bottle mouth caries for her expected child when discussing methods of infant feeding.
   c. Health teaching: A school nurse discusses hypoglycemia—its symptoms, causes, and treatment— of a child with diabetes mellitus who is beginning to make independent decisions about his or her disease and who has just experienced a hypoglycemic episode.
   d. Support/counseling: A pediatric nurse practitioner meets with children and their parents to help foster expression of feelings and thoughts after the death of a classmate from leukemia.
   e. Coordination/collaboration: A pediatric clinical specialist who practices in a small community hospital helps a family plan care for a child with cerebral palsy who needs surgery at a large medical center. Transportation, housing for the family, financial needs, community services for cerebral palsy are all planned for.
   f. Ethical decision making: A staff nurse on the infant-toddler surgical division at a large metropolitan children hospital is a member of an interdisciplinary team for a liver transplant patient and a primary nurse for two patients who were both born with biliary atresia and are both dying. She is instrumental in providing information to help decide which of the two patients will receive the transplant.
   g. Research: A pediatric clinical nurse specialist (CNS) sees differences in the recovery rate of children who are admitted with acute appendicitis. The CNS works with the staff nurse to identify differences in the care methods used and begins a clinical research project.
   h. Health care planning: A community health nurse is a member of the local nurses' association governmental affairs committee and speaks regularly with the congressman for the area where the community clinic is located.
3. *Response should include* the shift in focus from treatment of disease to health promotion (e.g., preventing folic acid deficiency has irradiated neural tube defects). Also discussed should be how roles in ambulatory care, prevention, and health teaching have expanded (e.g., nurse-managed asthma clinic). Home care and community health services should have changed in some way (e.g., home care staff nurses and community health staff nurses act as liaisons with hospital staff nurses). The nurse described should show a difference in independence and skilled technical expertise from 2000 to 2020. New examples of anticipatory guidance, child health and family assessment, discharge planning, and home care should be given. Collaborating with families to reach solutions should be mentioned. Ways to do more with fewer resources and less patient contact should be identified. How the nurse keeps abreast of developments should be delineated.

CHAPTER 30:   COMMUNITY-BASED NURSING CARE OF THE CHILD AND FAMILY

I. Learning Key Terms

1. q	2. l	3. h	4. c	5. g	6. f
7. e	8. m	9. i	10. j	11. k	12. p
13. d	14. b	15. o	16. a	17. n	

II. Reviewing Key Concepts and Content

18. a	19. c	20. b	21. d	22. b	23. c
24. c					

III. Thinking Critically

1. *Subjective:* Hold focus groups and tabulate the results. *Objective:* Examine records of churches— births, deaths, financial status.

2. Answers might include these or similar examples:
    a. *Family advocacy/caring:* Develop a coalition of families to address family violence.
    b. *Disease prevention/health promotion:* Develop a radio, television, and poster campaign to promote dental health.
    c. *Health teaching:* Develop a diabetes teaching tool for health professionals to use in a community where 80% of the population is Hispanic.
    d. *Support/counseling:* Facilitate a group for newly divorced people in a community with a high divorce rate.
    e. *Coordination/collaboration:* Establish the mechanism where city health officials meet on a regular basis with the goal to promote and improve the health and welfare of the citizens.
    f. *Ethical decision making:* Establish an ethics committee that is composed of citizens, town council members, and hospital executives of the local facilities, health department officials, social service organizations, religious leaders, and business owners.
    g. *Research:* Conduct a survey before and after participants attend a support group to determine whether the support group is an effective intervention for the community.
    h. *Health care planning:* A community health nurse is a member of the local nurses' association governmental affairs committee and speaks regularly with the congressman for the area where the community clinic is located.

CHAPTER 31: FAMILY INFLUENCES ON CHILD HEALTH PROMOTION

I. Learning Key Terms

1. g	2. d	3. h	4. f	5. e	6. b
7. i	8. j	9. a	10. c	11. d	12. e
13. b	14. c	15. a	16. g	17. h	18. f

II. Reviewing Key Concepts and Content

19. c	20. c	21. a	22. c	23. b	24. a
25. a	26. d	27. F	28. T	29. F	30. T
31. T	32. T	33. c	34. a	35. c	36. b

III. Thinking Critically

1. a. Promote physical survival and health of the children. (e.g., Reassure the parents as you examine each of the infants that they are healthy and that the parents are doing a good job.) Foster the skills and abilities necessary to be a self-sustaining adult. (e.g., Complete a family assessment. Using the assessment, identify the family's capabilities and look at basic attributes of the family, resources within the family, and family's perceptions of the situation.). Foster behavioral capabilities for maximizing cultural values and beliefs. (e.g., Assess the participation of the extended family for advice and assistance.)
    b. Immediate needs include emotional support during the stressful newborn period, positive reinforcement for correct parenting behaviors, education, and skill training for infant's needs.
    c. Establish a healthy family unit.
    d. Seek support from extended family, provide parenting instruction, attend support group for parents with twins, and identify community resources available for the family.
2. *Possible responses include:*
    a. *Natural consequences* are those that occur without any intervention, such as being late and missing dinner. These are effective only when they are meaningful. (e.g., Forgetting ballet slippers results in the child having to dance in stocking feet.)
    b. *Logical consequences* are those that are directly related to a rule such as not being allowed to play with another toy until the used ones are put away (e.g., not being permitted to visit a friend for 1 day after not coming home from that friend's house on time).
    c. *Unrelated consequences* are those that are imposed deliberately, such as no playing until homework is completed or the use of timeout. Withdrawing privileges is usually an unrelated consequence (e.g., no watching television at night until the pets are fed).
3. It usually takes the form of spanking and causes a dramatic short-term decrease in the behavior. However, the disadvantages include the following:
    * It teaches children that violence is acceptable.
    * The spanking is often a result of parental anger.
    * The spanking may physically harm the child.
    * Children become accustomed to spanking.
    * More severe corporal punishment may be needed each time.
    * Parents may resort to using paddles or other objects.
    * The punishment may interfere with effective parent-child interactions.
    * Child learns what they should not do—not what should be done.
    * Misbehavior is likely to occur when the parent is not around.
    * Punishment may interfere with the child's development of moral reasoning.

CHAPTER 32: SOCIAL, CULTURAL, AND RELIGIOUS INFLUENCES ON CHILD HEALTH PROMOTION

I. Learning Key Terms

1. e	2. b	3. i	4. c	5. h	6. d
7. a	8. g	9. f	10. j	11. k	12. l
13. m	14. n	15. o	16. t	17. p	18. q
19. r	20. s	21. u	22. v		

II. Reviewing Key Concepts and Content

23. b	24. d	25. d	26. a	27. b	28. a
29. b	30. a	31. d	32. e	33. d	34. a
35. f	36. c	37. b	38. f	39. e	40. d
41. b	42. a	43. c	44. d	45. d	46. a
47. c	48. a	49. b	50. b		

III. Thinking Critically

1. *Descriptions should include some of the following:*
   a. Hispanic: Find out who the primary caregiver is. The grandmother may be very involved and may actually control most of the feeding. If certain products are recommended, they may need to be written down for the head of the household, who may control their purchase. A relaxed view of time may necessitate reviewing medication schedule in relation to events such as leaving for work, eating a meal, or bedtime. Be aware that touching the infant during the instructional process may be particularly important if the family believes the "evil eye" symptoms will occur. Language comprehension should be assessed. Does the family prefer written instructions in English or Spanish? A set of both may be needed if family members differ in their command of English. A person may speak English well but may still need to read in Spanish. If the family member moves closer during the interaction, resist any inclination to pull away. In fact, during the instruction, the nurse should be positioned less than an arm's length from the patient and family members. Interpret indirect eye contact as evidence that the person feels as if you are displeased with something they have done. Allow the person time to vent and air concerns. Assess whether holidays are approaching that might interfere with recommendations about the bland diet. The nurse might want to discuss the concept of hot and cold imbalance in relation to the bland diet and to show awareness of the home remedies that might be recommended by the curandera(o). There may be some feeling that the illness is a punishment from God.

The child will be valued as a gift from God. The nurse should shake hands with the patient. It may also be appropriate to engage in an embrace if a relationship exists. The family may use spices in food but should have an ample supply of bland items such as rice.

   b. African-American: Time may be viewed differently and may need to be considered in terms of instruction about medications. Dairy foods may already be eliminated because some people of African ancestry may have a hereditary lactase deficiency. The natural forces of the seasons of the year and planet positions may be believed to affect the body processes, and supernatural forces may be part of the family's belief system. The illness may be seen as sent by God as punishment. Folk remedies may be used, and they may have a spiritual origin. Foods have properties of hot/cold and light/heavy and must be in harmony with the life cycle and bodily state. Children are valued as security in old age and viewed as gifts from God. Recent immigrants from Haiti may speak only Haitian Creole; language may need to be considered in giving written instructions. Family may resist dietary restrictions. Medication may be taken in relation to how the family perceives the severity of the illness. The foods may be quite spicy. If the family is Black Muslim, they may not eat many of the foods that are more traditional among many African-American families (e.g., pork, corn bread, collard greens).

   c. Asian-American: Health is viewed as a gift from parents and ancestors. Yin and yang—cold/hot energy forces—rule the world. Illness is caused by imbalance. Chi is innate energy. Family may use acupuncture, moxibustion, and herbs. Milk may be avoided because of hereditary lactose intolerance. Honor is very important. Self-reliance and self-restraint are valued. The family may not feel comfortable asking questions. Emotions may not be expressed openly. Rice is one bland food that is a staple in the diet. Depending on the geographic origin of the Asian ancestry, the food may be spicy.

2. a. "How did you travel to the clinic?"; "Do you prefer written instructions in English or Spanish?"; "Who usually cares for the child during the day?"

   b. Shake hands and provide a clear introduction. Sit down close to Noemi. Determine the need for a translator. Use pictures and models for more clear communication.

   c. Children are seen as gifts from God. Illness may be seen as a sign from God. The male is the dominant figure and influences many practices. Folk healing and remedies used by older family members may be tried. Perception of time may interfere with keeping appointments. Family is highly valued, and there is often a multigenerational family structure. Personal interests are often subordinated to family needs.

3. a. Assess each patient individually. Determine their particular cultural beliefs and practices. Use language resources specifically designed to greet and familiarize the family with procedures. Use a cultural reference manual that includes a brief description of the culture, their views on matters such as health, illness, and diet, and a list of interpreters and ethnic community services or other sources for quick reference.

   b. *Examples of acceptable responses:*
   Many cultural groups use shame to provide social controls. Children in these groups learn that anything is acceptable as long as one is not caught. This kind of orientation may keep the caregiver from applying concepts taught about discipline and limit setting in the education program.
   Some cultures perceive diarrhea as a cleansing of the body that is essential for health maintenance, and the caregiver may not want to use all of the techniques taught in the education program to stop diarrhea in gastroenteritis.

CHAPTER 33: DEVELOPMENTAL INFLUENCES ON CHILD HEALTH PROMOTION

I. Learning Key Terms

1. c	2. a	3. s	4. l	5. b	6. r
7. k	8. j	9. q	10. i	11. h	12. p
13. g	14. o	15. f	16. n	17. e	18. t
19. m	20. d				

II. Reviewing Key Concepts and Content

21. c	22. a	23. c	24. b	25. a	26. c
27. f	28. a	29. d	30. b	31. e	32. d
33. b	34. b	35. b	36. a	37. c	38. c
39. c	40. d	41. c	42. d	43. a	44. e
45. c	46. b	47. f	48. a	49. d	50. i
51. h	52. g	53. a	54. d	55. b	56. c
57. d	58. a	59. c	60. d	61. d	62. g
63. d	64. c	65. e	66. f	67. j	68. b
69. a	70. i	71. h	72. b	73. d	74. a

III. Thinking Critically

1. Factors should include watching television for 4 to 5 hours a day, family history of heart disease, aggressiveness, overweight, elevated cholesterol.
2. Strategies should be described that restrict the child's viewing of violent programs, increase the parents' awareness of the content of the shows that are viewed, help the child correlate consequences with the actions, point out subtle messages, and help the child explore alternatives to aggressive conflict resolution.
3. Outcomes described should include the child selecting more healthful snacks, watching television for about 1 hour per day, increasing physical activity, and exploring the possibility of adding out-of-the-home activities, such as scouting, sports, and music.

CHAPTER 34: COMMUNICATION AND HEALTH ASSESSMENT OF THE CHILD AND FAMILY

I. Learning Key Terms

1. d	2. k	3. e	4. c	5. h	6. f
7. b	8. i	9. g	10. a	11. j	

II. Reviewing Key Concepts and Content

12. c	13. b	14. d	15. b	16. d	17. F
18. T	19. T	20. T	21. F	22. b	23. a
24. c	25. d	26. d			

27. *Components of a pediatric health history:* identifying information, chief complaint, present illness, past history, review of systems, family medical history, psychosocial history, sexual history; it also may include a family history and a nutritional history.

28. b	29. c	30. a	31. d	32. c	33. b
34. c	35. d	36. a	37. b	38. c	

39. Present, anthropometry

III. Thinking Critically

1. *Responses should include the following:*
   a. Parents, as well as children, are involved, and the nurse must decide whether to address the adult or the child.
   b. Relationships with the child are often mediated via the parent, whereas with adults, the communication is usually with one person only. Refocusing may be needed more often with family communication, because family issues may surface during the communication

process if the parent is involved in the interview. Developmental stage and age must be considered. Play and nonverbal or abstract communication techniques may need to be used with families, whereas communication is usually solely verbal with adults.

c. The informant for the child may be the parent, whereas the adult usually is his or her own informant. If the child is the informant, little may be known of the birth history, milestones, and immunization status. Birth history, immunizations, growth and development, family assessment, and nutritional assessment are all included in every child's assessment. In the adult these are usually not included or not included with the same depth.

CHAPTER 35: PHYSICAL AND DEVELOPMENTAL ASSESSMENT OF THE CHILD

I. Learning Key Terms

1. h	2. k	3. r	4. j	5. f	6. q
7. i	8. p	9. c	10. g	11. o	12. e
13. n	14. b	15. m	16. a	17. l	18. d

II. Reviewing Key Concepts and Content

19. b   20. a   21. d
22. Body mass index, race, ethnicity, very-low-birth-weight
23. a   24. T   25. F   26. T   27. T   28. b
29. Apical, 1 full minute
30. d   31. c   32. a
33. Maxillary, ethmoid
34. **P**upils **E**qual, **R**ound, **R**eact to **L**ight and **A**ccommodation
35. b   36. d   37. b   38. d   39. b   40. a
41. c   42. c   43. b   44. d   45. d

III. Thinking Critically

1. In the infant the ear canal curves upward. In older children the ear canal curves downward and forward.
2. Cyanosis will appear bluish in light skin and ashen gray in dark skin. Pallor will show as a loss of rosy glow in light skin and ashen gray or yellowish in dark skin. Pallor is difficult to assess in dark skin. Erythema is easily seen in light skin but difficult to see except in the mouth or conjunctiva in dark skin. Do not rely on this sign in dark skin. Ecchymosis is purplish yellow-green in light skin. In dark skin it is difficult to see except in the mouth or conjunctiva. Jaundice is seen easily in light skin. In dark skin assess the sclera, palms, soles, and hard palate.

3. *Responses should include* asking the parent whether the child's performance was typical behavior, emphasizing the successful items first, failed items next, and finally the delayed items. If the behavior was not typical of the child, defer the discussion and reschedule testing. Do not rely on the Denver II, but rather assess the whole picture. Note the parents' response. Respond honestly to parents' questions, stressing the need for further developmental testing.

CHAPTER 36:   THE INFANT AND FAMILY

I. Learning Key Terms

1. h	2. f	3. j	4. g	5. k	6. b
7. e	8. a	9. i	10. c	11. l	12. d

II. Reviewing Key Concepts and Content

13. b	14. b	15. a	16. c	17. b	18. b
19. c	20. d	21. a	22. b	23. d	24. c
25. c	26. a	27. c	28. F	29. T	30. F
31. F	32. T				

III. Thinking Critically

1. *Descriptions should include the following:* lifts head off table when supine, sits erect momentarily, bears full weight on feet, transfers objects from hand to hand, rakes at a small object, bangs a cube on the table, produces vowel sounds and chained syllables, vocalizes four distinct vowel sounds, plays peekaboo, fears strangers when mother disappears, and imitates simple acts.
2. *Interventions should include the following:* ask few questions for factual information; remain nonjudgmental, and do not indicate guilt; comfort the members of the family as much as possible; allow parents to discuss the event and what took place when help arrived; allow the family to say good-bye to the infant; accompany the family to the car or arrange for someone to take them home; debrief the health care workers who dealt with the family; assure that home visits are to be made; provide literature about SIDS; assist parents in their understanding of the disease; provide a forum for parents to cope with their grief and other emotions related to their loss; listen actively; and use the specifics of each situation to plan individualized, flexible care.
3. *Responses should include the following:* assess home for electrical safety and instruct parents about maintaining a safe electrical environment; inform utility company in order to initiate emergency procedures in the event of a power outage; assess family structure and function and teach other support family members so that they can

participate fully in the care of the infant; avoid alarm compromises; parents should sleep in a different bed, but be able to respond in 30 seconds; check monitor periodically; signal interference.

CHAPTER 37: THE TODDLER AND FAMILY

I. Learning Key Terms

1. c   2. i   3. d   4. h   5. b   6. e
7. g   8. f   9. a

II. Reviewing Key Concepts and Content

10. c   11. b   12. c   13. a   14. a   15. c
16. d   17. d   18. d   19. b   20. a   21. c
22. d   23. b   24. a   25. d   26. c
27. a. *Foods:* hot dogs, nuts, dried beans, pits from fruits
    b. *Play objects:* anything with small parts
    c. *Common household objects:* thumbtacks, nails, screws, coins, jewelry, old refrigerators, storage chest
    d. *Electrical items:* outlets, garage doors, car windows

III. Thinking Critically

1. A few questions and clinical data from the following areas should be described: nutrition, sleep and activity, dental health, injury prevention, temperament, and psychologic development.
2. Gross motor development milestones include the ability to go up and down stairs alone, using both feet on each step; run fairly well with a wide stance; pick up objects without falling; kick a ball forward without overbalancing.
3. Fine motor development milestones include the ability to build a tower of six to seven cubes; align two or more cubes like a train; turn the pages of a book one at a time; imitate vertical and circular strokes when drawing; turn doorknobs; and unscrew lids.
4. Language development milestones include having a vocabulary of 300 words; using two- or three-word phrases; using the pronouns I, me, and you; understanding directional commands; giving first name; verbalizing the need for toileting; and talking incessantly.
5. Negativism contributes to the toddler's acquisition of a sense of autonomy by the assertion of self-control and serving as an attempt to control the environment and a way to increase independence.

CHAPTER 38: THE PRESCHOOLER AND FAMILY

I. Learning Key Terms

1. h   2. p   3. g   4. o   5. u   6. w
7. f   8. n   9. e   10. t   11. m   12. d
13. l   14. x   15. v   16. c   17. s   18. k
19. b   20. r   21. j   22. a   23. q   24. i

II. Reviewing Key Concepts and Content

25. 3, 5   26. 2.3 kg/5 lb   27. b   28. c   29. d
30. T   31. T   32. F   33. F   34. d   35. a
36. a   37. c

III. Thinking Critically

1. The child will need some preparation for this new preschool experience. One cannot guarantee that the child will have less trouble adjusting than a child who has never attended day care. A change such as this, although not drastic, could cause disruption because of differences in the programs, as well as differences between the day care "caregiver" and the preschool "teacher" and styles used by each. The amount and quality of the attention may differ from the day care to the preschool. The preschool may have more expectations for the child to be independent and autonomous than the day care center does.
2. *An example:* The mother will verbalize at least five strategies that can be used to help prepare her child for the preschool experience.
3. *Possible responses might include:* visit the school ahead of time, introduce the child and the teacher, begin to talk about the new school, refer to the new school in a positive way, and maintain confidence on the first day.
4. Characteristics that indicate that the child is ready for preschool include social maturity, good attention span, and academic readiness.

CHAPTER 39: THE SCHOOL-AGE CHILD AND FAMILY

I. Learning Key Terms

1. g   2. k   3. h   4. j   5. f   6. d
7. a   8. b   9. e   10. l   11. c   12. i

II. Reviewing Key Concepts and Content

13. c
14. Shedding the first deciduous tooth; puberty, with the acquisition of permanent teeth

15. T   16. F   17. T   18. F   19. T   20. F
21. 9/10; 12/13   22. a   23. c   24. d   25. d
26. d   27. c   28. b
29. Hygiene, nutrition, exercise, recreation, sleep, safety

III. Thinking Critically

1. *Response should include* nutritional assessment and his knowledge and use of safety precautions when riding his bike.
2. *Response should include* support for the mother by reassuring her that her child is healthy and that playing soccer will allow him to increase strength and develop motor skill performance.
3. *Response should outline the information about* nutrition related to good lifelong dietary habits.
4. *Response should include* ideas about how to give the child recognition and positive feedback for his accomplishments.

CHAPTER 40:   THE ADOLESCENT AND FAMILY

I. Learning Key Terms

1. e   2. o   3. f   4. q   5. p   6. g
7. d   8. h   9. n   10. c   11. b   12. m
13. i   14. a   15. j   16. l   17. k

II. Reviewing Key Concepts and Content

18. 10½ to 15 years; 12 years and 9½ months
19. a   20. c
21. Pubertal delay
22. b   23. b
24. 2, 8; 15, 55; 4, 12; 15, 65
25. c   26. d   27. a   28. d   29. d   30. a
31. d   32. d   33. c   34. a   35. d   36. d
37. a   38. d   39. b   40. c   41. b   42. c
43. Primary amenorrhea
44. Secondary amenorrhea
45. c   46. d

III. Thinking Critically

1. Nonlean body mass, primarily fat, increases in adolescence. Fatty tissue deposition is more pronounced in girls, particularly in the regions over the thigh, hips, buttocks, and breast tissue. Using the 95th percentile as the top of the normal range, nutritional counseling to prevent additional weight gain and/or eating disorders should be instituted whenever there is concern.
2. A sense of group identity is essential to the later development of personal identity. Younger adolescents must resolve questions concerning relationships with peer groups before they are able to resolve questions about who they are in relation to the family and society. Peer groups serve as a strong support to the adolescent, individually and collectively, providing a sense of belonging and a feeling of strength and power. They form a transitional world between dependence and autonomy.
3. Show respect for the adolescent's privacy; show honest and sincere interest in the adolescent's beliefs and feelings; and listen without interrupting the adolescent.
4. Benefits include exercise for growing muscles and interactions with peers; "socially acceptable" means to enjoy stimulation and conflict.
5. Reasons include the emphasis on slimness as a standard for beauty and femininity and increased family stress.
6. Behavior modification programs that include consistency in approach, involvement of all team members, continuity of caregivers, clear communication among team, clear communications with the patient, and support of patient are most effective.
7. Factors that might be noted include a disturbed family situation, economic stresses, family disintegration, medical problems, psychiatric illness, abandonment, or alcoholism. Adolescent girls make more unsuccessful suicide attempts than boys and are likely to ingest pills as the method.

CHAPTER 41:   CHRONIC ILLNESS, DISABILITY, AND END-OF-LIFE CARE

I. Learning Key Terms

1. i   2. q   3. h   4. m   5. g   6. p
7. j   8. r   9. f   10. e   11. k   12. d
13. o   14. a   15. l   16. c   17. n   18. b

II. Reviewing Key Concepts and Content

19. b   20. d
21. Recipients of care
22. Silent in care
23. Managers of care
24. Monitors of care
25. Support the family's coping and/or promote the family's optimum functioning throughout the child's life
26. *Possible strategies* include providing education regarding what can reasonably be expected of the child, assistance in identifying the child's strength, praise for a parental job well done, and finding respite care so that parents can renew their energies.

27. a
28. *Possible tasks include* accept the child's condition; manage the child's condition on a day-to-day basis; meet the child's normal developmental needs; meet the developmental needs of other family members; cope with ongoing stress and periodic crises; assist family members to manage their feelings; educate others about the child's conditions; and establish a support system.
29. d   30. b   31. d   32. d
33. Shock/denial, adjustment, and reintegration/acknowledgment
34. d   35. c   36. c   37. b   38. d   39. b
40. c
41. *Possible answers include* loss of senses, confusion, muscle weakness, loss of bowel and bladder control, difficulty swallowing, change in respiratory pattern, and weak/slow pulse.
42. d   43. c   44. c   45. a   46. d   47. c

III. Thinking Critically

1. *Responses should include the following:*
   - Using the development approach emphasizes the child's abilities and strengths rather than his or her disability. Under the developmental model, attention is directed to the child's functional development, changes, and adaptation to the environment.
   - Families are supported in their natural caregiving and decision-making roles by building on their unique strengths as individuals.
   - By applying the principles of normalization, the environment for the child is normalized and humanized.
   - The school has now become an essential component of the child's overall physical, intellectual, and social development.
2. Assessment aids in evaluating the individual's ability to cope with various aspects of the crisis and identifies possible areas for intervention.
3. Children between the ages of 3 years and 5 years see death as a departure. They may recognize the fact of physical death but do not separate it from living abilities. They view death as temporary and gradual.
4. A preschooler is likely to perceive illness as punishment for past thoughts or actions.
5. Developmentally the adolescent's task is to establish an identity by finding out who he is, what his purpose is, and where he belongs. Any suggestion of being different, or of not being at all, is a tremendous threat to accomplishing this task. The adolescent's concern is for the present much more than the past or the future.

CHAPTER 42:   COGNITIVE AND SENSORY IMPAIRMENT

I. Learning Key Terms

1. v	2. j	3. u	4. k	5. i	6. l
7. h	8. m	9. g	10. n	11. t	12. f
13. o	14. e	15. s	16. d	17. p	18. c
19. b	20. q	21. w	22. a	23. r	

II. Reviewing Key Concepts and Content

24. b   25. d   26. c   27. a   28. b   29. d
30. Task analysis is the process of breaking a skill into its components; it is used when teaching mentally retarded children to help them master one part of the skill at a time, beginning with the parts the child has mastered already. Each task is separated into its necessary components and each step is taught completely before proceeding to the next activity.
31. c   32. b   33. a   34. c   35. b   36. d
37. b   38. a   39. d   40. h   41. f   42. d
43. c   44. g   45. b   46. e   47. a   48. d
49. b
50. Blindism is the self-stimulatory activity that develops to compensate for inadequate stimulation; it may retard the blind child's social acceptance.
51. *Possible strategies* include the following: talk to child about everything that is occurring; emphasize aspects of procedures that are felt/heard; approach the child with identifying information; explain sounds; encourage parents to room in; encourage parents' participation; bring familiar objects from home; orient child to surroundings. (If the child has sight on admission but will lose sight during hospitalization [e.g., as a result of eye surgery], point out significant aspects of the room's layout and practice ambulation with eyes closed before the procedure.)
52. b   53. b

III. Thinking Critically

1. *Responses should include the following nursing interventions:* ensure that the child has appropriate toys for entertainment; place the child in a room with other children of the same approximate developmental age; treat the child with dignity and respect; explain procedures using methods of communication appropriate for the child's cognitive level; focus on growth-promoting experiences for the child.
2. The hearing-impaired child is often unable to proceed past parallel play within a group, because of an inability to follow the direction of

cooperative play. Also, a hearing deficit may not allow the child to interpret enough of the conversation to join in. As a result, the hearing-impaired child may stay on the periphery or avoid social interaction altogether.

3. Speech is learned through a multisensory approach, and the usual mechanisms are not available to the deaf child.

4. *Responses should include the following:* avoid excessive eye strain when doing close work; periodically look into the distance to relax the muscles of accommodation; use proper lighting; light should not be glaring or cast shadows on reading material; get sufficient amounts of rest and nutrition; have eyes checked at least yearly by a licensed optometrist or ophthalmologist; teach safety regarding common eye injuries.

CHAPTER 43: FAMILY-CENTERED HOME CARE

I. Learning Key Terms

1. d   2. e   3. c   4. f   5. a   6. g
7. b

II. Reviewing Key Concepts and Content

8. less   9. d   10. a   11. c   12. c   13. d
14. d   15. c

III. Thinking Critically

1. *Responses should address* the medical, nursing and health maintenance needs of the child; financial, psychosocial, and educational issues of the child and family, as well as assessing needs and resources; planning for comprehensive care; coordinating services and referrals; monitoring and evaluating service; and providing administrative support and advocacy.

2. *Essential features of collaborative relationships in the home care setting include the following:* communication, dialog, active listening, awareness and acceptance of difference, and negotiation.

3. *Strategies for conflict resolution include* showing respect for parental preference and contacting the supervisor/case manager for help with problem solving.

CHAPTER 44: REACTION TO ILLNESS AND HOSPITALIZATION

I. Learning Key Terms

1. e   2. b   3. d   4. a   5. c

II. Reviewing Key Concepts and Content

6. b   7. b   8. c   9. a   10. b   11. a
12. d   13. c
14. *Possible answers:* Hospitalization may present opportunities for the child to master stress and feel competent in his or her coping abilities. There may be new socialization experiences. The child's interpersonal relationships may be broadened. Nursing strategies should be aimed at maximizing these benefits.
15. b   16. c   17. a   18. d   19. a   20. c
21. c   22. b   23. c   24. b   25. T   26. T
27. F   28. T   29. F   30. T   31. F   32. T
33. Question the child.
Use pain-rating scales.
Evaluate behavior and physiologic changes.
Secure (encourage) parent's involvement.
Take cause of pain into account.
Take action and evaluate results.
34. d   35. a   36. b   37. d   38. c   39. a
40. c   41. a   42. d   43. d   44. c

III. Thinking Critically

1. Recognize that family members know the child best and are most aware of the child's needs. Welcome unlimited family presence. Encourage family to bring other significant family members to visit. Arrange for family members to have a meal together.

2. *Some recommended toys for a 4-year-old child include the following:* large puzzles, blocks, dress-up materials, puppets, crayons, scissors and paper.

3. Be positive in your approach to the child. Be honest with the child. Convey to the child the behaviors expected. Be consistent in expectations and relationships with the child. Treat the child fairly, and help the child feel this. Encourage parents to maintain a truthful relationship with the child. Make certain the child has a call light or other signal device within reach.

4. *Suitable pain assessment scales include:* "Oucher," numeric scale, poker chip tool, word graphic rating scale, visual analogue scale, and color tool.

CHAPTER 45:   PEDIATRIC VARIATIONS OF NURSING INTERVENTIONS

I. Learning Key Terms

1. n   2. e   3. m   4. d   5. f   6. g
7. c   8. l   9. h   10. k   11. b   12. i
13. a   14. j

II. Reviewing Key Concepts and Content

15. d   16. d   17. c
18. *Possible supportive strategies include the following:* Expect success. Have extra supplies handy. Involve the child. Provide distraction. Allow expression of feelings. Praise the child. Use play in preparation of and after the procedure.
19. a. Give a toddler a push-pull toy.
    b. Touch or kick Mylar balloons.
    c. Make creative objects out of syringes.
    d. Practice band instruments.
    e. Move the patient's bed to the playroom.
    f. Put toys at the bottom of bath container.
    g. Make freezer pops using the child's favorite juice.

20. a   21. b   22. c   23. a   24. c   25. b
26. a   27. a   28. b   29. c   30. d   31. b
32. d   33. b   34. a   35. a   36. c   37. d
38. b   39. c   40. b   41. d   42. c   43. a

III. Thinking Critically

1. Help parents understand the purpose of the restraint, how to remove and reapply them, as well as the signs of complication from their use, and help parents soothe and calm the child.
2. Restraints should be checked every 2 hours to ensure that they are accomplishing their purpose; that they are applied correctly; and that they do not impair circulation, sensation, or skin integrity; and to ensure that the restraints are secured to the bed or crib frame, not the side rails.
3. The patient is dressed in a lightweight shirt and placed in a postural drainage position; then the nurse gently but firmly strikes the chest wall with a cupped hand. A popping hollow sound should be heard, not a slapping sound. The procedure should be done over the rib cage only and should be painless. Percussion can be performed with a soft circular mask or a percussion cup marked especially for the purpose of aiding the loosening of secretions.

CHAPTER 46:   RESPIRATORY DYSFUNCTION

I. Learning Key Terms

1. g   2. f   3. m   4. e   5. l   6. k
7. d   8. j   9. b   10. i   11. c   12. h
13. n   14. a

II. Reviewing Key Concepts and Content

15. b   16. c   17. c   18. b   19. b   20. c
21. d   22. a   23. c   24. a   25. b   26. a
27. a   28. c   29. c   30. d   31. c   32. a
33. b   34. c   35. b   36. d   37. b   38. c
39. d   40. c   41. b   42. d   43. d   44. a
45. c   46. b   47. c   48. d   49. b   50. d
51. b
52. Restlessness, tachypnea, tachycardia, diaphoresis
53. d   54. c   55. a   56. a   57. h   58. c
59. b   60. e   61. f   62. g   63. d   64. a
65. d

III. Thinking Critically

1. Monitor respiration; auscultate lungs; observe color of skin and mucous membranes; observe for presence of hoarseness, stridor, and cough; monitor heart rate and regularity; and observe behavior.
2. The goal of such treatment is to decrease the edema of the respiratory tract.
3. Child sweats profusely, remains sitting upright, and refuses to lie down. A child who suddenly becomes agitated or suddenly becomes quiet may be seriously hypoxic.
4. a. *Respiratory symptoms* include obstruction of bronchioles and bronchi with abnormally thick mucus.
   b. *Large, bulky, frothy, foul-smelling stools* occur because of a lack of trypsin, amylase, and lipase, resulting in large amounts of undigested food excreted in the stool.
   c. *Voracious appetite* occurs because so little food is absorbed from intestines that hunger continues and the child is stimulated to eat more.
   d. *Weight loss* occurs because appetite cannot compensate for great amount of fecal waste.
   e. *Anemia and bruising* result from an inability to absorb fat-soluble vitamins.
5. The child may return to school. There is no need for isolation because the disease is almost always noninfectious in children. Child should refrain from vigorous activity/sports and be protected from stress during the active stage of primary tuberculosis.

CHAPTER 47: GASTROINTESTINAL DYSFUNCTION

I. Learning Key Terms

1. h   2. g   3. n   4. e   5. m   6. f
7. l   8. d   9. k   10. c   11. o   12. j
13. b   14. i   15. a

II. Reviewing Key Concepts and Content

16. c   17. d   18. a   19. b
20. Major nutritional deficiencies include inadequate protein for growth; inadequate calories for energy and growth; poor digestibility of many of the bulky natural, unprocessed foods, especially for infants; and deficiencies of vitamin B_6, niacin, riboflavin, vitamin D, iron, calcium, and zinc. Strict vegetarian diets also require supplements of vitamin B_{12} and vitamin D.
21. c   22. b   23. d   24. c   25. c   26. c
27. d
28. Isotonic
29. Hypotonic, less
30. Hypertonic, loss, intake, greater
31. b   32. c   33. c   34. b   35. c   36. d
37. b   38. c   39. d   40. a   41. d   42. d
43. c
44. Inducing vomiting, counteracting the toxin with activated charcoal, performing gastric lavage, increasing bowel motility, and administering antidote
45. d   46. c   47. a   48. c
49. Handwashing
50. a   51. b   52. e   53. d   54. c   55. c
56. d   57. b   58. c   59. b   60. d   61. a
62. a   63. a   64. c   65. a   66. b   67. d
68. d   69. c   70. d
71. Assessment, support respiratory system; other supportive measures; gastric decontamination with assessment; monitoring and supportive measures; family support; prevention of recurrence
72. a   73. T   74. T   75. T   76. F

III. Thinking Critically

1. *Assessment should include* accurate history of bowel habits; diet and events that may be associated with the onset of constipation; drugs or other substances that the child may be taking; and consistency, color, frequency, and other characteristics of the stool.
2. *The stages of repair for Hirschsprung disease* include creation of a temporary colostomy, surgical correction by "pulling through bowel," and closure of the colostomy.
3. *Responses should include the following:* position infant prone with head elevated at 30 degrees for 24 hours a day, maintain position with a body harness or leave flat/prone, and do not put in supine position.
4. Pathology: Ulcerative colitis (UC) is a chronic inflammatory reaction involving the mucosa and submucosa of the large intestine. Mucosa becomes hyperemic and edematous with patchy granulation that bleeds easily and leads to superficial ulceration. Crohn's disease (CD) affects the terminal ileum and involves all layers of the bowel wall. Edema and inflammation progress to deep ulceration with fissure and obstruction.
   - Rectal bleeding: common in UC; uncommon in CD.
   - Diarrhea: often severe in UC; moderate to absent in CD.
   - Pain: less frequent in UC; common in CD.
   - Anorexia: mild to moderate in UC; can be severe in CD.
   - Weight loss: moderate in UC; severe in CD.
   - Growth retardation: usually mild in UC; often pronounced in CD.

CHAPTER 48: CARDIOVASCULAR DYSFUNCTION

I. Learning Key Terms

1. o   2. r   3. v   4. n   5. p   6. m
7. l   8. w   9. q   10. k   11. t   12. e
13. d   14. u   15. f   16. c   17. j   18. a
19. g   20. s   21. b   22. h   23. i

II. Reviewing Key Concepts and Content

24. b   25. a   26. d   27. a   28. c   29. b
30. *The most significant complications* include stroke, seizures, tamponade, and death. The patient may also suffer loss of circulation to the affected extremity, dysrhythmias, hemorrhage, cardiac perforation, hematoma, hypovolemia and dehydration, hypoglycemia in infants, and changes in the temperature and color of the affected extremity.
31. d   32. b   33. d   34. b   35. c   36. b
37. c   38. d   39. c   40. d   41. b   42. b
43. c   44. d   45. c   46. d   47. b   48. c
49. d   50. a   51. d   52. a   53. d   54. b
55. c   56. b   57. c   58. b   59. d   60. c
61. Perform only as needed. Avoid vagal stimulation (cardiac dysrhythmias) and laryngospasm; perform intermittently only, maintain for no more than 5 seconds. Administer supplemental oxygen before and after the procedure and monitor heart rate for changes in rhythm/rate. Position the child

to permit assessment of color, use of accessory muscles, and how the procedure was tolerated.

62. a 63. b 64. d 65. d 66. d
67. *Possible complications: Cardiac*—congestive heart failure, low cardiac output, dysrhythmias, tamponade; *Respiratory*—atelectasis, pulmonary edema, pleural effusions, pneumothorax; *Neurologic*—seizures, cerebrovascular accident, cerebral edema, neurologic deficits; *Infectious disease*—infections; *Hematologic*—anemia, postoperative bleeding; *Other:* postpericardiotomy syndrome (i.e., fever leukocytosis, friction rub, pericardial and pleural effusions).
68. a 69. d 70. b 71. c 72. b 73. c
74. b

III. Thinking Critically

1. *Responses should include the following clinical manifestations:* growth retardation; feeding difficulty; dyspnea; weak cry, cyanosis; and dry, hot skin.
2. *Components of a child's history that could indicate a high risk for congenital heart disease include the following:* maternal rubella; poor nutrition; maternal insulin-dependent diabetes; maternal age over 40 years; maternal alcoholism; a sibling or parent with a congenital heart defect; a chromosomal aberration, especially Down syndrome or other noncardiac congenital anomalies.
3. Digitalis improves cardiac functioning by increasing cardiac output, decreasing heart size, decreasing venous pressure, and decreasing edema. Diuretics remove accumulated fluid and sodium, thereby decreasing the work of the heart.
4. *Responses should include the following:* encourage parents to express their fears and concerns regarding the child's cardiac defects and physical symptoms; encourage family to participate in child's care; encourage family to include others in child's care to prevent exhaustion; and assist family in determining appropriate physical activity.

CHAPTER 49: HEMATOLOGIC AND IMMUNOLOGIC DYSFUNCTION

I. Learning Key Terms

1. e 2. c 3. a 4. f 5. b
6. d

II. Reviewing Key Concepts and Content

7. Iron deficiency
8. a 9. a 10. d 11. d 12. b 13. d

14. b 15. d
16. Idiopathic thrombocytopenic purpura
17. c 18. c 19. d 20. d 21. d 22. d
23. d 24. c 25. d 26. a

III. Thinking Critically

1. Analyze the drug and dosage and administer medication on a regular schedule. Suggest changes to prevent rather than treat pain after it occurs.
2. Apply pressure to area of bleeding for 10 to 15 minutes to allow for clot formation. Immobilize and elevate area above the level of the heart to decrease blood flow. Apply cold to promote vasoconstriction.
3. Provide meticulous skin care, especially in the mouth and perianal regions because they are prone to ulceration. Change position frequently to stimulate circulation and relieve pressure. Encourage adequate calorie/protein intake to prevent negative nitrogen balance.
4. Wear gloves and wash hands carefully; wear gowns, masks, and eye protection. Use needle precautions, and use precautions with trash and linen.

CHAPTER 50: GENITOURINARY DYSFUNCTION

I. Learning Key Terms

1. q 2. a 3. j 4. i 5. l 6. h
7. b 8. p 9. k 10. c 11. o 12. f
13. d 14. n 15. g 16. m 17. e

II. Reviewing Key Concepts and Content

18. d 19. a 20. b 21. b 22. a 23. c
24. c 25. c 26. b 27. a 28. c 29. b
30. b
31. Hemodialysis, peritoneal dialysis, hemofiltration
32. Hemodialysis
33. Peritoneal
34. Peritonitis
35. Fluid overload, surgical procedures
36. a

III. Thinking Critically

1. *Interventions should include the following:* offer a nutritious diet; limit salt during edematous phase; enlist the aid of the child and parents in formulation of a diet; provide a cheerful, relaxed environment during meals; provide special and preferred foods; serve food in an attractive manner; serve small quantities.
2. *Response should include the following:* maintain bed rest, balance rest and activity when

ambulating, plan and provide quiet activities, instruct the child to rest when fatigued, and allow for periods of uninterrupted sleep.
3. *Response should include the following:* encourage the parents to visit, spend time with the child, provide opportunities for the child to socialize with other children who have no infection, and provide appropriate play activities.
4. Protein is restricted in children with acute renal failure to prevent the accumulation of nitrogenous wastes.
5. *Nursing interventions should include the following:* assess home situation, teach the family home care, help the family acquire needed drugs and equipment, assist family in problem solving and diet planning, prepare the child and family for home hemodialysis and/or kidney transplantation, maintain periodic contact with family, and refer the family to special agencies and support groups.

CHAPTER 51: CEREBRAL DYSFUNCTION

I. Learning Key Terms

1. k   2. f   3. l   4. g   5. i   6. e
7. h   8. j   9. b   10. d   11. a   12. c

II. Reviewing Key Concepts and Content

13. c   14. b   15. a   16. c   17. c   18. d
19. c   20. a   21. b   22. d   23. c   24. a
25. b   26. d   27. c   28. c   29. b   30. a
31. d   32. c   33. a

III. Thinking Critically

1. *Assessment parameters should include* vital signs, pupillary reactions, and level of consciousness. *Interventions should include the following:* elevate head of bed 15 to 30 degrees, avoid positions or activities that increase intracranial pressure (ICP), prevent constipation, minimize emotional stress and crying, prevent or relieve pain, schedule disturbing procedures to take advantage of therapies that reduce ICP, and monitor ICP.
2. Assure parents that everything possible is being done to treat the child; continue to repeat this message frequently.
3. *Assessment data should include* a description of the child's behavior before and during a seizure, the age of onset of the first seizure, the usual time at which seizures occur, any factors that precipitate seizures, any sensory phenomena that the child can describe, duration and progression of the seizure, and postictal feelings and behavior.
4. *Interventions should include the following:* position the child on the unoperated side to prevent

pressure on the shunt valve; keep the child flat to prevent too rapid reduction of intracranial fluid; manage pain with Tylenol, Tylenol with codeine, or opiates; monitor neurologic status, vital signs, abdominal girth, and hydration status; monitor for infection of operative site; and inspect incision site for leakage.

CHAPTER 52: ENDOCRINE DYSFUNCTION

I. Learning Key Words

1. e   2. j   3. d   4. n   5. i   6. m
7. k   8. c   9. l   10. g   11. b   12. h
13. a   14. f

II. Reviewing Key Concepts and Content

15. The cell, the target cells or end organs, the environment
16. h   17. e   18. j   19. f   20. b   21. g
22. c   23. k   24. d   25. i   26. a   27. c
28. a   29. c   30. c
31. Acromegaly results from hypersecretion of growth hormone that occurs after epiphyseal closure. If hypersecretion occurs before epiphyseal closure, the disorder is called pituitary hyperfunction, and physical features do not become distorted as in acromegaly.
32. c   33. a   34. c   35. b   36. b   37. d
38. b   39. c   40. d   41. d   42. b   43. c
44. c   45. d   46. b

III. Thinking Critically

1. *Clinical manifestations of hypopituitarism include* short stature but proportional height and weight, well-nourished appearance, a tendency to be relatively inactive and to shun aggressive sports, retarded bone-age proportional to height-age, and eruption of permanent teeth is delayed and teeth are overcrowded and malpositioned. Sexual development is delayed but normal.
2. *Clinical manifestations of diabetes insipidus include* polyuria, polydipsia, irritability, and signs of dehydration.
3. *Expected symptoms include* irritability, shaky feeling, sweating, pallor, tremors, tachycardia, and shallow respirations.
4. *Treat hypoglycemia* by giving the child simple sugar followed by a complex carbohydrate and a protein.
5. The child will do the following:
   • Accept teaching provided
   • Demonstrate understanding of disease and its therapy
   • Demonstrate understanding of meal planning

- Demonstrate knowledge of and ability to administer insulin
- Demonstrate ability to test blood glucose level and urine
- Demonstrate understanding of proper hygiene
- Demonstrate understanding of importance of exercise regimen
- Demonstrate understanding of management of hyperglycemia and hypoglycemia
- Keep records of insulin administration and testing procedures
- Engage in self-management

CHAPTER 53: INTEGUMENTARY DYSFUNCTION

I. Learning Key Terms

1. i	2. r	3. h	4. q	5. g	6. s
7. p	8. f	9. b	10. o	11. e	12. y
13. n	14. d	15. m	16. c	17. t	18. x
19. l	20. v	21. a	22. k	23. u	24. w
25. j	26. cc	27. nn	28. bb	29. jj	30. aa
31. ii	32. z	33. mm	34. dd	35. hh	36. ee
37. ll	38. gg	39. kk	40. ff		

II. Reviewing Key Concepts and Content

41. c	42. c	43. a	44. d	45. b	46. b
47. d	48. d	49. a	50. b	51. T	52. d
53. c	54. c	55. d	56. d		

57. Thermal, electrical, chemical
58. Hot water scald

59. a	60. b	61. d	62. a	63. c	64. c
65. b	66. d	67. a	68. b	69. a	70. c
71. d	72. c	73. a	74. b		

III. Thinking Critically

1. *Possible responses:*
   - Administer soaks, baths, or lotions to provide a soothing film that reduces external stimuli.
   - Apply topical corticosteroids to affected area to provide a palliative antiinflammatory effect.
   - Employ restraint devices and scrupulous hygiene to prevent autoinoculation and secondary infection.
   - Apply intermittent wet dressing to help cool the skin by evaporation and relieve itching/inflammation; cleanse the areas by loosening and removing crusts and debris.
   - Apply occlusive dressings to increase the penetration of the medication and promote moisture retention.
2. *Possible diagnoses include the following:* impaired skin integrity related to eczematous lesions, high risk for infection related to risk of secondary infection of primary lesions, altered family

processes related to child's discomfort and lengthy therapy.
3. *Suggested interventions include the following:* use superabsorbent disposable diapers, change diapers as soon as they become wet or soiled, expose the area to light and air, do not use rubber pants or cloth diapers, clean the area well after each soiling, use an occlusive ointment, and avoid overwashing the skin.
4. School-age children are more susceptible because of their social nature and their proximity to other children.
5. Infection is a leading cause of death in the patient with thermal injury and is a serious complication. Adhering to sterile technique lessens the chance of infection.

CHAPTER 54: MUSCULOSKELETAL OR ARTICULAR DYSFUNCTION

I. Learning Key Terms

1. g	2. o	3. f	4. h	5. n	6. e
7. d	8. i	9. m	10. c	11. l	12. j
13. a	14. k	15. b			

II. Reviewing Key Concepts and Content

16. d	17. d	18. b	19. l	20. j	21. k
22. a	23. b	24. d	25. c	26. e	27. f
28. g	29. h	30. i	31. d	32. a	

33. Lordosis, kyphosis

34. d	35. a	36. b	37. d	38. a	39. c
40. a					

III. Thinking Critically

1. *Instructions to parents should include the following:*
   - Keep the extremity elevated on pillows for the first day.
   - Avoid indenting the cast until it is thoroughly dry.
   - Encourage frequent rest periods for a few days, keeping the injured extremity elevated while resting.
   - Do not allow child to put anything in the cast.
   - Keep a clear path for ambulation.
   - Use crutches correctly.
2. The nurse needs to understand the function of the traction. Check desired line of pull frequently to maintain alignment and check function of component parts. Make sure ropes move freely through pulleys and that weights hang freely. Maintain total body alignment, bed position and traction.
3. *Clinical signs include the following:* hip laxity on the affected side, asymmetry in the length of the

femurs, asymmetry of the thigh and gluteal fold, and broadening of the perineum.

4. Accentuate positive aspects of the adolescent's appearance; encourage the adolescent to wear attractive clothes and hairstyle; emphasize the positive long-term outcome of the surgery; help devise ways to deal with the reactions of others.

CHAPTER 55: NEUROMUSCULAR OR MUSCULAR DYSFUNCTION

I. Learning Key Terms

1. f	2. k	3. g	4. c	5. j	6. d
7. b	8. h	9. a	10. i	11. e	

II. Reviewing Key Concepts and Content

12. a	13. c	14. d	15. d	16. b	17. c
18. a	19. c	20. c	21. b	22. a	23. d
24. b	25. d	26. d			

III. Thinking Critically

1. The child will do the following:
   - Acquire mobility within personal capabilities
   - Be protected from injury
   - Acquire communication skills or use appropriate assistive devices
   - Exhibit signs of adequate rest and optimum nutritional intake
   - Be cared for by a family exhibiting adaptation to accommodate special needs child
   - Engage in self-help activities
   - Receive appropriate education
   - Develop a positive self-image
   - Receive appropriate care if hospitalized

2. *Suggested interventions include the following:* help parents develop a balance between limiting the child's activity because of muscular weakness and allowing the child to accomplish goals independently (refer to Chapter 41).

3. *Interventions aimed at preventing the complications of Guillain-Barré syndrome include the following:* observe for difficulty swallowing and respiratory involvement; monitor vital signs frequently; monitor level of consciousness; maintain good postural alignment; change position frequently; perform passive range of motion every 4 hours; ensure adequate nutrition; provide bowel and bladder care to prevent constipation and urine retention.

4. *Nursing goals include the following:* stabilize the entire spinal column with a rigid cervical collar with supportive blocks on a rigid backboard. Ensure airway patency and continually assess neurologic function to prevent further deterioration. Prevent complications and maintain bodily functions.

NOTES

NOTES

NOTES

NOTES

NOTES

NOTES

NOTES

NOTES

NOTES

NOTES